ULTIMATE INTIMACY

ULTIMATE INTIMACY

THE PSYCHODYNAMICS OF JEWISH MYSTICISM

Mortimer Ostow

with contributions by

Jacob A. Arlow *Martin Bergmann*
Eleanor Galenson *David J. Halperin*
Moshe Idel *Peter B. Neubauer*
Elliot R. Wolfson

Routledge
Taylor & Francis Group
LONDON AND NEW YORK

First published 1995 by
Karnac Books Ltd.

2 Park Square, Milton Park, Abingdon, Oxfordshire OX14 4RN
52 Vanderbilt Avenue, New York, NY 10017

Routledge is an imprint of the Taylor & Francis Group, an informa business

First issued in hardback 2019

British Library Cataloguing in Publication Data

Ostow, Mortimer
Ultimate Intimacy: Psychodynamics of
Jewish Mysticism
I. Title
296.712019

ISBN: 978-1-85575-105-7 (pbk)
ISBN: 978-0-367-32947-1 (hbk)

This book is dedicated to
the memory of my friend, companion, and teacher,
Gerson D. Cohen,
who introduced me to Kabbalah,
and to my study companions,
Ismar Schorsch and Stanley Schachter

CONTENTS

MYSTICISM AND PROPHECY

ESOTERIC MYSTICISM, *MERKAVAH* AND *HEKHALOT*

METHODOLOGY

SEX AND GENDER IN THE KABBALAH

EPILOGUE

CONTRIBUTORS

MORTIMER OSTOW, M.D., Med.Sc.D., Sandrow Visiting Professor Emeritus of Pastoral Psychiatry, Jewish Theological Seminary of America; President, Psychoanalytic Research and Development Fund; Attending Psychiatrist, Montefiore Medical Center, New York City.

JACOB A. ARLOW, M.D., Past President, American Psychoanalytic Association; Former Editor-in-Chief, *Psychoanalytic Quarterly*; Clinical Professor of Psychiatry, New York University College of Medicine.

MARTIN BERGMANN, Clinical Professor of Psychology, New York University Post-Doctoral Program; Training and Supervising Analyst, New York Freudian Society.

ELEANOR GALENSON, M.D., Clinical Professor of Psychiatry, Mt. Sinai School of Medicine; member, New York Psychoanalytic Society.

DAVID J. HALPERIN, Ph.D., Professor of Religious Studies, University of North Carolina; author of *The Faces of the Chariot: Early Jewish Responses to Ezekiel's Vision*, and *The Merkabah in Rabbinic Literature.*

MOSHE IDEL, Ph.D., Max Cooper Professor of Jewish Thought, Hebrew University of Jerusalem; author of *Hasidism: Between Ecstasy and Magic*, and *Kabbalah: New Perspectives.*

PETER B. NEUBAUER, M.D., Clinical Professor of Psychiatry, New York University; Editor, *Psychoanalytic Study of the Child.*

ELLIOT R. WOLFSON, Ph.D., Professor of Hebrew & Judaic Studies, New York University; author of *Through a Speculum That Shines: Vision and Imagination in Medieval Jewish Mysticism*, and the *Book of the Pomegranate: Moses de León's Sefer ha'Rimmon.*

PREFACE

Regularly in essays, books, and lectures on Jewish mysticism, the author will observe that the material is so strange and irrational that it invites psychological analysis. From his point of view, the psychoanalyst easily recognizes familiar dynamic formulations and myths and eagerly explores mystical materials for the universals of human fantasy and for the sources of irrational thoughts and behaviour; for information on methods of inducing alterations of behaviour; and for the universals that characterize the relationship between the individual and his community.

It is the purpose of this book to introduce the psychoanalytic study of the Kabbalah as a serious discipline. This is not a text on the subject, but rather a collection of essays with some commentaries, each of which is intended to illustrate the applicability of psychodynamic concepts to Jewish mysticism and thereby to serve as an introduction.

I should like to make clear to the reader that this endeavour is not intended as an attempt to reduce Kabbalah to a mental deviation or to explain it away. These studies were undertaken because, since it evolved, Kabbalah has been a powerful force in the life of the Jewish people. We should like to learn how and why it has developed, how it has acquired its power, and whether there is any prospect that it will become less or more potent an agent for alleviating or creating turbulence for the Jewish people in the future, both of which it did in the past.

Obviously, mysticism is no less important in the history of other peoples. But the subject is so large that to master it in the case of even one culture is a striking achievement. We limit ourselves here to Jewish mysticism and to only a few aspects of it, in order to make some degree of control of the subject possible.

We start with an introductory chapter, in which I review briefly, for the reader who is new to mysticism, its dimensions, and also suggest some psychodynamic formulations. The second chapter deals with the subject of apocalypse because, in my view, what I have called the "apocalyptic complex" lies at the heart of mysticism. The third chapter, by David J. Halperin, presents an example of prophetic mysticism as exemplified in the book of Ezekiel. The fourth chapter deals with esotericism, and the fifth with *hekhalot* and *merkavah* mysticism. Thereafter, Halperin contributes a chapter on methodology. There follow two chapters, one by Moshe Idel and a second by Elliot Wolfson, on sexuality in mediaeval Kabbalah. We have comments on chapter three by Martin Bergmann, on chapter four by Eleanor Galenson, on chapters four and five by Halperin, on chapter seven by Jacob Arlow, and on chapter eight by Peter Neubauer. In a series of introductions and some comments, I try to integrate these several components and set them all into a common framework.

The chapters attributed in the Table of Contents to Professors Halperin and Wolfson do not properly indicate their true contributions to this volume. They have generously and promptly reviewed my own essays and introductions, helped me to formulate some of my ideas, pointed out errors, and suggested relevant literature and observations. More importantly, they encouraged me to carry out this enterprise. I am greatly indebted to them, as well as to my other colleagues who share their wisdom and experience with us in this volume. Despite their efforts, the reader will doubtless encounter errors, and statements and opinions that are controversial. For these, of course, I take full responsibility.

I should like to take this opportunity to thank my secretary, Antoinette D. Flynn, for her faithful transcription of this often difficult text.

Finally I should like to thank Cesare Sacerdoti, publisher of Karnac, who conceived of this book and encouraged me to put it together.

EDITORIAL NOTE

A note about transliteration and spelling: Some of the Hebrew and Aramaic texts that our essays address are quoted in the original but rendered here in transliteration—that is, English letters reproducing approximately the sound of the original. In most cases, individual letters in English correspond approximately in sound to letters in the Hebrew alphabet. Problems arise in the case where two Hebrew letters correspond to the same sound in English, and also in the case of those Hebrew letters that correspond to no single English letter. For that reason, transliteration codes are used in scholarly publications. Many scholars use their own codes. I have not attempted to impose a uniform code on the essays in this book, preferring to let each author's essay conform to the code that he has been using in all of his work.

The differences among the codes are seldom problematic. By and large, ambiguity arises with respect to two situations: The *ch* sound, as it appears in the German word *ich*, is indicated in modern Hebrew by the letters *chet* and *chaf*. Most current, scholarly transliteration codes render the first by *ḥ*, and the second by *kh*. (In this volume we are using either *ḥ* for *chet* or *h* to represent both its corresponding letter, *heh*, and the *chet*.) Again, two Hebrew letters, *aleph* and *ayin*, are unvoiced. They are indicated in scholarly transliteration by orthographic signs that are not letters, resembling ' [a final quotation mark] for *aleph* and ' [an initial quotation mark] for the *ayin*. The *vav*, which is sounded as a *v*, is often transliterated as *w* to distinguish it from the *veth*, which is also sounded *v*. The *ts* sound, as in *tsadik*, is usually transliterated as ṣ or ẓ. Here we have omitted the subscripts that distinguish these from the same letter pronounced conventionally. Both *kaf* and *kuf* are pronounced and transliterated *k*; some authors use *q* for *kuf*.

The Hebrew alphabet consists only of consonants, and therefore consonants identify the root meaning of the word, while vowels, prefixes, and suffixes indicate its inflections. Although consonants were necessarily always pronounced with vowels, a consistent vowel orthography was not established before the sixth century C.E. The pronunciation of the vowels in modern Israeli Sefardic Hebrew differs in some respects from their pronunciation in Ashkenazic Hebrew. When the vowel sounds are reproduced in transliteration in scholarly texts, generally the Sefardic usage is given. The rendering of these sounds into English is generally by phonetically equivalent vowels. Scholarly papers that deal with ancient texts often omit all vowel symbols in transliteration, except for some consonants that also have vowel significance—*aleph*, *heh*, *vav*, and *yod*. Scholarly papers that deal with Hebrew grammar transliterate the vowel sounds punctiliously. Otherwise, the vowel sounds are usually rendered into recognizable and reasonably unambiguous English vowel letters.

It follows that transliteration is not necessarily consistent from author to author, from Ashkenazic to Sefardic, or even from one non-Hebrew language (e.g. German) to another (e.g. English). Accordingly, the reader will notice inconsistencies in usage in the transliteration of certain Hebrew names, depending upon which author is quoted. For example, the adjective derived from the name Sabbatai Sevi, is given as Sabbat*ian* by Scholem and Idel and Wolfson, but Sabbat*ean* by Y. Liebes. The celebrated second-century Tanna (scholar of the Mishnaic period) *Akiva* may also be referred to as *Aqiba*, *Akiba*, or *Aqiva*, depending upon which transliteration code is used. Again, Scholem and

Halperin speak of the *merkabah*, whereas Idel speaks of the *merkavah* (*b* and *v* are both represented by the same Hebrew letter, *beth*; it is pronounced *b* when it contains a dot—*dagesh*—and *v* otherwise). Note the two spellings *sefirah* and *sephirah*.

It will be helpful to remember that the suffix *-im* signifies the masculine plural and *-ot* or *-oth* the feminine plural. Words ending in *-ah* are usually feminine singular, e.g. *sefirah* (singular) and *sefirot* (plural).

At the end of the book I have provided a glossary of some of the less familiar Hebrew and Aramaic terms that appear in the text.

PROLOGUE

CHAPTER ONE

Dimensions of mysticism

Definitions

The reader without specialized knowledge of mysticism will expect this book to open with a helpful definition. The student of mysticism, on the other hand, will know that no definition of mysticism will do justice to the breadth and diversity of the phenomena that the term comprises and wonder what the term psychodynamics implies.

Philology does not help us much to delineate the profile of mysticism. The root of the word is said to be associated with the Greek word *muein*, which literally means "closing", with respect to the lips and the eyes. The word was used in connection with the rituals of initiation into Greek mystery religions, and the word "mystery" is said to be derived from it. Mysticism shares many concepts with the religious mysteries of the ancients, primarily the effort of the individual to achieve union with a universal being (Kerenyi, 1955, p. 33).

While theoretically it is desirable to initiate the study of behavioural phenomena with definitions for the purpose of achieving clarity, in my experience it is usually best to leave definitions to the end of the study—and one often concludes then that definitions are impossible.

However, as an initial approximation, I think that Evelyn Underhill's definition is probably as useful as any. "Mysticism", she says (1964),

> according to its historical and psychological definitions, is the direct intuition or experience of God; and a mystic is a person who has, to a greater or lesser degree, such a direct experience—one whose religion and life are centered, not merely on an accepted belief or practice, but on that which he regards as first hand personal knowledge. [pp. 9f.]

Here is Idel's definition (1988b):

> I consider a phenomenon to be of a mystical nature when there is achieved a contact with the Divine, differing from the common religious experiences cultivated in a certain religion both in its intensity and in its spiritual impact. Accordingly, the interest in ecstatic and unitive experiences as they occur in Kabbalistic literature are conspicuously mystical. I also, however, consider certain types of experiences as mystical even when they differ substantially from the previous type of mysticism: I refer to theurgical performance of the commandments as this appears in certain texts. [p. xviii]

Psychodynamics is a discipline that strives to detect regularities in mental processes in the sense that sequences and cause-and-effect relationships can be recognized. In order to do so, it is useful to assume the existence of intervening forces and counterforces that do not become conscious. Since the regularities of mental life seem to prevail fairly universally, one can attempt to "understand" behaviour—especially non-rational behaviour—among individuals and communities that one knows only from public information.

That mysticism has prevailed widely and still does, both in historical times and in geographical space, encourages us to infer that both its visible manifestations and the unconscious mental processes that underlie the visible are represented fairly uniformly in mankind. It will be even more interesting if, apprehending what these unconscious determining mental processes are, we can establish relations between mysticism and other behaviours that share these processes. If we are successful in discerning the mental dynamics, then we shall be able not only to understand mysticism better, but also to detect congruent, derivative, and correlated behaviours. Prediction in the area of human behaviour is not generally successful, even though we can all recall instances in which our forecasts proved correct. Informed anticipation probably characterizes better what we can hope to achieve.

Dimensions of mysticism

What are the things that we would wish to know about mysticism or about the individual varieties of mysticism that we shall encounter here—that is, what are its dimensions?

First we must distinguish between individual mystical experiences and practices on the one hand and group mystical movements on the other. How are these related, what do they share, and how do they differ? Second, what is the mystical experience? It is this experience that is said to be the defining characteristic of mysticism. The mystic declares that his experience is not susceptible of being described in words in the familiar categories of reason. It is *sui generis* and not definable. Essentially, the mystic feels that he is at one with a universal entity: the religious mystic feels himself united in some way (*unio mystica* in the Christian religion and *d'vekuth* [adhesion] among Jews) with his God; the secular mystic, with the universe or with nature. This feeling of unity may occur in a clearly demarcated mystical trance, or as an aspect of one's feeling as one goes about the business of one's daily life, or both. We would wish to know on what occasions the discrete mystical experience appears and what determines conversion to a continuing mystical frame of mind. Obviously, the openness to mystical conversion reflects a previous discontent and unhappiness. However, the specific nature of this unhappiness is seldom clear, nor does it appear to be the same for all individuals and on all occasions.

Some people, both in contemporary life and in accounts recorded in history, make strenuous efforts to induce the experience, while others describe being suddenly and surprisingly overwhelmed by it. The literature of mysticism records techniques for trance induction, strikingly similar even in dissimilar cultures. Most of these invoke purification rituals, such as bathing and changing into clean clothes; ascetic abstentions, mainly from food, drink, sexual contact, and sleep; solitude or isolation from stimuli, for example by remaining in seclusion for days and weeks, often with the eyes closed (cf. the Greek *muein*, to which I referred above, signifying "closing of eyes and lips"); meditation on a fixed image or endlessly repeated recitation of a mantra; and a fixed, often submissive posture, such as sitting with the head resting on the knees (Idel, 1988b; Scholem, 1941, p. 49).

We would wish to know what behavioural consequences flow from the mystical experience, either concurrently or subsequently. Actually, we should not assume that behaviour that follows the mystical experience or the onset of the mystical conversion is necessarily caused by it. It is conceivable that the same frame of mind that induced one, induced the other as well. Most commonly, the mystic, if his overt behaviour changes at all—and often no change is visible—will exhibit a new or increased degree of self-control, self-denial, submissiveness, and other forms of conduct that are generally considered moral. In some instances, quite the contrary is observed: a defiance of conventional standards and an overthrow of accepted values and norms. The Sabbatian messianic mystical movement of the seventeenth century and the Frankist mystical movement of the eighteenth century exhibited this Jewishly perverse heresy. In either case, the individual mystic can become the leader of a movement, conventional in the former instance or deviant or heretical in the latter.

We must also take into account the mental content associated with the mystical experience or mood. Here, too, we encounter a good deal of variation. In many instances the mystic describes a sudden or gradual onset of a novel consciousness of an exhilarating concern with, or approach to, the pervasive object of desire, usually some form or aspect of a deity. In other, more dramatic accounts, we read of a sudden visual or auditory experience that carries with it a profound conviction of reality—typically a hallucinatory vision of, or encounter with, a supernatural figure. This encounter then becomes an organizing personal myth that provides a presumably realistic explanation for the dramatic changes that have occurred.

One does not encounter reports of spiritual experiences very often in the psychoanalytic literature, perhaps because psychoanalysts do not listen for them. Yet I found that when I started to listen, the material was there.

PATIENT A

> A is an intelligent, active, moderately successful businesswoman in her mid-thirties, who reported to me that shortly after arriving in Aspen, Colorado, she experienced three "epiphanies". The first was the image of a small circle inside a larger concentric circle, suggesting a bull's eye. The image was accompanied by the words, "going steady, inside and out". The next day, while riding in a car, almost recumbent because she was not feeling well, she saw a tall aspen tree shaped like an "S" and she heard the words, "we're not perfect". A few minutes later she saw two such trees intertwined and heard the words, "forever together". A few days after these experiences, she dreamed of flying, crashing, going to see a doctor, and not being prepared for an examination. In the session in which she reported these epiphanies and dreams, she talked about Einstein's discoveries, and did he have manic-depressive disease, she wondered. On other similar occasions she reported overly ambitious and impractical ideas for new business ventures.

This was a manic-depressive woman who had had a number of attacks of manic thinking and behaviour in the past. She was at this point fairly well controlled by medication and psychotherapy, but she normally functioned at a hypomanic level. (Hypomania is a normal condition, short of mania, which is pathological. Like mania, it is characterized by euphoria, by a plethora of psychic energy, by creativity, ambition, self-confidence, vigour, and activity. Because of their unusual energy and creativity, hypomanics can operate in the world successfully, whereas manics become too disorganized, self-defeating, or psychotic to accomplish anything. Some individuals may function on a hypomanic level indefinitely and lead fairly gratifying lives of accomplishment. Others have a tendency to regress to mania or depression and may require fairly constant adjustment of medication.) Patient A proved to be an unstable hypomanic, but like many hypomanics, missed her euphoria when medication suppressed it. The level of hypomanic activity that she enjoyed left her vulnerable to manic flights.

What I was seeing in this session was the report of an incipient relapse into mania—incipient but controlled. The patient reported unusual experiences but remained able to function and had not become psychotic. What was the occasion for this relapse? In the first place, she had become aroused by what promised to be a potential romance. Many of her manic attacks in the past had been similarly initiated by romantic opportunities. I suspect that this episode might have been precipitated also by the hypoxia of mountain sickness, physiological effects of which appeared at the same time.

In this, as in previous attacks, she felt suddenly reinvigorated, inspired, and enthusiastic. She was open to revelations, "epiphanies". She became obsessed with certain overarching principles governing the universe, harmonies, vibrations, the possibility of clairvoyance and prediction. In this episode she was interested in Einstein's contribution to understanding the nature of the cosmos, and whether he shared her illness.

But look at the content of these materials. It deals with two issues. The first is union: "going steady inside and out" and "forever together". During this episode, she telephoned her mother one or more times each day. The second is disease and deficiency: "we're not perfect" and the dream about going to see a physician. In her dream, she was not prepared for an examination. The examination dream is a well-known phenomenon in psychoanalysis. In my experience, many of these examination dreams anticipate a medical examination with some anxiety because of fear that an illness will be uncovered. The dreams of flying and crashing represent symbolically her awareness that she was "high" and might "crash" into depression, as she had in the past.

The iconography, concentric circles and trees, reminds one of similar diagrams of the *Sefiroth*, the hypothetical supreme Godhead of the Kabbalah (Scholem, 1974, p. 109; 1991, pp. 42ff.).

We should also note that this "spiritual" thinking, with mystical overtones, is associated with regression to an irrational approach to reality, the patient concerning herself seriously with numerology (also a kabbalistic modality), prophecy, astrology, and the like. This state of mind was induced by a manic regression to a mild psychotic state.

Patient B

B is an unmarried woman, also in her mid-thirties, whose time is occupied with philanthropy and trying to find a husband. The only concern with the preternatural that she exhibits is a readiness to take seriously the currently popular modalities for circumventing reality such as those I mentioned above, and including astrology, clairvoyance, metempsychosis, fortune telling. This is a very pleasant, agreeable, and affable person with a moderate depressive tendency, which is easily controlled with medication. She is not especially volatile.

On one occasion she went out of town to a large charity event. She left home a few days early, together with a woman friend and the latter's two children, ages 10 and 12. They all stayed in an isolated cabin. The moon was full, and B tried to create a "religious ritual". She was of Protestant background but not actively religious or church-going. She purchased 15 crosses, some holy water, and a "glow-in-the-dark nativity scene". At one point that night she left the cottage with the two children, and they lay on the ground looking up at the stars and "meditating". I do not have the content of her meditation.

The next morning they all left and proceeded to the charity event for which they had come. There she became involved in what promised to become a romantic liaison with a married man. I suggested that in both of these activities she was trying to undo her loneliness, to become close to someone else. The major trauma of her childhood had been the mysterious and still unexplained disappearance of her father when she was about 8. Was she, I wondered, craving reunion with her father? She replied that she had recently seen a photograph of herself sitting on her father's lap, laughing very hard. Actually, she thinks about her father many times every day. Whenever she visits a new "psychic", the first question she asks was what had happened to her father.

It seems to me likely that her "religious" meditation on the ground under the stars, after she had acquired these religious items, can be interpreted as an attempt to communicate in a preternatural way with a non-material, supernal being, who represented her missing father. The feeling of union with a cosmic presence was not clearly enunciated here.

Patient C

C is an unmarried, successful Jewish businessman in his middle thirties, a man with many interests, skills, and friends. He is active not only in business but also in philanthropy and in athletics. For the most part his interests are limited to the here-and-now, the practical, the mundane. He almost prides himself on taking no interest in religion, nor any credence in the non-rational or magical. Yet, when he passes the neighbourhood of the cemetery where his father is buried, he will drive in and spend some time at the grave. He had loved his father but didn't grieve visibly to any prominent degree when his father died.

Recently, he had visited the ruins at Machu Picchu. "It was very moving", he said upon his return, "really cheering. I like being around ruins. What they were able to accomplish 500 years ago! I find architecture the most moving of the art forms. I have an increased desire to travel to ruins. The older things are, the more fascinated I am by them. Perhaps I have an affinity for isolation." He listed some archaeological ruins that he had visited, including ruins in Israel.

The night following that session, he dreamed of being among buildings that reminded him of these ruins at Machu Picchu. There was some action that was irrelevant to the subject of our concern. The dream concluded with his meeting with two older men whom he liked and respected, both contemporaries of his father, both seriously concerned with Israel.

Before going to bed that night he had been thinking about the recent bombing of the headquarters of Jewish organizations in Buenos Aires and the almost simultaneous fighting between Jews and Arabs in the Gaza Strip. "There seems to be no place in the world where Jews are safe", he concluded.

I find a clear correlation between C's propensity for solitary rumination among ruins of a past civilization that symbolize his personal past, and at his father's grave in the cemetery. His yearning for his father became evident in the dream. He associates himself with historic Israel. He alternates between active party-going and dating on the one hand, and solitary rumination on the other. It is here that his spirituality appears, his yearning for union, nominally with his father as he knew him as an adult, but actually with a larger entity from the past, for historic Israel and the parents of his early infancy, whom historic Israel represents. I see here a mystical element that C himself would probably not consciously recognize. Subsequently, an unconscious mystical tendency appeared in his analysis, reported below in the essay on *merkavah* mysticism.

While mysticism profoundly affects individual mystics, the group mystical movement exerts important and enduring influences upon the entire community. What is it that precipitates the mystical movement? Sometimes the movement appears in the wake of a specific event. For example, the Sabbatian movement is generally attributed to the distress that followed the exile from Spain and the pogroms of 1648. On the other hand, not all severe persecutions have been followed by the appearance of mystical communities. (On this controversy, see Scholem, 1973, p. 128.) As in the case of individuals, a community that is content is not likely to be susceptible to mystical influences. But the nature of the discontent that favours such susceptibility is not obvious, and probably not uniform.

Group mysticism is necessarily a more complex matter than individual mysticism. In addition to all the parameters that characterize the latter, we must take into account others that pertain to issues of group psychology, the relation of the individual to the group, the determination of group behaviour, and the influence of the leader. It is my impression that mystical groups usually exhibit the characteristics of fundamentalist groups. They tend, for example, to respond to a forceful, charismatic leader. They subscribe to a uniform set of beliefs. They vigorously suppress dissidence. As they gain following and power, they tend to become politically active and aggressive.

The individual who is a member of a mystical group not only experiences his own mystical impressions, but also participates in group mysticism—probably a related but different phenomenon. In addition, he sees himself now as a committed member of a group, which to a greater or lesser extent determines his thoughts and feelings.

The group and all of its members subscribe to a mystical doctrine, an attitude towards the universe, towards society, towards other individuals. This doctrine often includes a group memory of a special encounter, usually a mystic or legendary memory of a preternatural experience of a hypothetical progenitor or a current leader of the group. Sometimes it is not an account of an event, but, rather, an idiosyncratic way of reinterpreting a group scripture, as was true of the Spanish Kabbalists.

The group itself has to be understood in its relation to its surrounding community. The former often comprises a segment of the latter, which is different in one way or another—for example, elite versus populist, learned versus unlettered, religiously observant versus less observant. Generally, the mystical movement purports to encourage even greater observance of orthodox doctrine and practice. Whatever deviations are introduced may, in certain circumstances, amount to a dissidence from or rebellion against the dominant culture. In fact, though, the leaders sometimes justify these deviations by claiming that they are restoring the original archaic religious forms that had been discarded. The evolution of the mystical group may therefore represent a sociologically significant rather than simply a religious event.

Esotericism is an aspect of the mystical group that is fairly specific to group mysticism, though not necessarily characteristic of all mystical groups. In many groups the common myth or doctrine is considered secret, not to be shared with others. As we shall see, in *merkavah* and *hekhaloth* mysticism, esotericism is a major issue. The great mystery religions enjoined vows of secrecy upon new members—vows that were so seriously observed that till this day we have only superficial ideas of the rituals. While the Christians speak of the mysteries of early Christianity, in fact their mysticism is largely exoteric.

What is the relation between mysticism and religion? Most mystical reports are issued under the auspices of religion. The mystic yearns for union with his God, whatever the god of his religion. And yet if the chief goal of the mystical experience is some form of union with a universal entity, one might imagine that purely secular individuals could report similar feelings. Freud (1930a) reports that in a letter, Romain Rolland described

> a feeling which he would like to call a sensation of "eternity", a feeling of something limitless, unbounded—as it were, "oceanic". This feeling, he adds, is a purely subjective fact, not an article of faith; it brings with it no assurance of personal immortality, but it is a source of religious energy which is seized upon by the various churches and religious systems, directed by them into particular channels, and doubtless also exhausted by them. One may, he thinks, rightly call oneself religious on the ground of this oceanic feeling alone, even if one rejects every belief and every illusion.

Religion seems to be the natural medium for the evolution of the mystical experience. It posits a supernatural world, a divinity that pervades the universe and invites love.

How, then, does mysticism differ from normative, conventional religion? Perhaps the difference is quantitative rather than qualitative: mysticism is an especially intense form of religion. Many mystical movements, originally deviations from orthodoxy, are subsequently accepted into the conventional church. Perhaps, as Romain Rolland says, mysticism provides the "religious energy seized upon by the various churches and religious systems". Mystics regard their approach to their religion the only valid one, while the normative institutions often fear it as deviant and sometimes heretical, which it sometimes is. The normative orthodox Jewish establishment struggled bitterly against the early Hasidim, going so far as to incite the Russian government to take legal steps against them. The normative orthodox Jew will observe *mitzvot* and prescribed prayer and conduct himself in accord with the standards of orthodox Judaism. If he is scholarly, he will delight in conventional study of Scripture and Talmud. If he is less scholarly, he will be content to attend services and fulfil the commandments of rabbinic Judaism. The Jewish mystic, on the other hand, though he will usually observe the same *mitzvot* and observe the same standards of conduct, is concerned with something additional: the achievement thereby of a sense of joyous closeness to God and enthusiasm [literally, "being possessed by a god"]. A normative Jew wishes to *serve* God and participate in the religious life of his community. The mystic wish is to *experience* God, whether alone or within the bosom of his mystical community.

Psychodynamic propositions

Obviously, I am condensing in these few pages a highly complex phenomenon about which untold numbers of books have been written. Adequately to describe mysticism, its core, and its many variants would require a work of large numbers of volumes. What I offer here is an orienting introduction to the observations that we make in the subsequent essays as we attempt to study these phenomena from a psychodynamic point of view. Illustrations of many of the statements made in this essay appear in the later ones.

How is it possible to formulate, with any degree of confidence, psychodynamic theories about the behaviour of people whom we have not seen, or of groups that we have not directly observed? Those of us who have had experience with psychoanalysis, whether as patients or as psychoanalysts (all psychoanalysts were once patients), know how much evidence is required to establish hypotheses with any degree of confidence. Yet Freud did attempt to create a discipline of "applied psychoanalysis", which employs hypotheses and theories that are derived from clinical experience with individuals and are then applied to evidence available in history and literature, in order to suggest some interesting and enlightening formulations about individuals or groups outside our immediate view. I refer, for example, to *Totem and Taboo* (1912), *Civilization and Its Discontents* (1930a), and *Moses and Monotheism* (1939a). These have not always gained credence, but they have contrived thought-provoking, novel, and edifying approaches to familiar ideas.

Using data and hypotheses derived from clinical experience does not mean that I am assuming that the mystical phenomena that we are discussing are pathological, or that mystics are mentally ill. The usefulness of pathology—and this applies to physiology as well as psychology—is that by its distortion of normal relations it demonstrates what normal function is. For example, study of the effects of brain injury or brain tumour upon behaviour and mental function helps us to understand the nature of that behaviour and function in the normal state and the role that specific regions of the brain play in controlling them. Let me stress that the manifestations of mysticism—except in the case of mentally ill individuals—may be unusual or anomalous, but not necessarily abnormal in the clinical sense.

What circumstances predispose an individual to mystical experience? I have treated a fair number of religious Jews, some orthodox, some conservative, and some reform, and encountered no mention of spirituality, much less of mysticism. The more observant are concerned with fulfilling *mitzvot*, satisfying religious obligations, and often spending time studying Talmud. They almost never spoke of the *experience* that accompanied these actions. If I raised the question of spiritual concerns, they would assure me that the performance of *mitzvot* was accompanied by appropriate religious feeling, devotion, submission to God, sense of obligation, but I do not recall that any of them mentioned that issue on their own. However, the issue of spirituality did occasionally come up, but indirectly and negatively—that is, by reports of its absence. These people would sometimes report that when they became depressed, they lost their *kavvanah*, their sense of personal, devotional involvement in prayer. I heard a similar report from a Christian clergyman whom I treated over a period of time for recurrent depression. He acknowledged feeling well when he did feel well. At times, however, he would complain about the absence of spiritual feeling. That would return as he began to relapse into depression and as he struggled against it. The distress that accompanied the struggle seemed to satisfy his feeling of guilt, so that he made no complaint in that state of mind. But when he became definitively depressed, all sense of spirit left. He spoke of feeling "screwed into the ground". From this case, and cases A and B, though we do not have enough data to prove a proposition, we do have enough to ask a question—namely, is a heightened sense of spirituality associated with a struggle against depression? I think I have enough clinical evidence to infer that frank melancholic depression precludes the spiritual feeling.

It is probably not extravagant to assume that the mystic is discontent with the world as he experiences it and is looking for an opportunity to replace this experience with another. If the spiritual sense that we have been discussing regularly disposes to the mystical adventure, then one kind of precipitating discontent may be the onset of a depressive process. Parenthetically, we should think of depression as the outcome of a depressive process, which becomes a static condition only when and if that process proceeds to its end, despite a struggle against it that may not be appreciated as such.

We have very little revealing autobiographical material or even non-idealized biographical material concerning mystics before relatively modern times. Elie Wiesel (1978) has published a small volume containing some biographical data of four Hasidic *Zadikim*, each of whom exhibited some evidence of what we would now call melancholia. He contends (p. 122) that melancholy occurred commonly among these Hasidic *Rebbeim*, including the *Baal Shem Tov* himself. The vignettes that Wiesel gives scarcely qualify as clinically reliable biographies, yet they demonstrate that the leaders exhibited some degree of affective lability, pronounced shifts of moods. Isaac Luria, the leader of the Lurianic mystical movement of Safed, is quoted as having said,

> Melancholia is, by itself, an exceedingly unpleasant quality of personality, particularly in the case of an individual whose intention is to acquire esoteric knowledge and experience the Holy Spirit. There is nothing that impedes mystical inspiration—even for someone who is otherwise worthy of it—as much as the quality of sadness. [Fine, 1984, p. 65]

In her classic work, *The Mystics of the Church*, Evelyn Underhill (1964) presents brief biographical notes concerning many of the recognized mystics of Christianity. In the case of a surprising number of them, she speaks of their unusual behaviour as "pathological" or "abnormal", and she gives evidence of their emotional volatility and, not infrequently, clear-cut episodes of depression.

None of this proves that all of the celebrated mystics exhibited this affective volatility, nor that it was needed for permitting the mystical experience. It is perhaps more relevant that some of the ecstatic and mystical trances described by the mystics themselves sound to the psychoanalyst like hysterical episodes or states of mind that we encounter at the onset of a psychotic process. It is these that Underhill designates as pathological.

In any case, we are dealing in both Wiesel's and Underhill's cases with mystical leaders, many of whom were involved in mystical ecstasies and trances. Are these episodes always the result of mood shifts? And does the same volatility occur as often among the followers of mystical movements?

The psychodynamics of the mystical experience

What can we say about the mystical experience itself? Its essence, as we observed, is the sense of union with a universal being or presence, the *unio mystica* of the Christian mystic and the *d'vekuth* of the Jewish mystic.[1] We recognize that state of mind—we encounter it in psychosis, especially at its onset—and we say that it signifies a loss of *ego boundaries*. It occurs frequently in the delirium caused by hallucinogenic drugs, and that is why these are used in some religions to elicit mystical experience. It occurs in some cases of epileptic seizures originating in dysfunction of the temporal lobe. The loss of ego boundaries is commonly accompanied by impairment of the ability to distinguish between reality and illusion or hallucination, by the loss of the capacity to test reality, by impairment of

[1] In his magisterial text on Jewish mysticism, Gershom Scholem (1941) affirmed this distinction. It would be blasphemous, he said, for a Jew to claim or even aspire to true union with God. However, his student, Moshe Idel, a contributor to this volume, demonstrates that the idea of union does occur in the Kabbalah (1988b, p. 60).

the sense of reality, by inappropriate sensations of familiarity or strangeness, naturalness or unnaturalness, by illusions of size, of visual brightness, of auditory loudness or timbre, and by synaesthesias. (Synaesthesia is the illusory apperception in two modalities of a stimulus delivered in one. For example, an audible tone may be experienced as a combination of both visual and auditory impressions.) These are all parameters of perception that seem to be disturbed together in psychosis and delirium. Regulation of these parameters is probably accomplished in the anterior portions of the temporal lobe (Ostow, 1969).

I see two important differences between the sensory alterations of the mystical experience and the analogous alterations of delirium and psychosis. First, in the latter two instances, the patient is not aware that his perception is altered. He enters into the illusion. The mystic, on the other hand, describes these sensations as real, but he recognizes them as ego-alien, as strange, unnatural. Second, in delirium and psychosis, the patient has no voluntary control over these sensory changes; they come and go independently of his volition. In the mystical state, on occasion, the subject will declare that he is overwhelmed by his experience and that he cannot control it. Most often, however, not only does the subject retain control, but he actively induces the experience and the sensations that accompany it.

On the one hand, because we know that these illusions can be induced or suppressed by chemical substances, we might assume that they are the result of an organic—that is, chemical or physiological—process. On the other, we know that they can be self-induced, as can the cognate feeling of depersonalization, the loss of "self-feeling", so that we experience ourselves as outside objects. We assume that in earliest mental function associated with an archaic kind of consciousness, the very young infant scarcely distinguishes between himself and his caretaker, between himself and his mother's breast. If that assumption is correct, then the sensation of union represents a regression to archaic mental function, facultative for the mystic, obligatory for the psychotic. The mystic would seem to be trying to reinstate his earliest sensations of unity with his mother, the state of mind that existed before the process of differentiation that we call separation-individuation, described by Margaret

Mahler (1967), in fact, to undo that differentiation. The psychoanalysts who comment on the mystical materials that follow in the subsequent essays compare the mystical mythology with the wishes and fantasies of small children. All three of the clinical cases I cited above yearned for reunion with the parent of early childhood. The image of the archaic mother is probably not gender-specific—that is, the archaic image of mother can be projected out as either a male or a female supernatural figure. Therefore, that the object of union in Judaism and Christianity is usually but not always male is not incompatible with the notion that it is the archaic mother that is sought.

While analysts speak of loss of ego boundaries in the mental state that accompanies the mystical experience and the inception of psychosis, I think it would be more helpful to emphasize the cause of the loss, namely, the inability to prevent the making of false connections. Modern neuropsychological research teaches us that many—if not all—mental processes involve an integration of particulate components. We perceive and think in modules. We learn, for example, in the case of vision, that some neurons in the occipital cortex respond to colour, others to boundaries, others to grids or recurrences, and so on. The visual experience is created by the integration of these individual percepts. I cite this integration as an example of the automatic tendency to make connections.

Schilder (1942) tried to discern the nature of archaic perception. He described perceptions as they occur in delirium, intoxication, schizophrenia, and other illnesses. Apparently, in these illnesses a mechanism that integrates the individual elementary components of perception is inactivated. Von Uexkull (1921), one of the distinguished founders of ethology, inferred from his observations that among the lower animals perceived size, intensity, and distance are functions of the animal's interest in the object. Instinctual interest supersedes the influence of reality. As Tinbergen (1951) puts it, "The animal's perceptual world is constantly changing and depends on the particular instinctive activity that is brought into play" (p. 37).

Archaic perception, then, is particulate and fragmentary. We are compelled to infer the operation of a mechanism that synthesizes and integrates these individual perceptual elements so as to construct a coherent, meaningful, and reasonably accurate image of the immediate environment. Herman Nunberg (1955) spoke of the *synthetic function* of the ego: "The synthetic function of the ego thus manifests itself in an assimilation of internal and external elements, in reconciling conflicting ideas, uniting contrasts, and in activating mental creativity" (p. 151). The ego's function tends to establish a cause-and-effect relationship: "the need for causality", Nunberg calls it.

But this integration is not sufficient for human apperception. We require still a third apperceptive mechanism—namely, a mechanism that regulates the synthetic function and the need for causality. In psychosis the tendency to integrate and to unify becomes hyperactive and makes connections that are not realistic. The paranoid patient interprets random events as elements of a conspiracy to harm him. The delirious patient may find it impossible to separate out the several perceptual modalities, so that he therefore perceives colour together with a sound, sound with colour, touch with odour, and so on. Human perception in this disordered state then becomes similar to that of lower animals—a collection of impressions, the parameters and immediacy of which are determined by instinctual need rather than by objective reality. We have a good deal of evidence to support the assumption that certain structures within the anterior portion of the temporal lobe perform the function of regulating the parameters of apperception so as to yield a realistic image of the environment (Ostow, 1955).

I have undertaken this excursion because it pertains directly to our topic. At the onset of a psychotic episode, the second regulatory device is disabled, so that apperception is freed from the constraints of reality and becomes subject to instinctual need, as we assume it is normally in lower animals and in the human infant. In paranoia, cause-and-effect assumptions run wild; the patient sees them everywhere as proofs of his delusions. There are no coincidences: everything refers to him. (We speak of *ideas of reference.*) In the fully developed psychotic state, the patient does not realize that his apperception has become distorted. He credits his impressions fully and will tolerate no correction. At the onset of the psychotic state, however, he may retain a certain amount of objectivity. Patient A told me that everything seemed connected. The comet colliding with Jupiter created vibrations that she could perceive here on earth.

The entire universe was unified by vibrations. Everything was ultimately knowable. Another patient (quoted in Ostow, 1969) told me:

> "I am so confused, I feel I don't know what's real and what isn't."
>
> "I feel as if I'm walking about in a dream."
>
> "It's what I imagine LSD to be like."
>
> "Everything is sort of heightened—all my perceptions."
>
> "I'm scared."
>
> "This thing yesterday with the job [she had just started a new and somewhat more demanding job on the previous day], it was the strangest experience. It seemed to me as if the whole thing were set up for me—to show me certain things, to try me out. I felt that one customer represented me. It seemed like such a disorderly place—like my mind."
>
> "I saw all kinds of erotic images. Saks meant sex, and a steeple in a picture seemed like a penis."
>
> "Everything got tied up together. Everything fitted in so—it didn't seem *real.*"

Now these impressions of all-encompassing unity, of unusual size, intensity, brilliance, noise or silence, stillness or movement, real or unreal, familiar or unfamiliar, synaesthesia, often appear individually or together during the mystical experience. The experience of spirituality and of transcendence, of the "oceanic feeling", it seems to me, expresses, whether in larval or fully developed form, the sense of a loosening of ties with the immediate material world and of becoming united with the universe and all of its contents—both in time and in space. (The word *"olam"* refers to both the spatial and temporal universe. The *Kaddish*, to my mind one of the most spiritual of our liturgies, contains the word *"olam"* five times—twice in its spatial sense and three in its temporal sense.)

From these considerations, we come to the conclusion that the mystical experience is built upon two simultaneous regressions: one is the yearning regressively to reunite with the image of the parent of early childhood; and the other is the regression of ego function to an unrestrained tendency to synthesize and integrate, so that the individual loses his sense of individuality and seems to merge into the universe. The ego regression permits the illusion of the reunion. (Peter Neubauer, in his discussion of Wolfson's paper below, raises the question of the possibility of a progressive rather than regressive spirituality by means of sublimation. If he is correct, we shall have to develop criteria to distinguish between the regressive and the progressive spiritual experience.)

Acquisition of the ability to make distinctions, to discern individual entities from within a melange of colours and shapes and shades, is a developmental step. The myth of creation, as represented by the very beginning of Genesis, may be interpreted as a metaphor of individual psychic development. It tells us that the world came into being for each of us as we acquired the ability to discern distinctive qualities and entities from the primordial *tohu vavohu*: light from darkness, day from night, terrestrial waters from celestial waters, and the intervening heaven, sea, and land, the varieties of vegetation, the celestial bodies one from the other, and the seasons that they govern, the varieties of animal life, lower and higher, and, finally, mankind.

Appreciation of reality permits us, in the cognitive mode, to comprehend, to make inferences and predictions. In the affective and instinctual mode, it confronts us with the apparent implications of reality for gratification or disappointment, pleasure or frustration. In the presence of unremitting pain and distress, we are naturally tempted to alter our mode of mental function in the direction of undoing the developmental step that permits us to appreciate reality, and regressing to the earlier mode in which we see no boundaries between ourselves and the universe around us. Even though we do not surrender the ability to make cognitive distinctions in normal, facultative mystical states, we revert to the *feeling* of pre-individual unity. We can speculate that that regression results in the recapitulation of the infant's earliest awareness of the feeling of union with mother. Psychic individuation is achieved only by virtue of maturation.

We speak below of chaos. *Tohu vavohu* in Genesis 1 refers to primordial chaos, the utter absence of order and differentiation. This is the paradigm of apocalyptic destruction, and these same words are used in this sense in the apocalyptic scenarios of Isa. 34:11 and Jer. 4:23–27 (against Edom in the former instance and against Jerusalem in the latter).

The ego regression that we encounter in its most pronounced form in the trance state—but also to a certain extent associated with the mystical frame of mind of whatever degree—works another change that favours mysticism. Psychoanalysts who treat schizophrenic patients observe that they lose contact with real people in the real world and attend primarily to words and pictures—transferring the stamp of reality to these. Images and symbols replace reality. This phenomenon must be considered a consequence of the ego regression associated with psychosis. As they become real objects, words, symbols, numbers, and images lose their symbolic valence.

Scholem (1941, pp. 8ff.) suggests that mysticism can be considered the third and final stage of the evolution of religion. In its first phase, man sees the universe inhabited by a series of gods who represent various animal and human and natural characteristics, and who are easily accessible to man. Man does not distinguish between myth and reality. The second phase of religious evolution is marked by the acknowledgement of a transcendent God, utterly different from and scarcely accessible by man. He is worshipped not by imitation or by symbols of natural events such as fertilization, or by human sacrifice, but by behaviour that is deemed virtuous because it strengthens society. At a certain point, however, man becomes impatient with the remoteness, the abstract, invisible, and impalpable character of such a god, and alters basic religious ideas so as to attribute material and immediately perceptible qualities to the deity. God's qualities now become material rather than abstract. God's understanding, strength, wisdom, beauty, kingship, and so on become hypostases—that is, entities rather than abstractions.

The term "*Shekhinah*" is a case in point. It does not appear in the Tanakh. It is derived from the root "*shkhn*", which means "reside". At many points in the Scriptures God is spoken of as residing among the children of Israel, or in His Holy Tabernacle or Temple or city or Erez Yisrael. The word "*Shekhinah*" appears in the Talmud and other rabbinic texts, where it serves as a metaphor or symbol or allusion to God or His presence. However, in the kabbalistic texts the term becomes a hypostasized entity, which is considered a feminine aspect of God or sometimes the feminine element in the world of the divine *sefirot*, with varying degrees of independence. The mystic, here as elsewhere, prefers to interpret symbols as though they were the referents. From a verb indicating that God will reside somewhere, the mystic constructs a noun that implies a fully or partially separate divine entity.

I infer that this change is effected by the ego regression that I have been describing. Letters and numbers are no longer symbols but essences that possess potency to influence the deity and, through him, nature and the world. The attributing of potency to letters, numbers, and words, and the elaboration of techniques to use them for reaching and influencing God, create the possibility of a theurgic theology. By approaching God closely and influencing Him, one can begin to think of doing magic, including hurrying the advent of the Messiah. Many psychotics, too, believe that they can magically influence others and the world about them.

In general, the mystic lives in a world where words and thoughts and feelings have real consequences. Everything has a meaning. There are no meaningless movements or events. We are all elements of a unitary universe in which everything is connected to and influences everything else. Nothing is fortuitous or without consequence. We are never isolated or alone. We are embedded in a cosmic *matrix*—a word that is derived from *mater*, the mother, and the root of the word *material*. The ego regression helps us to alleviate our loneliness and feeling of isolation in a cold and inhospitable universe.

Just as we prefer continuity and regularity in our image of the universe about us, so we also prefer continuity and regularity in our view of our history. The quest for continuity reinforces our attachment to parents and children, which is primarily determined by our natural object love, based upon biological and psychological forces. But the sense of loyalty to ancestors and more remote descendants, though it can be seen as an extension of love for parents and children, can also be interpreted as extrapolating or continuing from the past and into the future aspects of ourselves. Within the current community, we see ourselves as threads in a fabric. We are elements in our community, but the mental image of the community is an extension of the mental image of ourselves. And the historic community provides continuity, both backwards and forwards, of our social selves.

As we observe below, apocalypse implies violent discontinuity—a reversion to chaos, which inevitably demands repair, undoing, rebirth. It is a regressive step of desperation taken when acknowledgement of reality becomes too painful to tolerate and when no reasonable response seems feasible. The striving for hypercontinuity, the rejection of individuality, individualism, and distinctiveness favours the mystical quest for union and the fundamentalist quest for social uniformity.

The trance and ecstatic states are the most dramatic forms of the mystical experience, although not all mystics describe them. The trance is a state of limited consciousness, of mental dissociation. The individual can respond appropriately to stimuli but seems unaware of anything other than the object of his concern at the moment. Perhaps it resembles the hypnotic state, but that depends upon the influence of an inducer, the hypnotist. The trance also resembles a state of hysteria in which aspects of behaviour and thought seem to be determined automatically and outside the individual's control. Nevertheless, when history, recent and past, free associations of the analytic hour, and concurrent dreams are available, the behaviour can often be understood as an appropriate response to a current situation. I am not really satisfied that this is an adequate explanation of the trance state, but I am afraid that we do not know too much more about it. In *Kabbalah: New Perspectives*, Idel (1988b) gives an extensive discussion of "mystical technique".

Ecstasy has been associated with mystical experiences ever since these have been recorded. It refers in general to a state of excessive excitement occurring as a result of the abandonment of self-control, in the course of which the subject becomes oblivious to normal concerns, insensitive to pain, and intent upon pleasure. It was said to have been induced in primitive and archaic religions and is described in the monotheistic religions of the Western world as well. The word "ecstasy", Greek in origin, was applied to the cultivated excitement of the Greek mystery religions (Angus, 1975, pp. 101ff.). In the trance state, the subject leaves the world of reality and focuses his mind on the extraordinarily gratifying sensation of union with his god. In the ecstatic state, the subject creates intense excitement by discarding ordinary restraints of self-control and dignity, and by subjecting himself to high-intensity stimulation, such as stimulating music and dancing. Ecstatic states are induced in the name of the deity and under the influence of the restriction of consciousness, as in the case of the trance, as the illusion of union is facilitated. The trance state is usually induced in solitude, ecstasy in a group setting.

The kabbalists employed still a third method of inducing a mystical state—namely, study and fantasy. The kabbalistic literature that we possess consists largely of extensive and intensive attempts to ferret out the secrets of the universe and the godhead by speculation and by reinterpretation of classical scripture. Kabbalists do not necessarily induce trances or ecstasies, although some do so—for example, Abulafia (Idel, 1988d). However, the kabbalists do create a feeling of personal contact with God. The process of study itself and the process of fantasy that accompanies it reorient the scholar, so that he sees his every activity as a direct interaction with God. Wolfson (1993a) argues that the theosophical ruminations contained in the *Zohar* are not merely speculative devices for expressing the knowable aspect of God, but a practical means for achieving a state of ecstasy, an experience of immediacy with God. Perhaps the exclusion or minimization or derogation of the ordinary stimuli of daily life permit the kabbalist to shrink his apperceptive world and to limit the sense of reality to the Divine Object of study. Speaking of the pietistic community of the Rhineland led by Rabbi Judah the Pietist, Ivan Marcus observes that they lived "in, but not of the other Jews" (Marcus, 1989). This expression felicitously expresses the fact that the mystic can participate in community life in terms of formal behaviour while his heart is with his mystical group and focused on his experience of communicating with his God.

Inasmuch as the mystic seems to be attempting to re-establish an earlier state of bliss with a parent surrogate, we are not surprised to find him intensifying his religious observance. He submits more intently to the will of God as that is transmitted to him. He observes all orthodox practices, not only out of genuine religious feeling, but also because he does not wish to be characterized as deviant. Trance states occur infrequently and ecstasies rarely, but the mystical attitude may prevail continuously over long periods of time. The Jewish Pietists of the Rhineland and the Egyptian followers of Abraham Maimuni, both of the thirteenth century, exaggerated their religious observances to the point that they were criticized and abused by their fellow Jews (Fenton, 1989; Marcus, 1989). The Spanish Kabbalists, on the other hand, showed little if any difference in external behaviour. What was special to them was how they thought and felt about what they did. Every piece of behaviour, no matter how mundane or prosaic, was experienced by them as an expression of devotion. Possibly this type of reinterpretation can be understood as still another though less dramatic alteration of the parameters of apperception that we mentioned above—namely, the ability to attach a sense of intimacy or worship to objects and activities that would ordinarily not carry these impressions at all, or would carry them to a lesser degree.

Far less common, but more consequential, has been the type of mystical union exemplified by the Sabbatian and Frankist heresies. Here the mystical union with God takes the form of identification, if not usurping, rather than submission. Psychoanalysts who treat children often encounter fears that the child will be destroyed or consumed by the parent—as, for example, in the Red Riding Hood story (where the wolf represents the "grandmother" whom in the story he supplants). But they also encounter fantasies in which the child sees himself as supplanting or consuming the parent, the *enfant terrible*. The mysticism that involves identification with God leads to overt antinomian rebellion against the religious community, usually with devastating results. Whereas the submissive attitude and posture suggest an antidepression manoeuvre, the usurping attitude in posture suggests an overcorrection from depression into its opposite—namely hypomanic or manic behaviour. Sabbatai Sevi was known to have oscillated between depression and mania. In the former state he was ineffectual; in the latter he became an antinomian, mystical messiah (Ostow, 1980; Scholem, 1973).

Most mystical accounts use the term *"rebirth"* to describe the feelings of pleasure and gratification that the mystical experience provides. We find that term or at least the concept in every true mystical system and in every mystical community and religion. William James (1902) spoke of the "twice born". "Born-again Christian" is the equivalent term used currently. The word is used to suggest the feeling of renewal, of the happy opportunity to start over. It implies the freedom from guilt and shame, from fear and anxiety; this feeling of freedom is assumed to exist in the newborn. In kabbalistic mysticism, which emphasizes not inner subjectivity but accounts of the nature of God, we find repeated references to birth, rebirth, pregnancy, growth, and maturation. Evidently, this concept is essential to mysticism.

The converse term, *"death"*, is encountered less frequently in mystical writing, but frequently enough to be recognized as a regular component of the mystical experience. Where it is not specified, in my opinion it is implied. The mystical experience is, in my view, a process of dying to the real world, which is the cause of pain and threat, and being reborn to a life of bliss in union with God (Idel, 1988b, pp. 65f.). The death–rebirth sequence is a special one, significant in psychology, both normal and pathological, as well as in many aspects of religion. We discuss it more fully in the following chapter.

Jewish mystical literature contains few subjective accounts of the mystical experience; the Christian literature contains many. Even where description of trances in the Jewish material are given, they are often given in the third person—that is, descriptions of another person's trance state. Among the Christian descriptions of the trance state, perhaps the most dramatic tell of the conversion of the subject from a negative attitude to religion to a positive one, or of conversion to a different religion. Perhaps the best-known of these mystical conversions is described by St. Paul (Acts 9:3–9; 12:3–16; 26:4–18)—namely, the account of his visual experience and conversion to the religion of Jesus that occurred on the road to Damascus. Augustine (Confessions 8:12) describes his conversion from a life of profligacy to a life of saintliness. In a contrite mood and submissive attitude, he obeys a child's voice instructing him to read. Taking up the Book of the Apostles, he read an admonition to give up his life of sensual gratification and to live a Christian life. Among modern authors, William James (1902) describes similar mystical conversions to the religious life (see especially his Lecture 9).

In all cases, the conversion is followed by an alteration in the individual's frame of mind and in his behaviour. He now becomes immersed in religion, and in some instances, as for example Paul and Augustine, he undertakes to preach to convert others, as though his personal experience endowed him with the privilege or obligation to bring others into the fold. In fact if we focus on acceptance of a "prophetic" mission, we can include the vocations of Isaiah (6), Jeremiah (1:4–10, 17–19), and Ezekiel (2, 3). (For a description of the psychodynamics of these vocation experiences, see Arlow, 1951.)

The accounts of the conversion experience impress the reader as unique and dramatic. However, examination reveals that they overlap with other experiences. The vocation of the prophets that I just mentioned is described as a mystical conversion experience. (The introduction to Halperin's chapter three discusses the relation between prophecy and mysticism at greater length.) Mystical experiences may occur to someone already religious, and they may move him, but they may result in no enduring change in behaviour or religious orientation.

It would be useful, I believe, to examine the several parameters of the conversion phenomenon individually—the abruptness, the mystical experience itself, the change in attitude and the prophetic mission. What is unique about the mystical conversion experience is the convergence of these elements.

With respect to the element of abruptness, we are accustomed to seeing alterations in frame of mind and attitude among family and friends, if not in ourselves, as we grow older, usually the result of maturation, of experience, of affiliation, that is, as a result of inner alterations and externally imposed influences. From day to day these changes are usually imperceptible; it is only over an extended period of time that we become aware of them. The psychiatrist, on the other hand, often sees striking changes occurring abruptly. The schizophrenic or manic-depressive in remission may relapse within a matter of days, hours, or even minutes. The relapse may occur as a result of some invisible inner psychological dynamic, as the result of an inner hormonal or metabolic change, as a result of some externally imposed trauma, or as the result of an unfortunate prescription of therapeutic medication. I do not claim that abruptness itself is pathognomonic of illness, but merely that in individuals ready for some major mental reorientation, the presentation of an adequate stimulus may suffice to induce it abruptly.

We have already examined the nature of the mystical experience. While in the case of most Jewish mystics we find continuing mystical attitudes, we do also encounter sharply demarcated incidents. The trance state is usually reported with a definite beginning and end.

With respect to the change in attitude, I believe that one can discern two elements—an antecedent feeling of distress, which is often a component of a depressive syndrome, and a distinct euphoria and vigour as an element of the mystical experience itself, which endures for some time thereafter, a rebirth. We have more to say about the subject of rebirth in the next essay. The rebirth experience sometimes leaves the subject with a sense of authority that he acquires as a result of submission to the higher authority, so that he may become a prophet of a new movement or merely a leader or teacher.

It is the combination of these elements, especially when they converge in a trance state, that creates the phenomenon that we call conversion.

Why the style of reporting personal experience flourished in the Christian but not the Jewish world is not self-evident. The Christians emphasized the acquisition of authority as a result of the event so that many of the mystics went on to organize mystical movements (see Underhill, 1964). The Jews, on the other hand, seemed to focus on the anxiety that anticipated the experience or accompanied it, reported as such, and also implied in the reluctance of the prophets to accept the vocation. *Merkavah* mystical literature especially emphasizes dangers. We encounter this issue again in chapter four, "Four Entered the Garden".

Mythology plays a role in many but not all mystical systems. When the mystical experience is considered an internal change, we hear little about theology—as is the case in most Christian mystical reports. The subject reports experiencing contact with Jesus or with God, the Father, but he ventures little original about either. In *merkavah* mysticism and mediaeval Kabbalah, the adept himself is less concerned with his own experiences than with the experience of the *merkavah* hero with whom he identifies in the former case, or the nature of the Godhead that fascinates him in the latter, or both. In both of these mystical systems, and in Gnosticism, which is related to the first, a bounteous mythology is created. We detect here an intense curiosity, which, in the absence of true knowledge, results in the elaboration of complex myths. In the case of Gnosticism and *merkavah* mysticism, these myths deal with the nature of God, with His appearance and dimensions, with the celestial hosts, angels, their appearance and dimensions, and with how a human might gain access to God and the dangers that he encounters in the effort to do so. In the mediaeval Kabbalah of Spain and later of Luria in Safed, these myths deal with God's qualities: *Sefirot*—that is, His wisdom, glory, power, love, justice, and so on—rather than on His physical appearance.

If we pursue the hypothesis about the mystical experience that we mentioned above—namely, that the mystic yearns to reestablish in an illusory way his earliest experiences with his mother or either parent (the currently correct expression is caregiver)—then these myths reconstruct early images of the parents. It does not seem to be too far afield to imagine that the infant's curiosity addresses itself to the parents' accessibility, physical appearance, and behaviour. Nunberg (1961) suggests that "infantile sexual curiosity is concerned mainly with these three questions: where do children come from; what is the difference between a boy and a girl; what are mother and father doing together?" "Usually", he continues, "answers to these questions are provided by the children themselves in the typical fantasies." In mystical mythology we find answers to these questions as though they were asked about God. We develop the theme of curiosity in the introduction to chapter four, "Four Entered the Garden".

Group mysticism

Turning now to the psychodynamics of group mysticism we encounter a higher order of complexity. On what occasions do groups become open to mystical reorientation?—apparently, when the group as a whole is subject to some kind of stress. It has not been easy to specify a kind of stress that is always followed by mystical enthusiasm, and certainly not to establish a correlation between the nature of the stress and the nature of the mystical response. Given any mystical movement, it is seldom difficult to point to an antecedent set of distressing circumstances: war, famine, persecution, oppression, social demoralization. Certainly Jewish history—even if we do not subscribe to what Baron calls the "lachrymose theory"—can always provide a reason for anxiety and sorrow.

There is one source of distress that has generally not been recognized in psychoanalytic literature to my knowledge, but that I think should be considered, and that is chaos, a state of disorder. Disorder means unpredictability, and it elicits anxiety based upon the inability to feel comfortable about the future. I refer not only to the danger of possible military assault from the outside or even hostility from within the community, but also to the hazards of starvation, disease, failure, humiliation, and the loss of those we love. For any degree of comfort, we must be able to expect with a reasonable degree of probability that there will always be food and shelter for one's family, a comfortable and stable home; that with reasonable precautions one will probably remain free of disease; that one will retain a recognized place in society; and that those we love will be with us for the foreseeable future. Any of the social traumas that I mentioned can create the anxiety of chaos—and that may be the common element.

In the United States today we see a progressive attenuation of the conventions, rules, and restraints that, even if illiberal and unjust, at least give the impression of order, predictability, and stability. The pendulum swings up and back between excessive social repression and control on the one hand, and, on the other, excessive repudiation of that order and structure. This repudiation exposes many individuals to a degree of chaos and unpredictability that they cannot easily tolerate. Not only does this corrective mechanism explain the conservative backlash that we are now seeing—for example, a militant Christian right and fundamentalism in all religious groups—it also explains the efflorescence of mystical impulse and pursuit, the return to a religion of the most fundamentalist kind, the popularity of nonrational interests and beliefs. These express the need for a return to the comfort and assurance, the regularity and predictability of the well-cared-for infant.

The recently popular scholarly and erudite religious studies include the study of mysticism. This interest can be at least partially attributed to a less-than-scholarly concern with the non-rational. I would guess that even the objective academic interest in these subjects is for many people not entirely unrelated to an unconscious quest for mystical reassurance.

Mystical movements, like other movements, are facilitated by active leadership. Leaders do not create the tendencies for mystical yearnings, but they do encourage and entrain it. They take advantage of a readiness that circumstance creates, and they mobilize and focus it.

I do not know that we can say very much about the qualities that make for effective mystical leadership. Certainly charisma can play an important role, but what is charisma for one culture may not be charisma for another. The probability of being accepted as a charismatic leader is increased if the individual demonstrates some unusual quality—a striking appearance, unusual verbal facility, remarkable capabilities such as an impressive memory. Capacity for logical thought and reasoning are not especially helpful. The leader who enunciates irrationalities or presents as facts what are clearly known not to be factual is often admired and respected because he validates the irrational hopes and desires and beliefs of potential followers. The more outrageous the leader, the greater his credibility. But these comments could be made about leadership in general, and certainly about leadership of fundamentalist movements. Many leaders are sincere; others seem to be dishonest and intentionally mislead.

The more recent the Jewish mystical movement, the more we know about it and about its leaders. The charisma of the Hasidic rebbeim is literally legendary. The Sabbatian and Frankist movements go by the names of their presumptive respective leaders. I say "presumptive" because Sabbatai Sevi was the nominal leader of the movement that is given his name; the actual leader was a charismatic young man, Nathan of Gaza. (For a discussion of the relation between Sevi's personality and his leadership, see Ostow, 1980.) The Ari, Isaac ben Solomon Luria, was the charismatic leader of the movement to which he gave his name. French and Spanish Kabbalists of the thirteenth century and thereabouts followed certain leading personalities, teachers who established schools of Kabbalah. But unique, compelling, charismatic leaders are not salient. The mystical community of the Hasidei Ashkenaz (the German pietists of the twelfth- and thirteenth-century Rhineland) was led successively by three individuals: Samuel ben Qalonimos, his son Judah (hehasid), and Judah's disciple Eleazar ben Judah of Worms (Marcus, 1981, 1989). Of the three, Judah taught and promoted a deviant (though not heretical) praxis, emphasizing the performance of the traditional and prescribed *mitzvot*, but to an extreme degree. He attracted followers, but most of the community found his teachings unreasonable and repudiated him. His father before him and Eleazar afterwards promoted a less extreme form of observance, and so did not suffer the rejection that he did. But the movement was soon eclipsed by Kabbalism.

Abraham Maimuni, the son of Maimonides and his successor as head of the Jewish community, taught a form of mysticism patterned after and strongly derivative from the local, contemporaneous Muslim mysticism of the Sufis. He, too, encountered a good deal of local opposition, but he modified his position so that his teaching persisted for some time (Fenton, 1989).

We do not have much knowledge of the leadership of prekabbalistic mysticism. Most of the material that we have is pseudo-epigraphic. Moreover, although we have some of the early literature, we do not have enough history to ascertain the dimensions of the various movements.

I think we learn that when the community is ready for promises and encouragement, the leader who can offer them will be followed, especially when he shows disdain for reality. However, a populace that is not so needy and desperate will judge more critically and reject would-be leaders who are not in tune with them.

The Hasidim are our contemporary Jewish mystics, and by observing them we may obtain some idea of the experience of being a member of a mystical group. What we find is something very similar to fundamentalism: uniformity in behaviour, beliefs, costume, worship service; subordination to a leader to whom remarkable qualities are attributed; focus on a specific scripture or rather a specific interpretation of the scripture; cultivation of a determined optimism; zealous separatism; deep fellowship; restriction of sexuality; rejection of science but not of technology; a view of themselves as the righteous and everybody outside the group as wicked; and conviction of a unique relation with God.

The mental regression required for the mystical frame of mind is encouraged by group membership. Group sanction replaces reality testing and lends the conviction of reality to non-realistic judgements. This effect prevails in ordinary contact among members of the group, strengthened by worship service, study, preaching, and teaching. But certain group activities possess even greater power to create mystical experience and to augment group cohesiveness. I refer here to the phenomena of group enthusiasm, group hysteria, group ecstasy, which we assume occurred in the Greek mystery religions and that we see now in American Christian revival meetings. The following comments of the Ari (Isaac Luria of sixteenth-century Safed, the architect of Lurianic Kabbalah) reflect the ideal of fellowship (Fine, 1984):

> Before an individual begins to pray in the synagogue . . . he must take upon himself the precept ". . . and thou shalt love they neighbor as thyself . . ." [Lev. 19:18]. And he should concentrate upon loving every member of the house of Israel as he loves himself, on account of which his prayer will ascend, bound up with all the prayers of Israel. By this means his soul will be able to rise above and effect *Tiqqun*.
>
> And especially when it comes to the love for one's associates who study Torah with one another, each and every person must bind himself to the others as if he were one limb within the body of this fellowship. This is particularly important when an individual possesses the knowledge and the mystical insight with which to understand and apprehend his friend's soul. And should there be one among them in distress, all must take it upon themselves to share his trouble, whether it has to do with some illness or with his children, God forbid. And they must all pray on his behalf. Likewise, in all one's prayers and petitions one should be mindful of his fellows. My teacher, of blessed memory, took great care to caution me about the love which we ought to bear toward our associates, the members of our brotherhood. [p. 66]

Psychoanalysts have offered some evidence that for the individual member, the group symbolizes the mother of infancy (Chasseguet-Smirgel, 1985; Scheidlinger, 1964, 1974). We speculated above that the mystic is trying to reinstate his early sense of unity with his mother. If that is true, then membership in a group reinforces the impression that he has achieved that reunion. The actual current unity of the group provides the feeling of infantile union and intimacy.

Esotericism, the need to preserve its secrets within the group, characterizes a number of mystical communities. As the mystic tries to escape from the distress of the real world in which he lives, with its disorder, unpredictability, lack of promise, he finds himself regressing to archaic yearnings—reaching back towards the infantile sense of union with mother, as we suggested above. Once initiated, this movement progresses with its own momentum. It is not a cognitively framed intention but, rather, an automatic process. Since it recreates a pre-verbal experience, its goal cannot be expressed in language except by allusion and metaphor, hence the "ineffability" of mystical experience. The sensations and the images associated with this regression are those of pre-verbal experiences with parents, including images of the parents' bodies, their physical characteristics and activities, and their ability to create and remove pleasure.

Such images have, of course, been abandoned in conventional religion with the evolution of monotheism. Paganism projected infantile images into the heavenly pantheon. The pagan gods represented individual qualities that children perceived in their parents and siblings and their own archaic fantasies and inclinations associated with infanticidal, incestuous, and murderous wishes. Worship of these gods included similar civilly disruptive acts of sexual license and human sacrifice. The Jewish religion abolished the concept of a god with human frailties and replaced it with a projection of the superego, a God, austere and majestic, unthreatened by rivalry, who demanded fear [*yir'ah*] as well as love [*ahavah*]. The mystic who starts within the monotheistic religion finds himself recreating these archaic images and tries to reconcile these with the monotheistic abstractions. For the Jewish mystic, God is divided into hypostases—the *En Sof*, the *Sefirot*, the *Shekhinah*, benign angels, malignant angels, the *sitra ahrah*. God has an anatomy; He has sex organs (see Cohen, 1982). The *Shekhinah* engages in sexual intercourse (see Idel, chapter seven, this volume). These notions are little if at all short of blasphemous in normative Jewish religion, and the mystic is engaged in a constant struggle to contain these images within orthodox theology—a struggle that sometimes fails, as in the case of the Sabbatean and Frankist heresies.

From the point of view of the individual, Hagigah (B.T.: Babylonian Talmud) 11b prescribes that the teaching of speculation about cosmogony, about Ezekiel's chariot vision, which ends with the visualization of God, and about sexual immorality must be stringently regulated and limited. Clearly it is feared that the dissemination of views on these subjects may subvert behavioural norms and group morale and morality. We return to this issue in chapter four, "Four Entered the Garden".

Esotericism makes a contribution to group cohesiveness. The secrets of the group, its beliefs, myths, and rituals, facilitate mutual loyalty among its members. They delineate the boundaries between inside and outside and discourage centrifugal adventure. The issue of secrecy, the need to restrict discussion of Kabbalistic theosophy, played an important role in the French and Spanish Kabbalistic circles of the thirteenth century (Idel, 1989a). Idel's researches on this matter have left me with the impression that the imperative for secrecy that Nahmanides and his followers demanded of Isaac the Blind and his followers in Gerona was based upon the fear that a competitive elite mystical community might be established. Of course, Nahmanides was adhering to *halakhah*, which clearly prohibits the dissemination of such esoteric doctrine. Other Jewish mystical circles did not hesitate to teach their own doctrines of Kabbalah to others in the hope of winning converts. Judah the Pietist and Abraham Maimuni, as well as Nathan of Gaza, attempted to spread their doctrines within their communities. I am not aware that esotericism played an important role in Christian mysticism. The conflict between esotericism and exotericism in contemporary Habad (Lubavitch Hasidism) is outlined by Rachel Elior (1993).

Sociological considerations

Mystical groups do not exist *in vacuo*. They precipitate out of a community matrix and they must relate to that matrix. We do not know anything of the complex intergroup dynamics that prevailed some 2000 years ago, when the earliest formulations of *merkavah* and *hekhaloth* mysticism began to appear. The literature speaks of those who "descended to the *merkavah*" but does not inform us how organized such a circle might have been. As we noted above, specific circles studied and created their own Kabbalah, and so we may surmise some rivalry. Sabbatianism created vigorous dissension within the Jewish community at large. The rise of Hasidism in the eighteenth century was strongly combated by opponents [*Mitnagdim*] who even invoked the participation of the Russian government. Today in the United States and in Israel we witness conflict and mutual disdain not only between the Hasidim and Mitnagdim, but also among the various Hasidic sects.

Like other fundamentalist groups, the Hasidim see themselves at odds with other Jews. When they acquire power of numbers or finance, they become more aggressive and try to impose their standards of religious observance upon others, as do the other Haredim—that is, right-wing orthodox. To a certain extent we may infer that the mystique of the group favours a separatism that is as aggressive as circumstances permit. But we cannot ignore another possibility—namely, that the mystical group isolates itself along already existing fault lines in the community.

Mystics are seekers. Their quest arises out of discontent. The reality in which they live and the community that sponsors that reality leaves some people without a feeling of confidence or comfort. They create a new universe for themselves and, by segregating themselves from the surrounding community, create their own social environment.

Most Jewish mystics have not been ready to declare open opposition to the orthodoxy within which they live. Yet their beliefs and feelings deviate from the historical norms. To whatever extent possible, they try to reinterpret classic texts so as to provide for their innovations, which they now present as more authentic than prevailing doctrine and praxis. Abraham

Maimuni affirmed that his mystical practice revived older forms that had been neglected. And yet there are differences, some of which, as we noted above, are plainly incompatible with classic forms. These differences reinforce the differences in social agenda between themselves and the others.

Other mystics declare themselves at odds with current orthodoxy. For example, the Sabbateans and Frankists claimed to have superseded it, and they reinterpreted classic texts in a way that were intended to justify their heresies.

Mystics generally attribute greater authority to their own personal or group experiences than to normative theology and practice. I would be inclined to look for an underlying antinomian tendency in all mystics and mystical movements.

BIBLIOGRAPHY

By way of further introduction to our study of the psychodynamics of Jewish mysticism, let me provide some orienting data.

First, what is "Kabbalah"? The word is derived from the verb *kabel*, which means "receive". Kabbalah, then, literally means "tradition". The Kabbalists contend that their mystical, theosophical, and theurgic systems were transmitted directly to Moses by God on the occasion of the divine revelation of Exod. 19 and 20. Rabbinic Judaism asserts that its Oral Law was transmitted then alongside the Torah or Written Law, and the Kabbalists claim that their esoteric doctrine accompanied both. The term "Kabbalah" is applied ambiguously to the totality of Jewish esoteric, mystical lore, and also to the systems of theosophy and theurgy that were devised and disseminated in mediaeval Provence and Catalonia and thence further abroad, and then to the Kabbalists of Safed in the sixteenth century, and subsequently incorporated with modifications into the doctrine of Hasidism. We have used the term in the latter sense in this book.

For those readers who are not familiar with the history and varieties of Jewish mysticism, let me provide a list of the major movements, together with some bibliography. For a general introduction to the field, one will do no better than Gershom Scholem's magisterial 1941 *Major Trends in Jewish Mysticism.* Scholem, the major twentieth-century scholar of Jewish mysticism who was largely responsible for promoting its study by canons of scientific scholarship, wrote a number of articles on the subject for the *Encyclopedia Judaica.* These were assembled and published in 1974 as a separate book, entitled simply *Kabbalah.* It is more concise than the original work, though it seems to cover the same ground and contains a more modern bibliography.

Although Scholem argues that there is no mysticism in the Tanakh, I would find it difficult to dismiss some of the prophetic passages as non-mystical. The first chapter of Ezekiel forms the basis for *merkavah* mysticism. The vocations of Isaiah, Jeremiah, and Ezekiel seem to me to qualify as mystical experiences, as noted above. Halperin's chapter in this volume takes up a mystical issue in Ezekiel, and the subject is further developed in his 1993 book, *Seeking Ezekiel: Text and Psychology*, from which our essay, somewhat revised, is taken.

The earliest esoteric material in Jewish mysticism appears as hints of "throne mysticism" in early apocalyptic texts, all apocryphal. Throne mysticism is based upon images of approaching God and visualizing Him while He is sitting on His throne. Starting probably during the first century C.E., comments appear in the Talmuds (*Babylonian* and *Jerusalem*) and Midrashim (extra- and post-Talmudic commentaries), referring to esotericism and the issue of secrecy. Chapter four, "Four Who Entered the Garden", gives an example of such material.

Beginning in the second and third centuries, Midrashim appear that describe mystical ascent (or, paradoxically, descent) to the *merkavah*, the throne chariot of the first chapter of Ezekiel, now a mystical seat of God. Related to this genre is the genre of *hekhaloth* (or "palatial chambers") mysticism. Again adepts attempt to ascend the various heavens to be able to view God seated on His throne among myriads of angels who are singing hymns of extravagant praise. These hymns are probably the precursors of the *Kedushah*, an antiphonic hymn of praise inserted into the *amidah*, the central liturgical piece of every synagogue service. Elements of these hymns appear also early in the *Shaharit*, the morning prayer, after the *Barekhu*, the call to worship. These materials are discussed in three small volumes:

1. *Apocalyptic and Merkavah Mysticism*, by Ithamar Gruenwald (1980);
2. *The Merkabah in Rabbinic Literature*, by David J. Halperin (1980);
3. *Jewish Gnosticism, Merkabah Mysticism and Talmudic Tradition*, by Gershom Scholem (1960).

David J. Halperin has also published a large compendium of Talmudic and Midrashic comments on Ezekiel's vision of the mystical throne chariot, the *merkavah*—a really impressive compilation and thematic organization of material from diverse sources. He attempts to confront the sources with each other and to reconcile them, and to draw psychological as well as historic and textual conclusions (Halperin, 1988a).

Kabbalah proper starts during the middle ages, reaching its full flowering in thirteenth-century Provence and Catalonia. It is primarily a theosophic study and doctrine in which the Deity is represented by a number of different entities, primarily the *En Sof*, a Divine Entity who cannot be delimited or circumscribed. The *En Sof*, though devoid of qualities or attributes, nevertheless, in its influence upon the universe, becomes manifest by ten of these. These are called *Sefirot* and are designated somewhat differently in different schools of Kabbalah, including for example: God's crown, wisdom, understanding, grace, judgement, beauty, eternity, glory, foundation, and kingship.

A brief, cryptic book, *Sefer Yezirah*, is attributed by modern scholars to a period between the third and sixth centuries. It reflects some aspects of *merkavah* and *hekhaloth* mysticism and anticipates Kabbalah.

Probably the oldest known source of Kabbalah is a terse, cryptic book, *Bahir*. The word means "clear", but the book is anything but clear. It appeared in southern France in the twelfth century. It developed the concept of the *Sefirot* from its earliest expression in *Sefer Yezirah* towards the form it took in later Kabbalah. The central text of the mediaeval Kabbalah appeared late in the thirteenth century in Castile. *Sefer Ha-Zohar*, the Book of Splendor, is pseudo-epigraphically attributed to the second-century sage, Simeon Bar Yohai, but it was probably the work of Rabbi Moses de León of Castile. The *Zohar* is a very long book. About half of it was translated into English by Harry Sperling and Maurice Simon. An anthology of texts, *The Wisdom of the Zohar*, was published in 1989, as an English translation, by David Goldstein, of the Hebrew translation (the original is in Aramaic) of Fischel Lachower and Isaiah Tishby, with extensive introductory and explanatory material by Tishby. For comprehensive and reliable discussions of Kabbalah, see Scholem's *Origins of the Kabbalah* (1962), and *On the Mystical Shape of the Godhead* (1991). Idel has elaborated upon and extended Scholem's insights with *Kabbalah, New Perspectives* (1988b).

In sixteenth-century Safed, Isaac Luria (1534–1572) known as the Ari [lion] taught a new and original version of Kabbalah, which elicited a widespread response. His Kabbalah is difficult and arcane, yet many were taken by his speculation that when God had created the world, He withdrew from a part of the cosmos, retracting Himself [*tsimtsum*], so to speak, so as to make room for the created world. A cosmic catastrophe caused the bursting of the vessels that contained the holy sparks [*shevirat ha-kelim*]. The world was then to be restored by a *tikkun olam* [cosmic repair], which could be effected by the religious acts of Israel—that is, study, worship, and *mitzvot*. The Ari himself wrote little, but his doctrines have been recorded by his student, Hayim Vital.

In 1665, a widespread Jewish messianic movement broke out all over Europe, North Africa, and the Middle East. Sabbatai Sevi, a Turkish Jew, probably manic-depressive, as Scholem (1973) cogently argues—under the influence of another, younger charismatic leader, Nathan of Gaza—had declared himself a messiah. The reasons for the readiness of the Jews from virtually all over the Jewish world to accept this claim and act on it by preparing to separate themselves from their homes to go to Palestine are not at all clear. Scholem discounts with reasonable arguments the idea that it was the effect of the Chmielnitzki pogroms of 1648. He attributes the readiness to accept Sabbatianism to the previous acceptance of Lurianic Kabbalah, with its rationalization of exile, that is, the dispersal of the holy sparks. The Lurianic Kabbalah, he says, satisfied the spiritual needs of the world-wide Jewish community. But Scholem does not explain why these spiritual needs became so much more peremptory at that point. Sevi invoked the message of Lurianic Kabbalah, which he used and abused and ultimately superseded. A fascinating and compelling account of this whole incident, together with its material and spiritual background, is given in Scholem's book *Sabbatai Sevi: The Mystical Messiah* (1973).

The major Jewish mystical movement of our times is, of course, the Hasidic movement. It began in mid-eighteenth-century Eastern Poland, initiated by Israel Baal Shem, and spread rapidly through Eastern Europe despite the bitter and sometimes violent opposition of the *mitnagdim*, and now flourishes in both Israel and the United States. The Hasidic doctrines are based upon Kabbalah, modified for the times and circumstances. Idel informs me that the Hasid internalizes the theosophy of the Kabbalists; what the Kabbalists posit as events in the cosmos, the Hasid apprehends within his own soul.

We know of many different Hasidic groups or dynasties which are not always on good terms with each other. The literature is voluminous. Here are some texts:

- *The Circle of the Baal Shem Tov. Studies in Hasidism*, by Abraham J. Heschel (1985);
- *The Zaddik. The Doctrine of the Zaddik According to the Writings of Rabbi Yaakov Yosef of Polnoy*, by Samuel H. Dresner (1960);
- *The World of a Hasidic Master. Levi Yitzhak of Berditchev*, by Samuel H. Dresner (1986);
- *The Paradoxical Ascent to God: The Kabbalistic Theosophy of Habad Hasidism*, by Rachel Elior (1993);
- *Hasidism: Between Ecstasy and Magic*, by Moshe Idel (1994).

Much of Hasidic spirituality is presented in the form of legends and parables. Several collections are well known:

- *The Hasidic Anthology. Tales and Teachings of the Hasidim*, by Lewis I. Newman (1934 & 1963);
- *Tales of the Hasidim* (Volume 1, *The Early Masters;* Volume 2, *The Late Masters*), by Martin Buber (1947 & 1975).

Joseph Dan has published an anthology of early and classic Hasidic texts:

- *The Teachings of Hasidism*, edited, with introduction and notes, by J. Dan and R. J. Milch (1983).

A collection of papers on Hasidism: *Essential Papers on Hasidism: Origins to Present*, has been edited and published by Gershon D. Hundert (1991).

Finally, a rich annotated bibliography on works about Jewish mysticism that exist in English has been published by Sheila A. Spector.

After this lengthy yet barely adequate introduction, we shall turn our attention to the study of apocalypse—a phenomenon different from but related to mysticism, as we shall see.

CHAPTER TWO

The apocalyptic complex

In the previous, introductory essay we considered a number of propositions regarding the psychodynamics of mysticism: the essential mystical quest, no matter how pursued, is psychologically the quest for reunion with the archaic mother; the trance is an altered state of consciousness, which may be induced in any of a number of ways and which facilitates the illusion of that union; in the mystical group, the individual achieves the illusion of being incorporated into the archetypal parent. In this essay I should like to demonstrate that mysticism is one of a number of individual and social phenomena that may be considered derivatives of what I propose to call the *apocalyptic complex.* Other derivatives of the apocalyptic complex include apocalypse proper, messianism, millenarianism, fundamentalism, religious cultism, and utopianism. That these phenomena are essentially different, one from the other,

---

Much of the material of this essay is taken from my paper, "Archetypes of Apocalypse in Dreams and Fantasies and in Religious Scripture", *Israel Journal of Psychiatry and Related Disciplines, 23* (1986) [2]: 107–122; *American Imago,* 43, 4: 307–334, 1986; *Conservative Judaism, 39,* 4: 42–55, Summer 1987.

is generally appreciated. Nevertheless, they do overlap. The Sabbatean movement was both mystical and messianic. In his magnificent *Pursuit of the Millennium* (1970), Norman Cohn gives examples of overlap of apocalypse, messianism, millenarianism, religious cultism, and political revolution. Some of the current Hasidic sects may be considered not only mystical but messianic and fundamentalist as well. I should like to present here the basic psychodynamic pattern of the apocalypse complex so that we can understand not only the origin of its various derivatives and how they relate to each other, but also the source of their power.

Most readers of this book will be familiar with the genre of apocalypse. It is a type of exhortatory writing that first appeared in the Jewish world, probably during or possibly shortly before the second century B.C.E., and continued to appear recurrently for several centuries thereafter, primarily in Christianity—and even into modern times (see Friedlaender, Holton, Marks, & Skolnikoff, 1985). The word itself is derived from the Greek *"apokalypsis"*, which means "unveiling" or "uncovering". Many scholars emphasize the component of revelation as the essential element of apocalypse. However, for others, the concept of the end of the world is central, and they include apocalypse in the genre of eschatology. The aspect of apocalypse that I find most useful as a basis for relating it to psychodynamics is its prediction of doom followed by the reassurance of survival and rebirth. The alternation of expectations of disaster and recovery, which is found in most early apocalypses and which I consider characteristic of the genre, relates apocalypse to other religious writings, for example Jewish prophecy, but also to some phenomena of mental life in health and illness.

Let us examine the second half of the Book of Daniel—that is, chapters 7–12, which conform to the pattern of the earliest apocalypses that we have. The apocalyptic scenarios in Daniel deal with the downfall of the Persian Empire, which succeeded the Babylonian, and the alleviation of the lot of the Jewish people. Scholars estimate that it was written during the first half of the second century B.C.E. as a heartening message for the Jews of the Seleucid Empire.

We find four separate "visions", as each revelation is designated. The first (chapter 7) is called a dream. These visions are symbolic demonstrations of what the future will bring, and they require interpretation by a supernatural creature, generally identified as an angel. Though they anticipate the future from the viewpoint of an author living at the time of the exile in Babylonia, nevertheless with respect to the probable time of the composition of the book, they record the past, and so present history masquerading as prophecy.

The visions were received in a trance state.

> "Only I, Daniel, saw this sight; the people who were with me did not see it but a great dread fell upon them and they fled to hide. I remained alone and I saw this great sight and I remained without strength and my own vigor was transformed into an adversary so that I could not retain my strength. I heard the sound of his words and when I heard the sound of his words I fell on my face in a torpor, and I remained prone. And a hand touched me and helped me to my hands and knees." [Dan. 10:7–10]
>
> "And he came to where I was standing and upon his approach I became terrified and fell on my face and he said, 'Understand mortal that the vision relates to the end of time.' Then as he spoke with me I fell into a torpor with my face to the ground. He touched me and helped me onto my feet. He said, 'I'm about to inform you of the events that will occur when wrath has come to an end, for this period is coming to an end.'" [Dan. 8:17–19]

The trance was presumably induced by conventional trance-inducing measures, such as we noted in chapter one.

> "In those days I, Daniel, behaved as though in mourning for three weeks of days. I ate no refined bread nor did meat or wine cross my lips nor did I anoint myself until the completion of three weeks of days." [Dan. 10:2,3]

The fact that the visions were experienced alongside a river reminds one of Ezekiel's position at the time of his *merkavah* vision (Ezek. 1:1). It is not clear whether the river had a significance in ancient times respecting supernatural communication that we no longer appreciate, or whether it was merely a stylistic convention for prophecy. (This use of river symbolism should be differentiated from Jacob's encountering an angel upon crossing the Jabbok. There, the angel represents the hazard of making a transition, returning home after a lengthy sojourn abroad.) Supernatural individuals appear in Daniel's visions. Some announce the vision; other interpret it; and the angel Michael will, at the end, rescue the Jewish people.

The visions include not only a symbolic enactment of future events, but also a description of God and His angels in the celestial court.

> "As I was looking, thrones were set in place and the Ancient of Days took His seat. His attire was white as snow and the hair of his head like clean fleece. His throne was surrounded by flames with wheels ablaze. A river of fire streamed forth and flowed before him. Thousands of thousands served him and myriads stood before him, the court was in session and the books were open." [Dan. 7:9,10]

One is reminded of Isaiah, chapter 6, and the details suggest Ezekiel, chapter 1. The description also anticipates the descriptions of the celestial court in the literature of *hekhalot* mysticism.

A few other features are not emphasized here but become salient in other apocalypses. The revelations, as we just noted, are given in arcane symbols and words. They require both decoding and interpretation. For example, the period of three and a half years is presented variously as "a period, periods, and half a period" (Dan. 7:25,12:7); "half a week" (of years) (Dan. 9:27); "2300 evenings and mornings", that is 1150 days (Dan. 8:14, 9:27, 12:7). Animals, familiar and strange, play the roles of people. Angels act as messengers, interpreters, protectors. We find one allusion to flight (Dan. 7:21), a staple of many subsequent apocalypses. A feature common to many other classical apocalypses—that is, vehicular travel through the universe, generally for the purpose of learning and understanding its nature—does not appear here. As the end of time approaches, in many apocalypses time and the processes of nature are arrested. The universe becomes unreal.

Much of mystical literature consists of reinterpretations of scriptural texts.

> "Between the first year of his reign (Darius son of Ahasuerus, of Medea) I, Daniel, studied books in order to ascertain the

number of years, according to the word of the Lord to Jeremiah the Prophet, the number of years that the desolation of Jerusalem would have to endure, 70 years." [Dan. 9:2]

"And while I was still engaged in prayer, the man Gabriel whom I had seen originally in a vision *flew* [v. supra] and reached me at about the time of the afternoon prayer and he understood and spoke to me saying, 'Daniel, I have come to grant you the understanding. At the beginning of your entreaties, a word was issued and I have come to tell it to you, because you are a precious person who understands words and interprets visions. Seventy weeks have been decreed for your people in your holy city to compensate for your transgression, to complete the measure of the sins and to expiate iniquity, to introduce eternal righteousness, to confirm prophetic vision and to anoint the Holy of Holies. Know and understand that from the time the word was issued to restore and rebuild Jerusalem until the anointing of the leader will require seven weeks, and for 62 weeks it will be restored, street and moat, though with distress. And after 62 weeks the Messiah will be cut down, and disappear and the hosts of a prince who has come will destroy the city and the sanctuary, but its end will come by flood, and destruction is decreed until the end of the war. During one week he will establish a covenant with a multitude, and for half a week sacrifice and offering will be terminated, and on the corner (of the altar) appalling abominations (will appear) until the decreed destruction will be poured out upon the violator.'" [Dan. 9:21–27]

The element of secrecy is represented here briefly.

"And you Daniel, keep these things secret and seal up the scroll until the end of time." [Dan. 12:4]

"I heard and I did not understand and I said, 'My Lord, what will be the outcome?' And he replied to me, 'Go, Daniel, because these things are secret and sealed until the end of time. Many will be purified and cleansed and refined, and the wicked will behave wickedly but the wicked will not understand, but the wise will understand.'" [Dan. 12:8–10]

In common parlance, "apocalypse" refers to catastrophic destruction, complete eradication. The major thrust of the Book of

Daniel is that ultimately disaster and defeat will befall the major empires that successively persecuted Israel.

What is not emphasized by many students of apocalypse is the importance of the ultimate rescue and vindication of the suffering population to whom the vision is directed. It is true that the message of survival and rebirth is often shorter and less salient than the message of destruction, but it is the main point, the source of comfort that justifies the entire endeavour.

> And at that time Michael the great prince who stands up for your people, will arise, and they will see a period of distress the like of which had never occurred from the time of the formation of the people until that time, and at that time your people will be rescued, all who are found recorded in the book. And many of those who sleep in the dust of the earth will awaken, some to life eternal and some to contempt and eternal degradation. And the wise will radiate like the radiance of the heavens and those who lead the multitudes to virtue will shine like the stars forever. [Dan. 12:1–3]

Clinical "apocalypses"

Having reviewed the form of the classical apocalypse, we can compare it with what I call the "clinical apocalypse". At the onset of a psychotic episode, the patient may believe that the world has changed, that there has been an abrupt discontinuity. In essence, this idea signifies the death of the patient's reality, which is equivalent to his self, while the new world represents his rebirth. Here is a classic description of an apocalyptic, psychotic delusional system, given by Freud in his discussion of the illness of Daniel Paul Schreber (Freud, 1911c), a German lawyer and judge in the late nineteenth century who became psychotic and subsequently described his experiences in a published memoir.

> At the climax of his illness, under the influence of visions which were "partly of a terrifying character, but partly, too, of an indescribable grandeur", Schreber became convinced of the imminence of a great catastrophe, of the end of the

> world. Voices told him that the work of the past 14,000 years had now come to nothing, and that the earth's allotted span was only 212 years more; and during the last part of his stay in Flechsig's clinic he believed that the period had already elapsed. He himself was "the only real man left alive" and the few human shapes that he still saw—the doctor, the attendants, the other patients—he explained as being "miracled up, cursorily improvised men". Occasionally the converse current of feeling also made itself apparent: a newspaper was put into his hands in which there was a report of his own death; he himself existed in a second, inferior shape, and in this second shape he one day quietly passed away. But the form of his delusion in which his ego was retained and the world sacrificed proved itself by far the more powerful. He had various theories of the cause of the catastrophe. At one time he had in mind a process of glaciation owing to the withdrawal of the sun; at another it was to be destruction by an earthquake, in the occurrence of which he, in his capacity of "seer of spirits", was to act a leading part, just as another seer was alleged to have done in the Lisbon earthquake of 1755. Or again, Flechsig [his psychiatrist] was the culprit, since through his magic arts he had sown fear and terror among men, had wrecked the foundations of religion, and spread abroad general nervous disorders and immorality, so that devastating pestilences had descended upon mankind. In any case the end of the world was the consequence of the conflict which had broken out between him and Flechsig, or, according to the aetiology adopted in the second phase of his delusion, of the indissoluble bond which had been formed between him and God; it was, in fact, the inevitable result of his illness.

The text makes clear that Schreber's delusional fantasies dealt with the conflict between his wish to be dead and his wish to be reborn. The death of the world replaced his own death. Despite Schreber's attempt to displace his wish to be dead onto the world, derivatives of the wish nevertheless appear in his delusional ideas that he had, in fact, died. Yet the new world represents an attempt at rebirth, though not a successful one.

In addition to the conflict between destructive and reconstructive forces that we find here and in profusion in the rest of the Schreber memoir and clinical record, other features of apocalypse are clearly represented: striking and terrifying visions and auditory experiences; the concept of the *seer*; numbers denominating the passage of time until "the end"; a villain; direct communication and an emotional bond between the individual and his god; a vision of God in His heavenly court; and a messianic mission by the patient.

But we do not have to turn to the abnormal to find clinical homologues to apocalypse. Dreams provide many such instances in some individuals who are scarcely mentally ill, if ill at all.

The following dream focuses on the need for revelation. It was reported by a Jewish woman, neither especially religious nor especially observant, but with a decent respect for the tradition and some intellectual interest in it. She is not mentally ill but is in psychoanalytic treatment because of some confusion about her aims and goals and because of a disturbing tendency towards mood swings, excessive in intensity and frequency.

> *"There was wilderness and rubble. We had walked for miles to get there. I walked with a band of followers. I was with a man with robes and a staff. The local people came to me. I asked about a structure like an old observation tower. It was cylindrical with a dome, high, at the edge of the town. An old priest, probably Christian. He believed that he was watching for the Messiah or Armageddon. Can I go up to ask him questions? Yes, but they kill people. I went upstairs inside the building. A man in robes met me. He had a dark beard. I had a manuscript that indicated that some old man would come and ask questions. I asked the questions, something about the staff. I can't remember the answers. He was not angry. He took me to a large window—an incredible view—you could see far off into the hills with the tower of stone. I was impressed that he had befriended me enough to show me this view."*

The dream starts in the "*wilderness and rubble*"—namely in the aftermath of apocalyptic destruction (note the reference to Armageddon). In other words, the patient is depressed. She is one of the "*band of followers*"—that is, she will achieve rebirth, recovery from her depression, within the context of a fraternal group. She describes a man with robes and a staff, and a Christian priest, both images of the archetypical sage of apocalyptic scriptures, and she also refers to a messiah. We find here a number of references to curiosity and revelation: an observation tower, the asking of questions, a manuscript, obscure answers, and an incredible view through a large window. The death–rebirth sequence appears here less prominently than the element of revelation. But it is represented in the initial hints of depression and the hope for a messiah. This dream illustrates the fact that the acquisition of secret information archetypically serves the interest of rebirth.

But let us look at the dream again to ascertain what especially fascinates the dreamer. Note especially the man with the staff, the cylindrical stone tower topped by a dome, and questions about the staff. The dream concludes: *"I was impressed that he had befriended me enough to show me this view."* It does not require much imagination to infer that this woman is curious about the leader's phallic equipment. Such an interpretation is reinforced by the fact that her father had exposed himself to her repeatedly when she was a child, occasionally deliberately, more often inadvertently. She recalls these experiences vividly. Evidently, in the context of her present depression, she recalls early revelations that excited her, and she hopes for a new revelation that will prove equally gratifying. It is likely that the actual revelation for which she hopes is a therapeutic revelation to be provided by her male psychoanalyst. She grew up and lives in an environment in which a man's virility is judged largely by his intelligence and ability to solve problems. Her analyst's perceptiveness and ingenuity in offering her insight into her difficulties gratifyingly reveals his virility to her.

But let us look at the dream still again. *"They kill people who ask questions."* When she asked the old man questions, he was not angry. She was gratified that he had befriended her enough to show her the incredible view. These features of the dream remind us that the search for secret knowledge is dangerous. We learn that from the Israelites' fear of God's revelation at Mount Sinai, as well as from many other instances in which excessively close approach to the Godhead proves fatal, as in the *Pardes* of Hagigah (see chapter three) and in the *Hekhaloth* texts. Curiosity that is too intrusive, an approach that is too bold, encounters anxiety, a consequence of regulation, that we attribute to conscience or superego. The attempt to evade death and to seek rebirth by the quest for revelation paradoxically invites further danger. Here I believe we have the psychodynamic basis of the fear of confrontation with divine secrets, except under certain protected circumstances.

In the following dream, based upon the images of the Book of Revelation, the disclosure of the secret saves the dreamer. This material is kindly provided by Dr Jacob A. Arlow.

> The patient has put his apartment up for sale. He is hoping to get enough money to enable him to leave his law practice and go to Hollywood to pursue a career in film. He intends either to write about film, to write scenarios, or perhaps even to produce. The patient has no experience or training in this field. To him, however, going to Hollywood means throwing off the shackles of inhibition and especially the proscriptions of the church regarding sexuality. In previous months, the patient has produced a great deal of psychoanalytic material of a frankly incestuous nature, coupled with thoughts of castration and damnation for sexual wishes, together with fear of authority figures. This material, however, has come out in an extremely isolated form. The patient repeats what he has learned as if it were a catechism. His insight is reduced to a formula, which is repudiated as such. The patient is most isolated in his productions. He gives hardly any details of day-to-day activities, conversations with other individuals, or fleeting fantasies, unless a specific inquiry is made about such items.
>
> Over the past weekend, preceding the Independence Day [July 4] holiday, the patient had as a weekend guest his only close friend. This is a man whom he has known from college days. Both are Catholics and lawyers with serious sexual problems. Both are dissatisfied with the practice of law and would like to leave it. The friend, Adolph, however, has two children and a wife and feels trapped. During their earlier years, the two would share sexual fantasies and giggle about "exploits" they had with girls. Although this is the patient's closest friend, he sees him perhaps once or twice a year. Adolph's wife is extremely withdrawn, as is their older child.

It is clear from the description that the patient and Adolph, who shared sexual fantasies and thoughts, both suffer the same kinds of inhibitions. Over the weekend, they went for a walk together and discussed their sexual inhibitions and the role of the Catholic Church in frightening them with eternal damnation for sexual transgression.

After his friend Adolph, Adolph's wife Sylvia, and the two children had left, the patient spent a quiet Fourth of July holiday reading a book that was essentially an interview with the Italian movie director, Fellini. On the night of 5–6 July, the patient had the following dream:

"My wife and I were somewhere up in the mountains in some small village. There were four people coming on horseback. They were knights like the Four Horsemen of the Apocalypse. They had stopped to tell us that there was going to be an earthquake and some of the area would be flooded. We were on a small island. They told us to move to a larger island, which we did. While we were there, the earth began to quake, fire began to flow and the small island where we had been was inundated with water. We were clinging close to the ground while the earth was shaking."

The patient stated that the dream must be traced to what he was reading in the Fellini interviews. Fellini spoke about the pervasive influence of the Catholic Church in Italian life. Its two-thousand-year-old influence pervades every aspect of Italian thought. Most particularly, however, Fellini emphasized the role of the Apocalypse. The ultimate vision of the Apocalypse is in the background of every Italian person's thinking, and, as such, it gives vibrancy to the lives of the Italians. Everything is lived against the background of the ultimate great struggle of the Judgement Day, when people will either be damned to eternal perdition or go to heaven with the angels, etc. Fellini felt, and the patient agreed, that it was the Church, not God, that introduced the idea of sexual pleasure as sin, making the apocalyptic vision one fraught with fear and trepidation.

Later in the session the patient quoted a further element from the Fellini interview. Fellini was questioned about the picture *8½* and Anita Ekberg. Fellini said he had not known Anita Ekberg, but when he saw a picture of her in an American film magazine, in which she was dressed in a skimpy leopard-skin, he exclaimed, "I hope to God I never run into her. I could never resist the temptation." In discussing this aspect of the material, the patient said, "There again is a woman as the devil, woman as the temptress and seductress."

To which I added that Anita Ekberg was noted for her large, sensuous breasts. The patient agreed, and I then reminded him of the sex play with his mother's "apples".

The patient had been in Italy ten years ago, he recalled, after the earthquake in southern Italy. He was at the Amalfi Drive and saw how the earth had just been torn apart by the quaking, how fragments of roads were separated from each other by dozens of yards as a result of the earthquake. He had also seen a mild eruption of a volcano in Sicily. The flowing lava connected with volcanic eruptions reminded him of visions of fire and brimstone in apocalyptic visions in the Bible in the Apocalypse of St. John.

The four knights in the dream were identified by the patient with the Four Horsemen of the Apocalypse. He could not, however, remember their names or exactly what they stood for, but he knew that they represented portents of great danger and ultimate destruction. In the dream, however, he was struck by the fact that the four horsemen were actually saviours and helpers. While discussing the four horsemen, the patient kept fondling his tie reassuringly.

I called the patient's attention to the fact that the four horsemen represented tremendous threats—conquest, war, famine, and death. It was when I mentioned Death and the Pale Rider on the white horse that the patient recalled the aspect of the Fellini interview that dealt with Anita Ekberg.

This material was used to demonstrate to the patient how, in spite of his advanced thinking, he still clings to the fear instilled in him by that part of the Catholic teaching about sex (incest) being a mortal sin, punishable by eternal damnation. This in spite of the fact that earlier in the session he supported Fellini's view that God really takes the total balance of man's deeds, good and evil, over the course of the seventy-or-so-year span and weighs man in the balance, but He would not condemn an individual just for one act of mortal sin, that it was the Church that introduced the idea of eternal perdition. In spite of all this, however, the patient, out of his own castration anxiety and guilt, still has to grapple with the fear of damnation (castration).

This case illustrates the prospect of destruction as punishment for sin. The patient, however, is not punished with the wicked, but escapes with the aid of the Four Horsemen, who, in the dream, abandon their classic role of portents of death and destruction and become helpers and rescuers. The reason that the threat fails is that, in view of his life-long masochism and depressive character, at Dr Arlow's suggestion, the patient had begun a programme of antidepression drug therapy with me a year earlier. His response to all medication had been positive but only temporary. On 22 June, 20 milligrams of fluoxetine (Prozac) had been prescribed, in addition to the 60 milligrams of methylphenidate (Ritalin) per day and the 0.5 milligrams of lorazepam (Ativan) three times a day that he had been taking. He had responded nicely to the fluoxetine. The dream, which occurred on 6 July, reflects the remedial effects of the latter in the patient's seeing himself as one of the saved rather than one of the doomed, and the Horsemen as friends rather than demons. This case illustrates the influence of mood on the outcome of the mythic drama as it is played out.

The number four appears commonly in apocalyptic dreams and in the true apocalypse; it is my impression that it symbolizes mother.

I propose the term "apocalyptic complex" for fantasies, dreams, illusions, beliefs, images that centre about the death--rebirth sequence or its reverse, even in the absence of the full apocalyptic syndrome. Many of these will contain, as components, revelation, travel, symbolism, numbers, confrontation with a deity, and so on. The apocalyptic complex then includes true apocalypse, along with other social phenomena such as messianism, millenarianism, and fundamentalism, as we see below. In classic religious literature, especially in the prophetic literature, predictions of doom alternate with comforting words that often allude specifically to rebirth. At the end of chapter 10, Isaiah announces, with an arboreal metaphor, the destruction of Assyria for its deadly harassment of Israel. The forest will be cut down. Continuing with the metaphor, in chapter 11 he promises that Israel will be reborn, that "a shoot will grow out of the stump of Jesse", the father of King David, and "a branch from its stock". A messianic rescuer will appear, who will destroy the enemy and initiate a utopian age.

As a clinician, I encounter alternations in mood to a limited extent in many people without serious mental illness, but much more frequently and importantly among patients with affective disease, such as manic-depressive illness, recurrent depression, depressive neurosis, borderline personality disorder, and attention deficit disorder, whether in adults or children. Such patients frequently report dreams in which the affective orientation alternates from destructiveness to constructiveness and back, from death to rebirth and sometimes the reverse.

In dreams that are concerned with the regulation of affect, the initial episode of the dream usually reflects the affective state of the dreamer. The dream then displays attempts to overcome or correct this affect deviation. Usually the last episode of the dream returns to the affect of the initial episode. Here is a dream of a woman with a propensity for mood swings somewhat more prominent than usual.

> *"The world was being flooded. The water was reddish and grayish. It was turbulent with white crests. I saw rocks and houses. People were drowning. We were on a high level, where there were white houses. I was on a boat—a nice boat, large with blond wood lacquer floors. There was a kitchen on the boat. I became concerned that it would capsize. We landed at a house on some land. We brought things onto the boat, glasses, no, plastic cups for fear that they might break, and food.*
>
> *What's the point of living if you're going to drown? I thought of suicide and became calmer. No, I said, there is always hope. If you die now, you eliminate hope.*

I saw some people drowning, some with hands raised, some protesting, some peacefully."

The dream starts on a depressive note: a flood, people drowning. The dreamer finds security on a boat, but her depressive tendency threatens her with the possibility of capsizing. She has the boat reach land, where she replenishes the food supply. But then the depressive mood reasserts itself in thoughts of suicide. She comforts herself with hope but sees others drowning. The dream reproduces an ancient myth, one version of which is expressed in the Noah's-Ark story. The latter ends, not as this dream ends, but with signs of rebirth, the dove's finding food and refuge, the actual landing of the Ark, and God's promise that He will never again attempt to destroy the world, and His instructions to man to produce progeny. He designates the rainbow as the eternal promise of rebirth.

The woman who reported this dream is the same woman who reported the dream about waiting for a revelation and a messiah. So when she is more hopeful, she expresses the quest for the revelation component of apocalypse, and when she is more depressed, she dreams of the death–rebirth sequence.

Apocalyptic archetypes

Clinical archetypes

The term "archetype" has become an indication of Jungian orientation. I intend no such implication here. What I describe is a series of images that appear widely, perhaps universally, in religious mythology, in creative works, in fantasy, in the hallucinations and delusions of the psychotic, and in everyone's dreams. Their appearance reveals a readiness to relate to other individuals and to the forces of nature in one of a limited number of stereotyped ways. Their origin can be debated. I would guess that they are formed when infantile experience is recorded and preserved by a hard-wired apparatus within the brain, with the resultant formation of relatively permanent paradigms or templates that are then used to recognize dangers and opportunities for gratification.

In dreams that conform to the apocalyptic complex we encounter the same archetypes that we find in classical apocalypses. Let me start by examining clinical material that I published in my book, *Drugs in Psychoanalysis and Psychotherapy* (Ostow, 1962). By using published data, I make it possible for the interested reader to learn considerably more about the patient, designated there by the initials XNZ, than I can present in this paper. I shall supplement this material with data obtained from patients recently or currently in treatment.

XNZ, a 37-year-old, married schizophrenic woman, volunteered two dreams during her second visit: One dream was of

> *a painting of a city that seemed* ***dead****—a ghost city. "It was painted in black and white and no human or animal figure appeared. All at once the doors of the houses opened and gaily dressed people came out, including my husband and me."*

I do not attempt to consider the personal, individual associations to any of the material that I present, since it is my purpose to call attention to universal archetypes. Here we have the typical *Weltuntergang* [world destruction] dream. The death of the world—that is, the patient's death projected onto the terrestrial canvas—is denoted by the desolation of the city, the absence of life and of colour. The desired *rebirth* is denoted by the opening of the doors and the appearance of people and colour.

A schizophrenic young man (GO), whose schizophrenia was under good control, omitted his medication one night and dreamed:

> *"I* ***watched*** *a movie that became* ***real life.*** *Grand Central Station was about to* ***explode*** *and* ***kill everyone*** *inside. A* ***great ball of fire.*** *It would pass from that building onto Park Avenue. I ran for my life.*
>
> *I watched it again. People were being led into a theatre innocently,* ***without knowledge of what's to come. They would die.*** *I watched from the second level.* ***Chaos.*** *No one had the authority to call the police. I ran out to Thirty-ninth Street.*

> *Swimming for my life. As fast as possible. Tough enemies with machine guns were firing indiscriminately.*
>
> *You appeared in the station. I was assured that chaos wouldn't break out again."*

On the following night he dreamed:

> *"My father and I tried to save our lives because the* ***world was about to end.*** *There was nowhere to go. Everybody would die. But no one was concerned.* ***We went to the boat shop to escape to the sea."***

The *Weltuntergang* patterns are obvious here, too, though here the process of destruction is exposed, rather than, as in the previous case, only the consequences. Accordingly, there is not sufficient resolution of the anguish to permit the expression of accomplished rebirth, though the hope for it is recorded. Notice the comment that a *lack of knowledge* contributed to the holocaust. Revelation would have saved the people.

The second of the two initial dreams reported by XNZ represented that:

> *The patient was driving very fast in an* ***automobile*** *with her husband. She was afraid of a* ***crash.*** *Suddenly she was* ***resting*** *on a* ***peaceful green*** *meadow.*

We recognize here again the death and rebirth images, the latter associated with the colour *green*, the symbol for vegetation. The death was not yet accomplished, but experienced in the dream violently as a crash. Another patient, very shortly after having recovered from a serious schizophrenic breakdown, recumbent during the session on my green analytic couch, found herself thinking of the Twenty-third psalm: "The Lord is my shepherd. I shall not want. He causes me to lie down in green pastures. He restores my soul." Notice that the green pastures in the Twenty-third psalm corresponds to the green meadow in XNZ's dream. Both represent not only revived vegetation, but also a tranquil and hospitable mother. In this thought of the Twenty-third psalm, the analyst was seen as a messianic deliverer: the messiah who *rescues* and *restores*. During the period of her acute illness she had believed that the world was being destroyed by a cataclysmic war between the United States and the Soviet Union.

I should like to draw attention in XNZ's second dream to the image of the *moving vehicle*. It, too, occurs commonly in apocalyptic dreams and represents, I believe, the patient's effort to escape from the scene of destruction and the anxiety created by the rage, to the Elysian fields that represent the tender mother. The vehicle, as a container, can be seen not only as a means of transportation, but as a symbol for mother's body, to which the individual wishes to be transported. In the dream, the rescuing vehicle itself escapes control, and not only fails to rescue the patient, but actually threatens her with destruction. That dream fragment is abruptly discontinued and replaced by the rebirth fantasy. In other dreams and fantasies, contrived when a patient has achieved better control, the vehicle successfully rescues him. A man (XM) who as a child feared that planes would fall from the skies and kill him, dreamed repeatedly of fear of plane crashes and fear of falling from a high place. A woman (GDU) whose child had wet himself at night, then came into her bed, dreamed:

> *"I was in a taxi. The driver went the wrong way. I got out. Some people got into the seat. One person hung onto the back window. I hung onto the fender. I have to get inside. Why is this guy riding on this part of the car? It's too dangerous. I, too, was sitting in a strange place."*

In another dream:

> *"I'm in a hot air balloon. It was too dangerous. I could die in the flame. But it was the only way to get someplace. Suddenly I was unable to breathe*, and I woke up."

These are only two of a long series of vehicular dreams presented by this patient, in most of which either she was excluded, or the ride was dangerous. That for her the vehicle represented her mother's body projected onto a terrestrial or cosmic backdrop is demonstrated by the following dream:

"On the floor I saw a kind of spaceship, a toy. The centre was a round dome with flat sides, like Saturn with its flat rings. Two bars came off at an angle and it was suspended by them. I picked it up. It was soft, not metal, like crocheting. It was too soft. It was not what I expected. I could not understand why I was intrigued by it. When I put it down, I couldn't understand why I had been so fascinated by it."

Here the spaceship, the cosmic vehicle, clearly takes the shape of the uterus, suspended by the fallopian tubes. The return to mother is frustrated, and the vehicle is disparaged as unworthy. The two bars also suggested the arms of the parent who carries the baby, as in the next dream.

That the movement of the vehicle symbolizes being carried by the parent is suggested by the following recollections of XNZ (Ostow, 1962):

> Shortly after her father died, when she was 11, she would be gripped by hypnagogic sensations of being "lifted by a pair of enormous arms and being rocked". In an even earlier fantasy, she saw herself "resting on an enormous white surface, like a sofa, very safe because the sides were too distant for anyone to approach". She associated this image with God. "No troubles could reach me, and there was plenty of room to explore." [p. 236]

The yearning to enter the mother's body again and be protected by her is precipitated by anxiety caused by the destructive wishes. I mentioned above the dreams of a schizophrenic young man, GO. These *Weltuntergang* dreams were immediately preceded by the following:

> "I had a nightmare. *I found myself in bed with my mother. We had no clothes on. She was insisting that I start sexual advances. I touch her breasts. I don't know whether she had anything on the lower part of her body."*

The dream starts with the patient's taking refuge with his mother. However his peremptory incestuous wish reasserts itself, and is terminated by the threat of apocalyptic destruction.

Returning to XNZ, later in her treatment she reported the following dream (p. 241):

> *"I was with mother at our home outdoors, in the evening. Suddenly the northern lights were in the sky, soft and lovely. I said, "How lovely!" They got more and more* ***colourful*** *and violent. They coloured the whole sky. Suddenly it was a great bomb attack with missiles. The sky was flooded with* ***falling objects.*** *I hurried her indoors. We were covered with ash and incurably contaminated by it. It was radioactive fallout. We got into the house. I tried to wash myself off."*

I shall ignore the obvious anal referents, though they occur not uncommonly in other apocalyptic material. The reason is that anality is neither necessary nor characteristic for apocalypse. Apocalypse may include any one or several of the psychosexual developmental phases. However the *colour* and *light* and *shimmering luminescence* occur characteristically in mystical fantasies, where they are associated with the expectation or experience of the gratification of the longed-for visualization and union with the Deity. The latter, though often designated as the father, is frequently described in terms more characteristic of the mother. In this dream, we see a reversal of the usual sequence. At the onset of the dream, the patient has already achieved idyllic reunion with the mother, to the accompaniment of the sense of luminescence and scintillation. However, that reunion is overtaken by the destructive impulses. Mother and she are both incurably contaminated. She is not able to *rescue* mother.

Light is also a very common symbol for rebirth, as dark portends danger and death. Fire combines rebirth with danger. It symbolizes what is infinitely attractive but may not be looked at—for example, the fiery area of God's genitals in the chariot vision of Ezekiel, chapter 1, and the image of God cited above from Dan. 7:9,10.

Notice the emphasis on *heavenly* events. It is the northern lights in the sky that please her. Then it is a group of *falling objects* that threaten and destroy her. In apocalyptic fantasies and dreams, the impulses are often projected out onto the cosmos, so that they are seen as imposed by cosmic forces onto human destiny. In my experience, when objects fall from the sky, they are usually seen as destructive; when they rise heavenward, they are usually protective and messianic. As an adolescent, XNZ entertained fantasies that:

> She was an *angel flying over* the city at night.

Here she identified with the messianic impulses that defended her against her destructive wishes and that she had projected out onto cosmic figures.

GDU reported a dream that resembled this northern-lights dream of XNZ:

> *"I got up at 1 a.m. It was very light because of an amusement park nearby that had bluish lights. It was like dawn. I thought I saw lightning, but it was yellowish, like firecrackers. They arched high and came down in a star burst, like a chrysanthemum. Up and down, one after the other. One came near me. It bounced like a tennis ball. We watched a long time. It must be the end of the day, and that's why they had fireworks."*

In another dream of the same night, the patient found herself driving past her mother's house, thereby confirming that the dream dealt with the complex of feelings centring about closeness to the mother, as was the case with XNZ.

Objects arching across the sky occurred commonly in her dreams. When the objects were rising, she felt comforted, and when they were falling, they created anxiety.

To illustrate the last point, I present another dream of hers:

> *"I was at home, watching the outside of a building with a man. There was a string of four children* ***swinging*** *out from a window. My son was at the end of the string. The man said it was dangerous. I reacted very calmly, "He's not falling." He slipped and* ***fell****, face-down onto the ground. The man said, "He was hurt." I rushed over, feeling guilty but powerless. Amazingly he was not hurt. It was so lucky. If there were rocks around, he could have hurt his eyes or his head."*

In another dream of that night:

> *she was hanging* ***streamers overhead*** *in a large room that would be used for dancing.*

Note here the features of something hanging overhead; the falling from a height; and threat of catastrophe. As a child, she had feared being attacked by birds flying overhead. The feeling of powerlessness in the dream is what I believed sparked the apocalyptic thinking in the first place.

> After mother's death, XNZ reported, I had a dream of two short Hebrew words; I thought it was a revelation: I felt the earth was only a temporary place and that I would soon join mother in Heaven, or wherever God was.

XNZ remembered a few Hebrew words from his minimal Hebrew-school education in childhood and could just about recognize Hebrew letters. In the dream, the ancient, traditional script was seen by her as the *revelation* of a *secret* that gave her the magical power to reunite with mother in her celestial home.

These archetypes are found not only in patient after patient among those that have the task of dissipating rage, but also in clear and unmistakable form in apocalyptic documents available to us. I cited the clinical references here to establish that classical archetypes appear spontaneously within the individual and invite the individual who is preoccupied with them to associate himself with groups in whose mythology and religious scriptures he recognizes them.

Classical archetypes

The various classical apocalypses differ from each other in detail, each having been written to respond to the anguish of a specific period and a specific place. The styles as well as the contents differ, the emphases, symbolism, and messages. Differences can be seen between the Jewish and the Christian apocalypses, and of some of them it is believed that they started out as Jewish pieces and were modified to apply to the Christian community. In the Book of Revelation, we can find some classical apocalyptic archetypes.

As the name of the book indicates, the text is given as a *revelation of a secret* hitherto withheld (see Rev. 1:1, 1:19, 4:1, 5:1). Both the content of the scripture and the meaning of its many symbolic statements have been mysteries, and both are here disclosed. The secret is transmitted from its Omniscient Source by an agent, who appears sometimes as the *author of the document* (Rev. 1:1, 1:19), at other times as a mysterious *wise person* or creature. In Revelation we find the phrase "One like a son of man" (Rev. 1:13), who reveals what has been hidden.

At a number of points (Rev. 1:13, 3:4, 19:8, 19:13) a *white robe* is specified as a garment that signifies purity. In the Book of Daniel (10:5), the angel who conveys the vision to Daniel is spoken of as *"clothed in linen"*.

The *massive disruption* that we associate with apocalyptic literature appears in a number of extensive accounts throughout Revelation, most of them vivid and dramatic. The *end of the world* as we know it is clearly described. The classical apocalyptic struggle between the forces of Good and the forces of Evil is given in Rev. 12:7–9 and Rev. 20:7–10.

> And there was a war in Heaven, Michael and his *angels* fighting with the *dragon*. And the dragon and his angels fought, and he did not prevail, neither was there found a place any more for him in Heaven. And the great dragon, the ancient serpent who is called Devil and Satan, was *cast out*, he who deceives the whole world was *cast out* onto the earth, and his angels were cast out with him. [Rev. 12:7–9]

Falling celestial objects recur many times throughout the book. Sometimes the objects fall, sometimes they are hurled down. Most of the time the fall is associated with destruction, as it is in the clinical material cited above. Let me quote one example:

> And the seven angels who had the seven trumpets prepared to blow them. And the first one blew his trumpet; and there was *hail* and *fire* mingled with *blood*, and it was *hurled to the earth*. And a third of the trees were *burnt up* and all the *green*

> *grass* was burnt up. And the second angel blew his trumpet; and something like a great mountain *burning with fire* was *hurled* into the sea. And a third of the ships were destroyed. And the third angel blew his trumpet; and a *great star, burning* like a torch *fell* from the heavens and it fell upon a third of the rivers and upon the springs of water. And the star is called by the name, "The Wormwood". And a third of the waters became wormwood, and many men died from the waters, because they were made bitter. [Rev. 8:6–11]

However, in the opposite mode, the "new Jerusalem" also descends from the heavens, but the descent is gentle rather than violent (see below).

Flying creatures appear frequently in Revelation; most of them are *angels*, but there are also eagles. Their intention may be either hostile or friendly.

Moving vehicles, which appeared so often in the clinical material, are seldom encountered in this apocalypse. We read of "the new Jerusalem descending out of heaven from God" (Rev. 21:2), and "a white cloud and on the cloud one like a son of man was enthroned" (Rev. 14:14), but movement is not expressly attributed to this cloud. In 3 Enoch a "fiery chariot" is specified as the vehicle for cosmic travel (Rev. 6:1). Many chariots are said to be provided for God in 3 Enoch, chapter 24. "A huge four-faced chariot of Cherubim" is described in another Gnostic text, the *Hypostasis of the Archons*. In the Jewish *Hekhaloth* text, *Hekhaloth Rabbati*, a carriage of fire is offered to the traveller to pass from the sixth to the seventh Hekhal (Rev. 23:1).

Though the specific references to vehicles are relatively few in Revelation, there is a good deal of movement through the heavens, not by vehicles, but with the help of eagles, angels, and other flying creatures. The author is carried by an angel (Rev. 17:3) to view the various apocalyptic events and portents. In other apocalypses—for example, in 1 Enoch—the author is transported through the entire cosmos to view its mysteries and portents, and the book contains many references to the transportation.

Since apocalypticists project from inside onto the cosmos, they focus primarily on the heavens. They seldom project their impulses and fears onto the depths of the seas and the ground, though occasionally they do. Therefore we encounter celestial events far more frequently than events originating below. Chthonic, demonic monsters are sometimes described as rising from the earth or the sea. In Revelation, two monsters are described, one arising out of the sea (Rev. 13:1) and one out of the earth (Rev. 13:11). In patients' dreams I have only infrequently encountered dangerous monsters arising out of the depths. The infant nursing at the breast looks upward to its mother's face, and to all adults, so long as the child is small.

The rebirth theme occurs in every apocalypse as the desired resolution of the problem created by the initiating humiliation and consequent rage. In Revelation, a resurrection of the dead is described in 11:11 and in 20:4; a birth is described in 12:1–5; and the new heaven, earth, and new holy city of Jerusalem replace their earthly predecessors, which were destroyed (Rev. 21:1–4).

> And I saw a *new heaven* and a *new earth*; for the first heaven and the first earth had passed away, and the sea was no more. And I saw the holy city, the *new Jerusalem*, descending out of heaven from God, prepared as a bride adorned for her husband. And I heard a great voice from the throne, saying, "Behold, the dwelling of God is with mankind. He will dwell with them, and they shall be his people, and God himself will be with them, and he will wipe away every tear from their eyes, and death shall be no more, neither mourning nor crying nor pain anymore. For the former things have passed away. . . ."

The remainder of chapter 21 and the first half of 22 describe the reconstructed Holy City.

Psychodynamics

From these considerations I conclude that apocalypse, whether classical or the apocalyptic complex, is not just a genre, a style of religious writing. Rather, I believe that it is the expression of a mental mechanism, perhaps universal, that seeks to regulate affect. When an individual is depressed, the mechanism strives to overcome the depression and replace it with euthymia (absence of mental pain) or euphoria. When an individual is too euphoric, too "high", this corrective mechanism acts to restore the mood to a median position. Depressive affect generates images of disorder, disease, death, or destruction. Euphoria generates images of survival and rebirth. For many people the regulation of affect is so efficient that one scarcely becomes aware of mood swings. For other individuals, however, mood regulation is inefficient and a constant challenge, and it is they who exhibit the apocalyptic complex.

These considerations are of more than academic or theoretical import. As everyone knows by now, powerful chemical substances in the brain regulate affect. When a patient, in the course of his mood swings, becomes fixed in a depressive excursion, an antidepression drug can free him to return to a euthymic position. Similarly, when the excursion takes the patient to a manic position, one of the antipsychosis tranquillizers can overcome that. When the pathology is excessive volatility rather than a unipolar deviation, control is more difficult, though often possible by a judiciously titrated combination of drugs of these two classes. The psychopharmacologist who takes the time and trouble to learn about dream interpretation and to examine his patients' fantasies and dreams in addition to their symptoms can find, in the dream manifestations of the apocalyptic complex, helpful clues to supplement and inform his clinical judgement.

Because the apocalyptic complex is the expression of a basic unconscious mechanism, it appears in many products of mental life, behaviour, fantasy, creative endeavours, as well as dreams. I have tried to demonstrate what I consider to be the impressive congruence between archetypes found in classical apocalypses and those found in the dreams of some individuals who are concerned with affect control.

In most of our mental life, we strive to maintain continuity. We wish to have ideas consistent with each other. We wish to maintain continuity in our love and social relations and in the way we live. We see our parents and ourselves and our children as a continuous chain. Apocalypse, on the other hand, means discontinuity, abrupt change. It is a fantasy of an end, a fundamental reorientation, a destruction of the old, and replacing it with the new. The death–rebirth sequence is the mechanism by which continuity is disrupted. It is perhaps a biological device for responding to a desperate situation.

We should note one important difference between the classical apocalypses on the one hand, and the dreams and delusions that I have reported on the other—namely, that the former, though they may have been created by individuals, have become important to the religious life of communities. In other words apocalypse may satisfy the needs of an individual or of a group, and often of both simultaneously.

How does a group come under the influence of apocalyptic thinking? Not all members of the group are equally concerned with affect regulation. Nevertheless, even those whose mood is fairly stable, who can retain a certain degree of equanimity under stress, may find themselves entrained, compelled to accept the apocalyptic mode under the influence of a minority that is noisy, demanding, and aggressive. We do not have accounts of group responses to ancient apocalypses, but we do have historical accounts of the reception of the Sabbatean movement and Hasidism. To be sure, neither of these is exclusively apocalyptic: the former is messianic, and the latter is mystical. But they both demonstrate the group dynamics involved in responding to a newly presented mystique that appeals powerfully to only a portion of the population while the others resist it.

Variants of the apocalyptic complex

Taking our cue from clinical experience, we can actually discern three different types of clinical apocalypse complex. First, the depressive state is especially likely to give rise to apocalyptic thinking. The patient, when he despairs of escaping from depression on his own, becomes angry and wishes harm either to himself or to others around him, with the conscious or unconscious hope that major alleviation will follow. Suicide will effect reunion with a dead parent, or save one's family from bankruptcy by means of insurance. Serious suffering will elicit rescue. Schreber's *Memoirs* is an apocalyptic plea for rescue.

In an apocalyptic complex of this first type, dreams will usually start with portrayals of disaster, death, disorder, or destruction. Then the dream will change or be replaced by another in which we see movement towards repair. However, the dominant depressive affect then reasserts itself as the dream or dream sequence terminates. The dream of the flood exemplifies this apocalyptic type.

I append here a letter that I received recently from a patient whom I had not seen for 17 years. He is a brilliant but manic-depressive businessman whose judgement was so warped by his illness that he was not able to retain the fruits of his intelligence and enterprise. He was usually more optimistic or more pessimistic than the situation warranted. Sometimes his investments worked out successfully, but in the long run he did not do well. At the time that he wrote this letter, he was mildly to moderately—not severely—depressed and was planning to return to consult with me.

> *Just to bring you up to date, November 1976 was one of my last visits to you after the major breakdown of my life. It's been downhill generally since then on every front—depression, finances, self-esteem, confidence. Today, after some very bad years I do not diagnose myself with true clinical depression. My condition is a deeply ingrained, growing pessimism about the world, my family and myself in these anni horribiles—now a major transition era—into the unknown. In my view, everything has gone wrong for me—family and finances. I was at first surprised and shocked. Suicide when I had a million dollar insurance policy was an option. I didn't take it—it lapsed. Suicide not good for a family anyway.*
>
> *No activity—no desires. I read, write for myself, mostly protesting that the world is blind. The Chaos Theory is very real to me. The Age of Enlightenment from the Declaration of Independence on. Life, liberty and the pursuit of happiness and progress is a dying idea. The new one is unknown but survival will be a different ball game. I refuse to renounce Judaism or the existence of a Creator or a force beyond human forces who probably does roll the dice and doesn't guarantee anything—but we who are about to die must salute him. I wish there may be something after life, but if it's nothing, let it really be nothing (Hamlet's worries). I cannot guess*

how my children and grandchildren will fare in the new world.

I must and can adopt to the increasing slings and arrows of outrageous fortune. Every now and then I need help. Playing golf, which I don't, isn't enough.

I come to see an old friend, a wise man—looking for a wise word that strikes a responsive chord. I respect your profession but feel it is much too early to talk of it as being in anything but its infancy. The young ones cannot cure the melancholy of the human condition.

P.S. I guess there is no wise word. Acceptance, for the saints. I'm not one. Play games, golf, bridge. Mostly for the young ones. I can't. I want some joy—impossible now. Happiness was never possible unless you go into "sublimation", religious trance, devotion and belief in anything and any field. Impossible. It seems like death or Alzheimer's Disease is the only solution.

One day, one hundred or one million years from now, there will be either a Messianic Era or apocalypse. Right now we're on the verge.

Note the sense of failure and futility and the contemplation of suicide. The universe is chaotic for him. He expresses ambivalence about thoughts of an after-life. He seeks a wise seer who will offer revelation, a "wise word", and he voices a faint hope for apocalyptic messianic rescue. He alternately accepts and rejects the possibility of belief and religion. However, he enclosed with his letter a copy of a speech given by Vaclav Havel on Independence Day, 1994, reprinted in the *New York Times*. I cite here one of Havel's closing paragraphs:

> What makes the "anthropic principle" and the "Gaia hypothesis" so inspiring? One simple thing: Both remind us of what we have long suspected, of what we have long projected into our forgotten myths and what perhaps has always lain dormant within us as archetypes. That is, the awareness of our being anchored in the Earth and the universe, the awareness that we are not here alone nor for ourselves alone but

that we are an integral part of higher, mysterious entities against whom it is not advisable to blaspheme.

We have in both the letter and to a lesser extent in Havel's speech affective disease, depression, apocalyptic thinking, and mysticism.

The second type of clinical apocalyptic complex occurs primarily in the case of psychotic individuals who are truly manic or schizophrenic. The patient who is too "high" anticipates being brought down by a powerful supernatural force, or by a conspiracy of enemies. These delusional, usually paranoid ideas express the unconscious influence of the control mechanism that is activated by the "high" state and acts to arrest it.

Manic-depressive businessmen are apt to come to grief when they succeed too well. The apocalyptic complex comes into action silently, punishing them for their presumption, by distorting their judgement and causing serious failure of the business venture in which they have characteristically overextended themselves. They soon crash into depression. The Promethean enterprise expresses the "rebirth" or hopeful, overly ambitious phase of the apocalyptic complex, while the subsequent crash, which sometimes leads to accomplished suicide, expresses the destructive phase. There is no revelation except the prophetic warnings of family and friends, which the subject rejects.

The dream of the young man (GO) in incestuous embrace with his mother illustrates this second type of apocalyptic complex. Here the dream starts with representation of the unacceptable desire. That phase is interrupted by a punitive, destructive interlude—the subsequent explosion in Grand Central Station. But the dream may not terminate before the initial Promethean drive reasserts itself, or at least until relief is found. This patient dreamed that he was saved by his analyst. The primary rebirth tendency reasserted itself in the rescue.

More dramatic and tragic are those instances in which a hitherto quiet and unobtrusive individual suddenly goes berserk and attacks others, often strangers, violently. Fury, psychotic dissociation and altered consciousness—as, for example, the trance state—may be engendered by the third type of apocalyptic complex, the result of the struggle between powerful depressive and antidepressive forces.

A young man was being treated for disabling mood swings. He was a decent, cultured, responsible person who harboured some racial antipathies, which he was sometimes able to acknowledge as unreasonable. On one occasion, disappointed by the inadequate effect of an antidepression medication, I withdrew it gradually. Within a few days, he abruptly became seriously agitated and had great difficulty controlling murderous impulses directed towards other races. Reinstating that drug and adding an antipsychosis tranquillizer promptly overcame this quasi-psychotic state and reinstituted normal self-control.

These variants of individual apocalyptic complex give us a clue to similar variants in the case of the group. Most classical apocalypse seems to be addressed to the misery of an oppressed population. It predicts the destruction of the enemy and the rebirth of the victims. That is true of both scriptural apocalypses that we have quoted—Daniel and Revelation. We see a homologue of the apocalyptic dreams and fantasies of the depressed individual.

Most prophetic threats of doom are addressed to a Promethean population, defying restraint and the accepted principles of morality dictated by religion. These are usually followed by messages of comfort. Previously, I quoted the beginning of chapter 11 of Isaiah, promising messianic rescue of Israel. Assyria will be destroyed, but only after it carries out God's design:

> Assyria, the rod of my anger, that hold the staff of my fury in their hand. I send them against the wicked people, I charge him against the people of my anger to take booty and spoil, to turn it into mire of the streets that is trampled underfoot. [Isa. 10:5,6]

The prophet then continues with the observation that Assyria does not realize that it is merely an agent in the hands of God but has overbearing ambitions.

> Therefore so says the Lord, God of Hosts, my people who dwell in Zion do not fear Assyria who beat you with a staff and raises his rod above you like the Egyptians. Because shortly my anger will subside. [Isa. 10:24,25]

> The Lord God of Zion will lop off the crowns of the trees with an axe; the tall ones will be cut down and the high ones will be laid low. And he shall cut down the thickets of the forest with iron and he will fell the Lebanon with superior strength. [Isa. 10:33,34]

Then follows the messianic rebirth of Assyria's victims, Israel:

> And a stalk shall grow out of the stock of Jesse and a shoot will sprout from his roots. And the spirit of the Lord will rest upon him, a spirit of wisdom and understanding, a spirit of counsel and strength, a spirit of knowledge and fear of the Lord. And his discernment will flow from his fear of the Lord; he will not judge merely by what he sees nor decide on the basis of what he hears. He will judge the poor with righteousness and decide justly for the humble of the land; he will beat rebellious territories with the rod of his mouth and with the spirit of his lips he will destroy the wicked. Justice will be the girdle for his loins and fidelity the girdle for his hips. And the wolf shall dwell with the sheep and the leopard shall lie down with the kid; and the calf and the young lion and the young of the cattle will mingle, and a small child shall lead them. And the cow and the bear shall graze, and their young will couch together, and the lion will eat straw like the ox. And the young child will play on the hole of the viper and the infant will pass his hand over the den of the adder. No one shall do evil or destroy on the whole of my holy mountain for the earth will be filled with the knowledge of the Lord as the waters cover the sea. [Isa. 11:1–9]

The well-known verses describing the ingathering of Israel follow.

The most dangerous of the social apocalypses are homologues of the third clinical type: fury generated by the conflict between depressive and antidepressive forces. They incite the millenarian adventure, such as those detailed by Norman Cohn in the *Pursuit of the Millennium* (1970), and such as the Nazi Holocaust. We see the venting of fury upon others in order to achieve inner tranquillity, which never comes so long as the instigating depressive threat continues. Such apocalypses frequently end in suicidal behaviour, though not necessarily before widespread damage has been done. This is active apocalypse as distinguished from expectant apocalypse. The apocalyptic group effects the destruction, rather than merely hoping for it or fearing it. Millenarian apocalypse is exploited as a divine justification for murder and other forms of criminal behaviour visited upon others who are designated as the enemy of the Lord.

Mysticism and the apocalyptic complex

I have included this essay on apocalypse in our study of mysticism because the two overlap. Mysticism may be seen as a member of the group of phenomena that conform to the general pattern of the apocalyptic complex.

In the case of many apocalypses, the revelation is a mystical experience, usually a trance experience, as we observed above in the case of Daniel. The author announces that he has had a kind of immediate experience of the deity, or of a supernatural agent—the same experience as that to which the mystic aspires: a view, a voice, a feeling of presence. For those who subscribe to the apocalypse, it becomes an orienting and venerated scripture—absolute and unchallengeable. The Jewish mystic also orients himself around a fixed scripture. It may be the Torah and Talmud that he reinterprets to extract its "hidden secrets". It may be the *Zohar* or other Kabbalistic documents that contain these secrets. Apocalypse clearly demonstrates the death and rebirth duality. That duality is less visible in mysticism, but in my opinion it is intrinsic and essential to it. For the mystic, the rebirth is achieved either by the initiating mystical experience, or by entering the mystical life, or by both—that is, the mystical life itself provides important gratification. The mystical experience is the first, and the mystical life is a second rebirth component. In addition to individual rebirth, the *tikkun* of Lurianic Kabbalah promises literally to restore the state of perfection of the universe, which had been destroyed by the bursting of the vessels.

The antecedent death phase is less visible in mysticism. In apocalypse we find two elements representing death: the miserable state of the world that causes the pain and the wish for its destruction. And there are two rebirths: the gratification of gaining the hope for and the anticipated reconstruction of the real world. The same is true of mysticism. Just as we can discern two types of rebirth experience, we can also discern two types of death experience: the first is the dismal state of the world in which the mystic lives and from which he wishes to extricate himself; and the second is his turning his back on the normative experience of the real world, or on a major portion of it, or derogating it mentally while investing his enthusiasm and vital interests in a sacralized experience of it. In the dualities of both apocalypse and mysticism, each component has two elements, the chaos of the world as perceived and the wish to turn away from it in the case of the former, and the psychic reorientation and the action taken subsequently to reconstruct the broken world in the case of the latter. As I noted above, Idel (1988, pp. 65f.) quotes mystics to the effect that union with the Godhead necessarily involves annihilation of the self.

These last comments about the death–rebirth duality turn our attention from the formal similarity between apocalypse and mysticism to the psychic similarities. In each case, the world of sorrow and pain, frustration and disappointment, is also the world of reality, which the mature individual is forced to confront. However, we each have a threshold beyond which we give up and regress to the psychic state of early childhood, when we looked to our parents for comfort and protection. In apocalypse, a divine or semi-divine redeemer is promised. The receiver of the revelation may be permitted to ascend in a vehicle to the Most High. In dreams such ascents are interpretable as voyages back to mother or father. In apocalyptic communities, a charismatic leader takes over. The mystic, too, seeks return to mother or father, but by the medium of immediate but symbolic experience, the experience of reunion and identification. In the mystical group, the charismatic leader serves as an intermediary between the individual and the deity—psychologically, even if not designated as such by religious doctrine—and almost literally as a parent figure. The Hasidic rebbe is a case in point.

This discussion obviously brings us to another member of the apocalyptic complex, messianism. In most apocalypses, salvation is brought about at the hands of a supernatural rescuer, a saviour. Most messianic pretenders describe their experiences of vocation, their being called to their mission, as a mystical experience. They are informed of their mission by a supernatural figure who appears to them in a trance, or by way of other mystical communication. Sabbatai Sevi declared himself the messiah when he interpreted a message voiced by his companion and "manager", Nathan of Gaza. Sabbatai reported that Nathan had fainted and "A voice went forth from his mouth, saying [Hos. 6:2], 'After two days he will revive us, and the third day he will raise us up and we shall live in his sight'—and this was all" (Scholem, 1973). In classical apocalypses we encounter supernatural figures, some of whom communicate the apocalypse, some of whom interpret it, and others promise to save. As we observed above, similar functionaries are found in apocalyptic dreams.

Fundamentalism can also be understood as a member of the apocalyptic complex. Many fundamentalists believe in apocalypse. They credit an inerrant scripture. The essential element of fundamentalism is the integration of the individual into the group, obliterating his own identity in order to enjoy the sense of union with the others. Like the mystic and the apocalyptic, the fundamentalist derogates the world of external reality and replaces it with the separatist reality of his community and the scripture, interpretation of scripture, and religion of that community. A community, as we mentioned above, represents the mother. The process of rejecting the outside world and finding renewal within the group again demonstrates the death–rebirth succession.

The belligerent millenarian who is usually both apocalyptic and fundamentalist attempts to rush the *end of days*—the *eschaton*—by his attacks on unbelievers. His apocalyptic death–rebirth scenario is obvious. The union with the religious parent surrogate, in his mind, depends upon eliminating the symbolic sibling. The psychology of the utopian can be understood in the same way, though he is less dangerous and less belligerent.

Assuming the correctness of these hypotheses, we must wonder how it is determined which variant of the apocalyptic complex will be selected by the population at risk. Presumably the choice is determined by environmental factors—political, psychological, economic—as well as by morale and the nature of the leadership.

From the arguments that we have considered here, I believe that mysticism can be understood as one variant of the apocalyptic complex. It responds to a harsh and intransigent reality, but the psychodynamic pattern and characteristic archetypes are probably determined ultimately by biologically based behavioural tendencies.

MYSTICISM AND PROPHECY

CHAPTER THREE

INTRODUCTION

Prophecy is an institution of religious leadership that appeared in ancient Israel during and after the conquest of Canaan and continued until the first part of the Persian period. The early popular prophets, such as Samuel, Elijah, and Elisha, contributed to the consolidation of the commonwealth. Their actions are recorded even more fully than their words. The later or classical prophets are known primarily by their words, though we have some biographical data too. The best known are Isaiah, Jeremiah, and Ezekiel. It is with Ezekiel that Halperin's essay is concerned.

Although apocalyptic appeared perhaps three centuries after the presumed termination of the age of prophecy and is considered by scholars to be a very different phenomenon, I believe that prophecy can easily be subsumed within the category of the apocalyptic complex. Our sources are meagre, but there seems to be some evidence for a gradual evolution from prophecy to classical apocalyptic, as common sense would suggest, rather than an abrupt cessation of the one and, after an interval, the inception of the other (Hanson, 1979).

But whether or not that proposition can be demonstrated, we can find in classical prophecy unmistakable components of the apocalyptic complex. The prophets in their oratory warn of catastrophe, sometimes as punishment for sinful behaviour, sometimes as the consequence of unwise political or military adventure. But alternatively they assure Israel of survival and rebirth: "Comfort ye, comfort ye, My people, says your God" (Isa. 40:1). And Ezekiel's prophecy of the rebirth of the dried bones is more dramatic, if less well known (Ezek. 37). As a contribution to the reassurance of Israel, the prophets occasionally foretell the downfall of the oppressing enemy empire.

Every prophecy is presented as a revelation given to the prophet by the Lord. The revelation deals with the current status of things, with prevailing immorality and presumptuousness, or, on the other hand, with despair resulting from oppression; but it tells us also that the former will be punished and that Israel will be delivered from the latter.

A prophet may be called to prophecy by a specific event—often a trance experience such as those described in Isaiah, chapter 6, and Ezekiel, chapter 2, or speak of the "end of days" of Isaiah, chapter 2. The prophet may describe a journey accomplished by supernatural means—for example, Ezekiel, chapter 8—and a vehicle that travels through the heavens, as in Ezekiel, chapter 1.

My point is that classical prophecy and classical apocalypse can easily be distinguished one from the other, but they both contain elements that classify them as members of what I have called the apocalyptic complex—and from that conclusion I infer that they share a common psychodynamic structure.

If we look at the trance experiences as reported in the biblical text, we shall have little reason to question their mystical nature. Repeatedly, Ezekiel describes the visions that he receives. He falls to the ground overwhelmed. A spirit enters him. The hand of the Lord comes upon him. He is transported in spirit from one place to another. When the word of the Lord comes to him, he begins to prophesy: the actual vocation to prophecy is given in chapters 2 and 3.

A similar description of vocation to prophecy is given in Isaiah, chapter 6—namely, a vision of the Divine Presence, profoundly moving visual and auditory experiences, hearing the voice of the Lord, and finally the direct assignment to prophesy. The similar commissioning of Jeremiah is given in chapter 1. Each account describes an oral experience. Ezekiel is instructed to eat God's words in the form of a material scroll. Isaiah is touched on the lips with a live coal by a seraph. Jeremiah is touched on the mouth directly by God. God's word is placed literally in the mouth of the prophet. In each case, the prophet resists the assignment. A splendid psychoanalytic study of this vocation experience is given by Jacob Arlow (1951). Arlow draws attention to the transmission of authority by the oral route, the prophet's ambivalence, and the role of the death–rebirth mechanism.

> The consecration of the prophet is a temporary schizophrenoid abandonment of reality and withdrawal of object libido. A schizophrenic tries in vain to re-establish these ties by involving his fellow man in the distorted relations of his delusions. The prophet, however, through his mission, succeeds in re-establishing the emotional bond with the world of reality because his message truly corresponds to a deep emotional reality waiting to be stirred in the soul of his contemporaries. The apocalyptic dream of Isaiah of an era of universal peace, when "nation shall not lift up sword against nation", is a true representation of the aspirations of humanity.

Without saying so explicitly, Arlow clearly places prophecy in the domain of the apocalyptic complex. He also compares the "heightened narcissism" of the prophet to a hypomanic state.

The reader will recall, too, that in chapter one I noted the fact that whereas in the case of most mystics the outcome of the mystical trance state is a submissive, subordinate, self-effacing posture, in the case of others the mystic emerges from the trance state as a teacher and leader. These are the mystical leaders whose roles in history have been recorded, whereas the former group are seldom remembered as individuals. Dynamically, we may say that the leaders emerged from the trance state, the state of union with the image of the archaic parent, identified with the Divinity and with the parent whom He represents. The individual, self-effacing mystic sees himself as clinging to a divine parent by obedience and unusually intense religious devotion. The prophet sees himself reborn by virtue of his identification with God; the rebirth of the individual mystic is achieved by his compliant righteousness.

Even though the mystical trance state results in the prophet's identification with God, his prophecy expresses his own views for which he claims divine sanction, and the affect is his too.

In chapter two I suggested that the trance is favoured by a state of affect disequilibrium—specifically, the state in which depressive and antidepressive tendencies struggle against each other. In my experience, that state also tends to generate anger. Therefore, trance and anger often occur together in prophetic literature. The anger becomes explicit in the experience of the prophetic vocation.

> And I said, how long oh Lord? And he said, until cities remain without inhabitants and houses without people and the ground will remain desolate. And the Lord shall remove the population and much of the land will be abandoned. [Isa. 6:11,12]

But that threat is immediately followed by the promise of rebirth:

> But a tenth will remain and repent and will be consumed like the terebinth and the oak whose trunk survives despite the loss of leaves, and that trunk is the holy seed. [Isa. 6:13]

For the individual mystic, the conflict is resolved in the euphoria of the *unio mystica*, while the destructive component is confined to the experience of rejecting the material and mundane.

We shall see that in *merkavah* and *hekhaloth* mysticism, the conflict itself is expressed directly in the fantasy. The questing mystic is punished for his presumption by the angels unless he can assure them of his religious worthiness and self-effacing intent.

David J. Halperin has recently published a book, *Seeking Ezekiel: Text and Psychology* (1993), in which he studies the Book of Ezekiel systematically from a psychoanalytic point of view. His carefully crafted study moves step by step to what seems to be a necessary and persuasive argument. He concludes principally that Ezekiel is dominated by "a dread and loathing of female sexuality". "Whatever one may say about the biblical God in general (or God in general), the God of Ezekiel was a creation of Ezekiel's own brain. This proposition follows inevitably from the work we have done here." Halperin also demonstrates clearly the rage generated in Ezekiel's mystical prophetic experience.

We have before us a brief segment of that book, somewhat revised for our purposes here. This segment demonstrates the power of psychoanalytic exegesis for explicating the many problems of text and content with which the book abounds. It also demonstrates clearly the destructive aspect of the prophet's mystical trance, his mystical identification with God, and a specific kind of mystical revelation—namely, penetrating secret sinful fantasies and longings, which may well have been projections onto others of his own secret desires. Professor Martin Bergmann provides a commentary from the point of view of the practising psychoanalyst. He discusses the psychodynamics of the prophet's relation to his God and emphasizes the sadomasochistic components.

Ezekiel and the Elders of Judah: The workings of a prophetic trance

David J. Halperin

INTRODUCTION

In the spring of 597 BC, Nebuchadnezzar, king of Babylon, subdued the rebellious kingdom of Judah and captured its capital, Jerusalem. He deported to Babylonia the more substantial persons of the kingdom. He left behind "the poorest of

---

The bulk of this paper originally appeared in David J. Halperin, *Seeking Ezekiel: Text and Psychology* (University Park, PA: Pennsylvania State University Press, 1993), pp. 58–73. I have lightly revised the material, and provided it with an introduction and a conclusion, for its present publication.

I am indebted to the following persons: Pamela E. Kinlaw, who served as my research assistant, helped me interpret Prov. 18:11–12. Daniel Merkur provided me with references on dreams in sequence; and, in a lecture of 17 March 1988, he pointed out the shamanistic seances described by Rasmussen and their interpretation. I owe to James H. Sanford the reference to the seance described by Bogoras. Mortimer Ostow called my attention to the potential importance of Jaazaniah's name in shaping Ezekiel's attitude towards the man; while Robert Segal stressed the importance of distinguishing between Ezekiel's hatred of Jaazaniah having been the people of the land", under a new king whom he had selected (2 Kings 24:14–17).[1]

Judah again rebelled. In 587 or 586, the Babylonians again captured Jerusalem, this time destroying the temple of the Judean God Yahweh along with the rest of the city; and, once again, Jews went into Babylonian exile.

Of the "prophets" of the time—self-proclaimed spokesmen for Yahweh, whose oracles eventually made their way into the canon of the Hebrew Bible—Jeremiah was among those Jews who stayed in Jerusalem until its final fall. His contemporary, Ezekiel, was among those exiled in the deportation of 597. Our concern here is with Ezekiel, and with the Biblical book that bears his name.

This document represents itself, with considerable plausibility, as Ezekiel's own account of the visions and messages he received from Yahweh over a period of at least 22 years, beginning in 593 BC[2] Its central concern is the city and temple Ezekiel left behind. The first half of the book (chapters 1–24) pounds across the idea that the city, drenched in blood and sin, is doomed, for its temple is corrupted beyond hope of reform. True to the prediction, both city and temple are destroyed (Ezek. 33:21–22). In the book's second half, Ezekiel promises their restoration (chapters 33–48) and turns his fury on such foreign powers as Tyre and Egypt (chapters 25–32).

All this is backed up by prophetic rhetoric, which is often gruesome and occasionally obscene (e.g. chapters 16 and 23) yet throughout powerfully effective. It is backed up also by bizarre visions (e.g. chapters 1, 8–11) and pantomimes (e.g. Ezek. 12:1–20). Ezekiel must perform strange operations on his own

---

unconscious or simply suppressed. My wife, Rose Shalom, M.D., directed me towards the discussions of sudden cardiac death in the medical literature and helped me interpret them. [D.J.H.]

[1] All Biblical quotations in this chapter are my own translations from the Hebrew.

[2] The commentaries of G. A. Cooke (1936), Walther Zimmerli (1969), and Moshe Greenberg (1983; to ch. 1–20 only) are the great Ezekiel commentaries of our century and must be consulted by all students of the text. William H. Brownlee's commentary on Ezek. 1–19 (1986) is a useful bibliographical resource. H. H. Rowley (1953–54) gives an excellent summary of approaches to the Book of Ezekiel in the first half of this century.

body (Ezek. 5:1–4). He must lie paralysed (Ezek. 4:1–8). He is obligated, until he protests, to bake his bread with human excrement (Ezek. 4:9–15). His tongue is bound, and his dumbness leaves him only when the temple is at last destroyed (Ezek. 3:22–27, 24:25–27, 33:21–22).

It is no wonder that Ezekiel has sometimes been thought a sick man (Lang, 1981, pp. 57–76). Moderns have occasionally tried to diagnose his illness. August Klostermann (1877) accounted for Ezekiel's peculiarities in terms of what the nineteenth century called "catalepsy". Edwin C. Broome (1946) attempted a psychoanalytic approach to these peculiarities; the outcome was a diagnosis of paranoid schizophrenia (cf. Jaspers, 1947). Biblical scholars have normally either dismissed Broome—often in the most disparaging terms—or ignored him altogether (Cassem, 1973; Davis, 1989, p. 66; Garfinkel, 1987, 1989; Howie, 1950, pp. 69–79). Psychoanalysts have occasionally adopted some of Broome's interpretations of passages from Ezekiel, while apparently remaining unaware that it was he who had first proposed them (Arlow, 1951; cf. Merkur, 1988).

For all its flaws (notably, its useless effort at diagnosis), Broome's psychoanalytic approach seems to me fundamentally sound. I have argued at some length that Ezekiel's book does, indeed, provide us with reliable clues to the psyche of its author: a marvellously gifted yet profoundly disturbed man, haunted by a pathological dread and loathing of female sexuality, and by a profound ambivalence towards a dominant male figure whose features he normally displaced onto his God (Halperin, 1993).

One of the cornerstones of this interpretation is the "temple vision" of Ezek. 8–11. Scholars have long recognized that this text is riddled with problems from beginning to end and have offered a wide variety of solutions to these problems. The most effective solution, in my opinion, is to see this vision as an authentic description, not of anything that actually went on in the Jerusalem temple, but of the psychic landscape of its author. This landscape can be most effectively mapped in psychoanalytic terms.

In the pages that follow, which are drawn from my longer study, I offer my theory of the reality that underlies Ezekiel 8–11. At this stage of the argument, I have not yet entered into the analysis of Ezekiel's symbolism and what this has to tell us about the psychology of its creator. My aim is, rather, to clarify the nature and some of the determinants of Ezekiel's visionary experience and how this experience interacted with the physical and social realities in the midst of which Ezekiel found himself. At the same time, my reconstruction of the reality behind the text must contribute to the elucidation of the text itself. To the extent to which I succeed in this goal—to which my reconstruction makes sense of textual problems that have baffled earlier expositors—to that extent we may trust that its representation of Ezekiel and his surroundings approximates the historical truth.

The chambers of imagination

Ezekiel 8:1 dates the vision described in the following chapters to "the sixth year, the sixth month, the fifth day of the month"—that is, some time in September, 592 BC (Greenberg, 1983, p. 8). Ezekiel sits in his house, the "elders of Judah" in attendance. A luminous human form appears to him and holds him transfixed. A "spirit", meanwhile, "lifted me up between earth and heaven and brought me to Jerusalem in visions of God" (Ezek. 8:1–3). Some time later, the spirit again lifts Ezekiel up and brings him back to Babylonia, "in the vision, in the spirit of God; and the vision I had seen lifted off me. And I spoke to the exiles all the words of Yahweh that he had shown me" (Ezek. 11:24–25).

In-between, the prophet has seen the temple of Jerusalem desecrated by a string of "abominations", each worse than the one before. An "image of jealousy, that incites jealousy", stands at the northern inner gate of the temple court. Seventy elders of Israel burn incense to images of unspeakable creatures inside a mysterious chamber. Women sit weeping for "Tammuz". A group of men stand outside the temple and prostrate themselves towards the rising sun (Ezek. 8:3–18).

Vengeance follows. A band of human-like beings passes through Jerusalem and slaughters the entire population, except for those "who sigh and cry over all the abominations that are done in their midst", and who have been set apart by a mark on their foreheads (chapter 9). One of these beings, the one who has made the mark, is sent to burn the city with coals of fire (Ezek.

10:2–7). The glory of Yahweh, until now resident in the temple, leaves the bronze cherubim on which it has been encamped and mounts a chariot carried by animate cherubim (Ezek. 10:3–4, 18).

The chariot pauses in its departure at the east gate of the temple (Ezek. 10:19), where it and Ezekiel encounter a band of sinful Jewish leaders. Ezekiel prophesies against them, with the result that one of them, Pelatiah ben Benaiah, drops dead (Ezek. 11:1–13). There follows an oracle, its relation to its context uncertain, which appears to defend the religious status of Ezekiel's fellow-exiles against the arrogant claims of the Jerusalemites (Ezek. 11:14–21). The chariot, Yahweh's glory on it, leaves Jerusalem and settles on "the mountain to the east of the city" (Ezek. 11:22–23). And Ezekiel is returned to Babylonia.

The scholars who have discussed this vision have normally focused on the "abominations" of chapter 8. Precisely what religious practices is Ezekiel describing? (See, e.g., Albright, 1942, pp. 165–168; Gaster, 1941.) To what extent does his account of them accurately represent cultic activity carried out in the Jerusalem temple during the last days of the kingdom of Judah? If Ezekiel's account is substantially accurate, as most have supposed, how are we to square it with the claim of the Second Book of Kings that King Josiah (640–609 BC) had earlier purged the temple worship of non-Yahwist elements; and with the same writer's failure to accuse Josiah's successors of having undone his reforms (2 Kings 23–25)? But if Ezekiel's vision is "pure fantasy"—as Yehezkel Kaufmann has powerfully argued (1960, pp. 428–432)—how are we to account for his intense conviction of its reality? How can we explain his hearers' evident willingness to believe him on this point?

In the course of elucidating this issue, the commentators have naturally had to grapple with the question of the nature of Ezekiel's experience and of his role in the events he describes. Most obviously, if he was physically in Babylonia, how did he know what was going on in the Jerusalem temple? How could he have brought about Pelatiah's death in Jerusalem? Some have gone so far as to suppose that Ezekiel was clairvoyant; or, alternatively, that the Babylonian setting of his book is a fiction, and that Ezekiel actually lived and preached in Palestine (see Lang, 1981, pp. 7–12, 75–76).

This latter alternative—which requires at least some editorial tampering with the text—brings us to a literary question posed by chapters 8–11, as indeed by the entire book of Ezekiel. To what extent is the account of the temple vision actually Ezekiel's work? How much of it was created by later writers? The very conservative stand Greenberg (1983) has taken on this question contrasts sharply with Zimmerli's (1969) willingness to identify many layers of editorial work in the vision and to identify an original core that is considerably shorter than the corresponding text that now appears in our Bibles.

Our present constraints will not allow us to enter into the details of this last issue. Yet our analysis of the visionary experience here described will suggest that the text as we have it is essentially trustworthy. The difficulties scholars have perceived in it are real, but they do not require that we peel away various inauthentic layers from an authentic core. Rather, they demand a fresh look at what Ezekiel meant to say, and at the situation reflected in his words.

Two postulates will guide us towards understanding the vision.

First, the "elders of Judah", mentioned at the beginning of the vision (and, by implication, at its end) are not merely part of the vision's framework. They are its audience. They are the objects of its accusations as well. It is they who appear as the twenty-five sun-worshippers of Ezek. 8:16 (called "elders" in Ezek. 9:6, according to the reading of the Masoretic Hebrew Text), and as the twenty-five "princes of the people" in Ezek. 11:1.[3] They appear also as the seventy elders of Ezek. 8:11; only here their number has been determined, not by the reality of the historical situation, but by the Pentateuchal tradition of the "seventy men of the elders of Israel" (Num. 11:16–17, 24–30). They crop up again and again in the vision, because they are

[3] The Masoretic text has "twenty-five" in both 8:16 and 11:1. The Greek version of the Septuagint reads "twenty" in 8:16, but supports the Masoretic Text in 11:1. I suggest that these numbers reflect the actual number of elders who sat before Ezekiel, which was between twenty and twenty-five. The variations—between the Septuagint's 8:16 and 11:1, between 8:16 according to the Masoretic Text and 8:16 according to the Septuagint—represent variant approximations to this actual number.

part of its environment. They are, indeed, its main exciting factor. That is why, within the vision, they are indestructible.

Second, the charges made against them are not only fantasy (as Kaufmann, 1960, has argued), but are explicitly stated to be fantasy. Only, Ezekiel will not acknowledge the fantasy as his own. He therefore projects it onto the elders, declaring that he is exposing *their* hidden wishes. The grounds for Ezekiel's erroneous conviction are to be elucidated—as I do in my book (Halperin, 1993)—along psychoanalytic lines.

The situation described in Ezek. 8:1—"I was in my house, the elders of Judah sitting before me"—recurs twice in the Book of Ezekiel. "Men of the elders of Israel came to me and sat before me" (Ezek. 14:1). "In the seventh year, in the fifth month, on the tenth of the month, men of the elders of Israel came to inquire of Yahweh, and they sat before me" (Ezek. 20:1).

Commentators have pointed out that this situation is stereotypic. Like so much in Ezekiel, it is reminiscent of the prophet stories in 1 and 2 Kings. Specifically, 2 Kings 6:32 represents Elisha as "sitting in his house, the elders sitting with him"; and the language of this passage is very suggestive of Ezekiel's (Carley, 1975, pp. 42–45). It does not follow, however, that we are dealing with a purely *literary* stereotype. The situation may have become a staple of prophet-narratives precisely because it tended to recur in real life. We have no reason to deny that on certain occasions Jewish elders did sit in Ezekiel's house while they consulted him, or that the Book of Ezekiel describes three such actual occasions.

Now, on the second and third of these occasions, Ezekiel interacts with his visitors in a violently hostile manner.

In Ezek. 14:3, Yahweh advises his prophet that

> these men have lifted up their idols upon their heart, and put the stumbling block of their iniquity before their faces [*he'elu gillulehem 'al libbam umikhshol 'awonam natenu nokhah penehem*]. Am I indeed to let them inquire of me?

Ezekiel must declare to them that anyone

> who lifts his idols upon his heart and puts the stumbling block of his iniquity before his face, and then comes to the prophet, I Yahweh have responded to him concerning it [?], according to the multitude of his idols. . . . I will set my face

> against that person, I will make him a sign and a subject of proverbs, and I will cut him off from my people. [Ezek. 14:4, 8][4]

The Israelites must therefore repent of their idols [*gillulekhem*], turn their faces away from all of their abominations [*to'abotekhem* (Ezek. 14:6)]. We can hardly doubt that Ezekiel indeed delivered this message with appropriate violence.

Notice that Ezekiel does not accuse the elders of actually having worshipped idols, performed iniquitous acts, or committed "abominations". Rather, they have *imagined* doing these things. They "have lifted their idols upon their hearts"—that is, admitted them to their thoughts. (The idiom is most clearly paralleled in Isa. 65:17, Jer. 51:50, and Ezek. 38:10. See also note 7, below.) When Ezekiel tells them to turn their faces away from their abominations, he is, as Greenberg says (1983, p. 248), using "a metaphor for disregarding what is only in the mind". Yet these imaginary abominations, whose nature is left entirely vague, merit the most ferocious retribution.

Ezekiel, whatever he may have believed, can hardly have had direct access to what the elders were thinking. We may suppose, if we wish, that he constructed his notions of their fantasied "abominations" by some process of inference—however confused and distorted—from what he had observed of their speech and behaviour. But there is another possibility, which better accords with a psychoanalytic approach to the "abominations" and which therefore draws strength from the ability of this approach to elucidate the details of Ezekiel, chapter 8 (Halperin, 1993). It is that the elders' imagined "abominations" were Ezekiel's own fantasies, which he projected onto them.

Yet the elders, being human, must occasionally have had thoughts of which their consciences disapproved. It is hardly fantastic to suppose that they may have felt Ezekiel's vague accusations to apply to them, and that they left his presence feeling guilty and chastened.

[4] Verses 7–8 largely repeat and expand verses 4–5, and both passages are cast in the style of the Pentateuchal source known as the "Holiness Code" (Lev. 17:20, for example). The repetitiousness and the use of language akin to that of the Holiness Code are both characteristic of Ezekiel (Carley, 1975, pp. 62–65). The meaning of *bah* in verse 4 is unclear, and the text uncertain.

Ezekiel's response to the inquiring elders in chapter 20 is no less hostile. As in chapter 14, Yahweh is indignant that such men have come to inquire of him (Ezek. 20:3, 31). He blames them for their ancestors' "abominations" (*to'abot*, in verse 4; this is the word used throughout chapter 8). He demands to know whether they are defiled in the ways of their ancestors, whether they go whoring after their ancestors' despicable things [*shiqqusehem*], whether they continue to offer child sacrifice "to this day" (verses 30–31).[5] "The thoughts that have crossed your minds[6]—that which you say, 'Let us be like the nations, like the families of the lands, serving wood and stone'—will certainly never come to pass" (verse 32).

Here again, Ezekiel claims to know what his visitors are thinking. These alleged thoughts are enough to provoke his accusation that the elders replicate the sins of their forbears—whose hearts and eyes went after abominations (verses 16, 24; cf. Num. 15:39), who could not bring themselves to cast away the sins they looked after and hankered for [*shiqquse 'enehem* (verses 7–8)]. It again appears, though not as clearly as in chapter 14, that Ezekiel's fury is directed against what the elders have imagined, not what they have done.

In blaming his audience for the sins of the Israelite ancestors, Ezekiel condemns himself together with them. We may read this as an admission that their sins are his. That is to say, the imaginings he condemns in the elders are really his own.

Can we extend these observations, by analogy, to chapters 8–11?

In these chapters, too, people's thoughts come under attack. This is clearest in Ezek. 11:1–13, where the "princes" Ezekiel

---

[5] I read verses 30–31 as a series of four questions, the first beginning with the interrogative *he* (Kautzsch, 1910, p. 296), each of the others with *waw*. This supposition softens, though it certainly does not eliminate, the seemingly implausible charge that the Babylonian exiles were practising child sacrifice (Greenberg, 1983, p. 387; Heider, 1985, pp. 373–374). Ezekiel insinuates it with a question (of the are-you-still-beating-your-wife variety), but does not assert it outright. I have argued (Halperin, 1993, pp. 167–172) that Ezekiel knew perfectly well that the elders were not sacrificing children, yet he was driven by his psychopathology to imagine that they *must* be doing so. His insinuating question represents a compromise between his fantasy and his awareness of reality.

[6] *Ha'olah 'al ruhakhem*; corresponding to *he'elu . . . 'al libbam* in 14:3.

denounces are said to be "the men who think iniquity [*hahoshebim 'awen*], and who give bad counsel concerning this city" (Ezek. 11:2).[7] "Bad counsel", it is true, would suggest that the "princes" not only "thought iniquity", but went on to translate their thought into persuasive speech. But Ezek. 11:5 indicates that they are blamed for their thoughts as well as for their speech. "Thus you have said, house of Israel", Ezekiel declares to them in Yahweh's name, "and I know the thoughts that have crossed your minds [*uma'alot ruhakhem ani yeda'tiha*]." This boast, of having unmasked the villains' secret musings, would have little point if these had already been publicly expressed.

We note that the language of this passage echoes that of chapters 14 and 20. *Ma'alot ruhakhem* corresponds to *ha'olah 'al ruhakhem* (Ezek. 20:32). The fragmentary denunciation of Ezek. 11:21, which does not fit very well with its present context and seems to be connected with Ezek. 11:1–13, is reminiscent of Ezek. 20:16.[8]

But I think 8:12 contains a more significant, if less obvious, reference to evil thoughts. The Hebrew text reads: *hara'ita ben adam asher ziqne bet yisra'el 'osim bahoshekh ish behadre maskito*. The Revised Standard Version reflects the nearly universal understanding of this passage: "Son of man, have you seen what the elders of the house of Israel are doing in the dark, every man in his room of pictures?"[9]

But, so understood, the text is difficult. Kaufmann (1960, p. 430) has pointed out that it appears to contradict the preceding

---

[7] *Ba'ir hazzot*; more commonly translated, "in this city" (e.g. Revised Standard Version [RSV]). I translate it as I do in accord with my belief (defended below, and in Halperin, 1993, pp. 73–79) that Ezekiel is addressing his fellow exiles.

[8] Cf. 11:21, *we'el leb shiqqusehem weto'abotehem libbam holekh*, with 20:16, *ahare gillulehem libbam holekh*.

[9] In a footnote, the RSV translators scrupulously record that the Hebrew has plural "rooms", as if each elder has not one but several "rooms of pictures". The Septuagint, which significantly differs from the Masoretic Text throughout 8:7–12, supports it here, omitting only the word *bahoshekh* ["in the dark"], for there is no reason to suppose that *en to koitoni to krypto auton* is anything but a guess at the meaning of *behadre maskito*.

verses, which have the elders gathered together in a single chamber. To maintain the conventional understanding, we must suppose that "the vision of the seventy elders all together seems to have been replaced by another of each in his private rooms" (Greenberg, 1983, p. 170), or that "the sinful form of devotion which the prophet saw practised in an assembly of the seventy elders took place also in individual houses" (Zimmerli, 1969, p. 242). Cooke, supposing that the locale must be the temple, wonders whether it is "likely that each of the seventy elders had a chamber to himself" (1936, p. 95). Zimmerli himself, following Carl Heinrich Cornill and Georg Fohrer, considers deleting the whole passage as a gloss. Clearly, there is a real problem here.

The crux of the problem, and the path to its solution, lie in the word *maskit*.

Outside our passage, the word occurs five times in the Hebrew Bible.[10] Two of these occurrences, Lev. 26:1 and Num. 33:52, plainly refer to some sort of idolatrous engravings. Prov. 25:11, using *maskiyyot* for a silver frame in which "golden apples" can be set, confirms that the word can mean a skilfully crafted object.

But the other two occurrences suggest another option. In Psalm 73:7, it is not easy to understand *maskiyyot lebab*—literally, "*maskiyyot* of the heart"—as anything other than "sinful imaginings" entertained by the wicked, which are followed (in

[10] Other derivatives of the root *sky* are not very helpful, since they are even more ambiguous than *maskit*. Job 38:36 uses *sekhwi* in parallelism with *tuhot*: "Who has placed wisdom in the *tuhot*? Who has given understanding to the *sekhwi*?" If *tuhot* here refers to human organs of thought or feeling (as appears from Psalm 51:8, its only other occurrence in the Bible), it is reasonable to suppose that *sekhwi* here is "mind" or "imagination". The context in Job, however, points to some sort of meteorological phenomenon. The Revised Standard Version translates accordingly. In Isa. 2:16, *sekhiyyot hahemdah* appear in a list of lofty things that are to be brought low on the day of Yahweh: cedars, mountains, towers, walls, and, in immediate parallelism, "ships of Tarshish". This implies they are some sort of structure. On the other hand, they are followed (verse 17) by *gabhut ha'adam* and *rum anashim*, which are best taken as referring to human pride. If *sekhiyyot hahemdah* are placed in the latter company, we might reasonably take them to be "splendid imaginings"—with a pejorative connotation, as we will see in connection with *maskit*.

verses 8–9) by arrogant and threatening speech.[11] (By contrast, the psalmist identifies himself in verse 1 with the "pure in heart", and claims in verse 13 that he has purified his heart.) In Prov. 18:11, "the wealth of a rich man is his strong city, and like a lofty wall *bemaskito*". The meaning of the last word is not absolutely clear from the context, but the common translation "in his imagination" suits it very well. This is reinforced by the preceding verse, which declares Yahweh's name to be the "strong tower" in which the righteous can find protection. The rich man's wealth, by contrast, is a fortress only in his fantasy.[12] In both of these passages, *maskit* has a negative connotation.

If we translate Ezek. 8:12 in accord with this second meaning of *maskit*, we get:

> Have you seen, son of man, that which the elders of the house of Israel do in the dark, *each in the chambers of his [wicked] imagination*? [or, more freely, "each in his own perverted fantasies"]. For they say, "Yahweh cannot see us, Yahweh has forsaken the land."

In other words, each of the elders—by which we will understand, each of the twenty-odd elders gathered before Ezekiel—is supposed to entertain secret fantasies in which he gathers with his fellows, in an august college of seventy, worshipping monstrosities in an eerie cave.

The parenthesis in the preceding sentence, of course, has got ahead of the argument. We have seen that, in chapters 14 and 20, Ezekiel accuses the elders who come to consult him of entertaining thoughts of ill-defined abominations. In chapters 8 and 11, he accuses *certain people who figure in his vision*, again, of entertaining wicked thoughts. I have asserted, but have not demonstrated, my belief that the villains of Ezek. 8:11 and 11:1 are visionary representations of the "elders of Judah" who sit

---

[11] In verse 11, these sinners "say, 'How can God know? Is there knowledge with the Most High?'" [*ekhah yada' el weyesh de'ah be'elyon*]. The parallel with Ezek. 8:12—"they say, 'Yahweh cannot see us, Yahweh has forsaken the land'"—is very striking.

[12] Pamela E. Kinlaw points out to me that Prov. 18:12 confirms this interpretation, declaring that the arrogance of "a man's heart" [*leb ish*] precedes catastrophe.

before Ezekiel in 8:1, and that it is these elders who supposedly indulge the "perverted fantasies" of Ezek. 8:12. My next task must be to demonstrate, first, that this understanding of the vision is plausible; and, second, that it is true.

Vision and audience

What exactly happens to Ezekiel when "the hand of the Lord Yahweh" falls upon him (Ezek. 8:1)?

> "I saw, and behold, an appearance like that of a man, fiery from the appearance of his loins downward; and, from the appearance of his loins upward, like the color of *hashmelah*.[13] He sent forth the likeness of a hand, and grasped me by the hair of my head. The spirit lifted me up between earth and heaven, and brought me to Jerusalem in visions of God" [Ezek. 8:2–3].

Most moderns, no doubt influenced by the apocryphal "Story of Bel and the Dragon" (which itself presumably reflects exegesis of this passage), have supposed that Ezekiel was carried to Jerusalem by the hair of his head. But the text does not say that (Greenberg, 1983, pp. 167, 195; Soleh, 1981, p. 282; Vogt, 1981, p. 40). Rather, the human-like figure holds Ezekiel transfixed. Thus transfixed, he feels the *ruah*—the Hebrew word can mean either "spirit" or "wind"—lifting and carrying him to Jerusalem (cf. Carley, 1975, pp. 13–37). We are thus assured that, in contrast to Ezek. 3:14–15 (which in many respects parallels our passage), Ezekiel's body does not follow the exalted wanderings of his spirit.[14] It remains in place—and, perhaps, remains active—in Babylonia even as Ezekiel's spirit is active in its imaginary Jerusalem.

---

[13] Following the Masoretic Text, but (1) reading, with the Septuagint, *ish* for *esh* as the fifth word of the verse; and (2) deleting, again with the Septuagint, the words *kemar'eh zohar* as a gloss on the cryptic *ke'en hahashmelah.* (I do not attempt to translate this last word. The Revised Standard Version guesses: "gleaming bronze".)

[14] Ezek. 3:14–15: "The spirit/wind [*ruah*] lifted me up and seized me, and I went [*wa'elekh*] bitter in the heat of my spirit [*bahamat ruhi*],

What sort of activity might we expect of Ezekiel's body? Ethnographic data on trance and related states allow for more than one option (Walsh, 1993). A seer may go into a complete trance and remain unable to describe his experiences until after the trance has passed. This is, admittedly, what Ezek. 11:25 would lead us to expect. But this verse would not exclude another scenario, familiar from reports of shamanistic seances, where the shaman continues to interact with—and, often, to rebuke—his audience, even while his spirit wanders through other worlds.

In one such seance, which Knud Rasmussen observed among the Iglulik, the shaman produces "sounds like those of trickling water, the rushing of wind, a stormy sea, the snuffling of walrus, the growling of bear". After the seance is over, the shaman's wife explains that these were the sounds of the route which the shaman, in the form of the Great Bear, has been exploring for his audience's benefit. In another episode, again reported by Rasmussen (from the Copper Inuit), the shaman visibly wrestles with the "Sea Woman" in the presence of his audience, while she speaks through his mouth and charges the audience with taboo violations. At the same time, the shaman apparently visualizes himself as being in the Sea Woman's watery home, for he is able to report that her lamp is once more turned the right way up (quoted in Merkur, 1985, pp. 95–101).

The Sea Woman's accusations of taboo violations immediately bring us into Ezekiel's mental world. So does Waldemar Bogoras's report of a seance among the Chukchee, where a female spirit, speaking through the mouth of a male shaman, reproaches one of the audience for mistreating bears. "Afterward she told another listener that she saw that in the last autumn he had killed a wild reindeer buck" (Bogoras, 1965, p. 459). The shaman thus "sees", in his trance, the sins committed by members of his audience. Still in trance, he rebukes them. This is very like the way I imagine the interaction between Ezekiel and the "elders of Judah".

Yahweh's hand being mighty upon me. And I came to the exiles at Tel Abib, who dwelt by the river Chebar." Ezekiel correctly fails to distinguish the "spirit" that carried him from his own. By shifting the source of activity from the "spirit" to himself (with his use of *wa'elekh*), he shows himself aware that his travel took place by normal locomotion.

If ethnographic evidence suggests that a seer may interact with his surroundings while his spirit wanders in visions, experimental evidence suggests that the surroundings are likely to influence the content of the visions. Leslie H. Farber and Charles Fisher (1943) found that the spontaneous dreams of a hypnotized subject "are influenced by his own unconscious needs and the interaction of these with the hypnotist and any other persons included in the hypnotic situation". With a woman present, for example, he may dream "of climbing a staircase; of a sewer pipe running through a tunnel; of driving a car around the left side of a mountain into a tunnel". The experiments of Robert Rubinstein, Jay Katz, and Richard Newman point in the same direction. "The experimental situation itself . . . emerges as a major determinant" of the contents of dreams experienced under hypnosis or (at the hypnotist's suggestion) the following night (Rubinstein, Katz, & Newman, 1957). These dreams express, albeit in concealed form (of which more below), "intense feelings about the hypnotist and the hypnotic situation" (Newman, Katz, & Rubinstein, 1960).

If we translate these findings into the biblical setting, we have a fairly clear picture of what might have been expected to happen when the hand of the Lord Yahweh fell on Ezekiel in the presence of the elders of Judah. He went into a trance. He experienced hallucinations that expressed both his prior unconscious concerns and his "intense feelings", conscious and unconscious, towards the elders who sat before him. On the authority of these hallucinations, he conveyed his feelings towards the elders both during the trance and afterwards. It is no surprise that these elders should be stimuli and subjects of his visions, as well as their audience.

Certain features of Ezekiel 8–11 become more intelligible if we suppose that this was indeed the case.

To begin with, there is the curious survival of a second-person address in the Masoretic Text of Ezek. 8:16. This passage describes the climax of the "abominations". Twenty-five men (twenty, according to the Septuagint) stand, their backs to the temple, their faces to the east: *wehemmah mishtahawitem qedmah lashshamesh* ["and they were ________, eastward toward the sun"]. The second Hebrew word in this phrase is unintelligible as it stands. Nearly all translators, from the Septuagint on, treat it as if it were the participle *mishtahawim*, "prostrating themselves". Yet the Hebrew text, impossibly, tacks a second-person plural suffix [*-tem*] onto the participle.

Admittedly, some manuscripts of the Masoretic Text do read *mishtahawim* (Cooke, 1936). But the more difficult reading is certainly ancient, for it is attested unequivocally in a midrash that the *Palestinian Talmud* attributes it to Rabbi Hiyya bar Abba.[15] The text of the midrash is corrupt but can easily be restored (Jastrow, 1950, *s.v. sht*). It explains the peculiar form as a hybrid, combining *mishtahawim* ["they were prostrating themselves"] with *mashhitim* ["they were laying waste"]. The men were simultaneously "prostrating themselves to the sun and laying waste to the temple".[16]

The mediaeval grammarian and Bible commentator David Kimhi (ca. 1160–1235) also saw the word as a hybrid and called attention to other examples of the same phenomenon: 1 Sam. 25:34 [*wtb'ty*]; Jer. 22:23 [*ysbty . . . mqnnty*]; and, most obviously relevant, Ezek. 9:8 [*wn's'r*].[17] (*Miqra'ot Gedolot*; Chomsky, 1933, pp. 85–87, 98–99; Talmage, 1975, pp. 95–96.) But he proposed a different explanation for it. Following Ibn Ezra, he suggested that it combined the participle *mishtahawim* ["they were prostrating themselves"] with the second-person plural perfect *hishtahawitem* ["you prostrated yourselves"]. Ezekiel, he explained,

---

[15] Sukkah 5:5 (55c). There were two scholars named Hiyya bar Abba: one lived at the beginning and one at the end of the third century A.D.

[16] The current text reads *mishtahawim* a second time, in place of *mashhitim*. This makes no sense and does nothing to explain the peculiarity of *mishtahawitem*. Rashi and Kimhi (in *Miqra'ot Gedolot*, *ad loc.*) cite the correct text. Their reading is supported by the Targum and by the derivative midrash in *Song Rabbah* 1:6, in which the citation of Lev. 22:25 ("their corruption [*moshhatam*] is in them") will make sense only if the midrash presupposes the interpretation *mishtahawitem* = *mishtahawim* + *mashhitim*.

[17] Most modern scholars—including the commentators who dismiss *mishtahawitem* as a scribal error—acknowledge that *wn's'r* in Ezek. 9:8 is a hybrid. They explain it, plausibly, as combining the variants *wa'eshsha'er* and *wenish'ar 'ani*, both of which mean "and I was left [alone]".

> found those men [in his vision] *prostrating themselves* to the sun; and he said to the men who had come [to consult him]: "Have you [also] *prostrated yourselves?*" [*Miqra'ot Gedolot*; Kimhi 1847, p. 380; Chomsky, 1952, pp. 171, 213–214; Talmage, 1975, pp. 95–96]

Following Kimhi's explanation of the form, William Brownlee (1986) has suggested that someone had written *wehishtahawitem* in the margin of Ezekiel, as an allusion to Deut. 11:16 and Josh. 23:16. This was then conflated with the text's *mishtahawim.*[18]

Most modern scholars have preferred simply to emend to *mishtahawim*, with the early translations and several Masoretic manuscripts. But it is difficult to imagine how, as a simple blunder, *mishtahawitem* could have survived. More likely, the earliest scribes knew what the strange suffix meant. By the time its meaning had been forgotten, it was too deeply rooted in the textual tradition to disappear entirely.

Kimhi, I believe, was on the right track. The word is indeed a hybrid, preserving a trace of a second-person variant that goes back to the speech of Ezekiel himself. But "you were prostrating yourselves" is better taken as an accusation than as a question. It is a "slip", in which Ezekiel reveals that the men he sees prostrating themselves to the sun are none other than his audience, the "elders of Judah" who have come to consult him.

I suggest that at one time two versions of Ezekiel's vision of the polluted temple were extant. One, more faithfully reproducing the actual occurrences of the seance, preserved the slips and apparent inconsistencies in the words of the ecstatic prophet; the other edited them away. It is not unthinkable that Ezekiel himself may have been this editor. The versions will then represent, not different writers, but the same man in greater or lesser control over the language of his originally unconscious productions.

The Septuagint translators will have had the more elegant and less original of the two versions before them. The scribes whose text ultimately gave rise to the Masoretic Text had both, and conflated them. This variation is thus akin to other diver-

---

[18] My teacher, the late Isaac Rabinowitz, explained the form as a combination of *mishtahawim* with *hishtahawayatam* ("their prostration"; cf. 2 Kings 5:18).

gences between the Masoretic Text and the Septuagint in Ezekiel 8, which, I have argued (Halperin, 1993), can be explained by the assumption that the former reflects the prophet's unconscious more directly than does the latter.

Pelatiah and Jaazaniah

This reconstruction of the link between the contents and the audience of Ezekiel's vision yields the key to a particularly puzzling feature of that vision. In Ezek. 11:1–13, Ezekiel prophesies against a group of twenty-five "princes of the people" who stand at the east gate of the temple; among them are two otherwise unknown individuals named Jaazaniah ben Azzur and Pelatiah ben Benaiah. Apparently as a consequence, "when I prophesied, Pelatiah ben Benaiah died. And I fell on my face, and I cried in a loud voice: 'Oh, Lord Yahweh! Are you making an utter end of the remnant of Israel?'" (verse 13).

The event as reported is difficult to square with the Babylonian setting of Ezekiel's book. This difficulty has driven some scholars either to credit Ezekiel with clairvoyance or to claim that Palestine was the true place of his activity (see above). Yehezkel Kaufmann (1960, p. 431) has solved the problem by simply denying that the event happened outside Ezekiel's imagination:

> The commentators have gratuitously verified Pelatiah's death, though it is not clear why this detail of the vision of 8–11 should be regarded as more real than the slaying of all the inhabitants of the city and its burning by celestial beings.

But this is unsatisfying. In chapter 9, not one but all of the sinners of Jerusalem are slain; just as, in chapter 37, not one but all of the dried-up skeletons to whom Ezekiel preaches are revived. Surely, in chapter 11, we would expect not one but all of the wicked "princes" to perish at Ezekiel's word. Why does Pelatiah alone die—unless something more than Ezekiel's fantasy is responsible for this detail?

A hypothesis offered by Louis Finkelstein (1940) will, with appropriate alteration, suit the data. The trance state described in chapters 8–11, Finkelstein thinks, revived in Ezekiel memories of a childhood visit to the temple with his father. It was then that Ezekiel saw the idolatrous rites that Josiah's successor Jehoiakim (609–598 BC), under Babylonian pressure, had introduced into the temple.

> Decades later, as a prophet in Babylonia, he reconstructed the scene, as vividly as though he were passing through it once again. He could identify the very places of these nefarious crimes, he could see the faces of the transgressing priests, he heard once again the voice of God calling for their destruction.

Pelatiah was among the idolaters Ezekiel had seen as a child. He was also among the "elders of Judah" who now came to consult him. "In his vision Ezekiel saw Pelatiah once more committing idol worship in the Temple. And as he was telling what he saw, Pelatiah fell down dead" (Finkelstein, 1940, 1.319, 2.688).

Against Finkelstein, I would speak of Ezekiel's fantasy of Pelatiah's iniquities in Jerusalem, not his memory of them. (There is no reason whatever to believe that Jehoiakim introduced idolatry into the temple; Halperin, 1993, pp. 47–56.) Childhood memories, indeed, are at the root of the vision of chapters 8–11, but only in very distorted form.[19] Apart from this, however, I find Finkelstein's reconstruction persuasive. Ezekiel gave Pelatiah ben Benaiah, with the rest of the elders, a role in his hallucinations of unspeakable deeds perpetrated in the temple. Ezekiel's hostility towards the elders as a group is, I have argued (Halperin, 1993), a displacement of his rage against the male figure who dominated his childhood. Pelatiah and his colleague Jaazaniah got an extra share of his hostility, for reasons that are uncertain but are perhaps partly linked to the fortuitous circumstance of their names.[20] Ezekiel's rage stirred

---

[19] "If his mother had been insulted before his eyes", says Finkelstein of little Ezekiel's experience in the temple, "Ezekiel could not have been more outraged." Finkelstein's choice of image is wonderfully perceptive.

[20] Pelatiah [*pelatyahu*] = "Yahweh has delivered"; Jaazaniah [*ya'azanyah(u)*] = "Yahweh gives ear". Both names will have had powerful resonances for Ezekiel. *Ya'azanyahu* recalls Ezekiel's infantile trauma of having cried unheard, his consequent sense of himself as mute (3:24–27;

up powerful and deadly emotions within Pelatiah, as a result of which he collapsed and died.

How could this have happened? Bible readers will recall the story of how Ananias and Sapphira similarly dropped dead in the face of Peter's rebukes (Acts 5:1–11). But a tale of this sort obviously cannot be used to confirm or to explain the death of Pelatiah. Fortunately, more up-to-date evidence is available.

In the late 1960s, George L. Engel collected 170 contemporary reports of people collapsing and dying when faced with emotional stress. The cause of death was occasionally known, and often assumed, to be heart failure. Most of these reports came from newspapers, but in 16 cases Engel was able himself to confirm their details (Engel, 1971). More recently, Bernard Lown and his colleagues have devoted a series of investigations into the phenomenon of "sudden cardiac death", and confirmed on both clinical and experimental grounds that it can be triggered by an emotional stress (De Silva & Lown, 1978; Lown, 1982, 1987, 1988; Lown et al., 1976; Reich, De Silva, et al., 1981; Verrier, Hagestad, & Lown, 1987).

Our concern here is not with Lown's formidable efforts to elucidate the physiological workings of the phenomenon, but with his and others' accounts of the psychological stresses that might trigger it. Engel found that, for men, the single most deadly category of stress is "personal danger or threat of injury, real or symbolic" (27%); while "loss of status or self-esteem" accounted for 6% of his total cases and for 9% of the males. (Ezekiel threatened Pelatiah with both.) Lown and his colleagues established that interpersonal conflicts, public humiliation (Reich, De Silva et al., 1981), and rage (Verrier et al., 1987) can all induce dangerous irregularities in the heart's rhythm. Lown

---

24:25–27, 33:21–22), and his conviction that God will shut his ears to his people's cries (8:18). *Pelatyahu* is from the same root as *palit*, "fugitive", which appears in 24:25–27 as a figure towards which Ezekiel looked for deliverance from his muteness, and which apparently served as an unconscious representation of his own infant self (Halperin, 1993, pp. 172–176, 194–199, 207–216, 231). We might speculate that Jaazaniah and Pelatiah, unlucky enough to bear names that expressed Ezekiel's unconscious longings, therefore became targets of his rage at the frustration of these longings. But we cannot judge the extent to which this motive may have been reinforced by others, presumably rooted in historical factors of which we know nothing.

makes the important point that the stress that triggers such irregularities need not in itself be life-threatening. Evoking a painful topic, or bringing a painful memory to consciousness for the first time, may work a deadly effect on the heart (Lown, 1987, 1988).

Lown et al. (1976) report a particularly dramatic case of a healthy 39-year-old man who suddenly collapsed in his home with a heart attack. Just before the attack, he and his two teenage daughters had been engaging in "much sexually provocative rough-housing, which was interrupted by the ring of the doorbell announcing the arrival of a neighbor. It was when one daughter answered the bell that he slumped to the floor. His last words were, 'I'm sorry.'" This man—who, according to the authors, had habitually repressed his aggression and sexuality—must surely have interpreted the doorbell to mean that someone was coming to condemn him for the unspeakable impulses he had allowed to emerge. He collapsed and nearly died.

In a similar way, we may well imagine that Ezekiel's sexually charged vision of the temple "abominations" (details in Halperin, 1993) evoked in Pelatiah long-repressed yearnings and terrors of his own. He then heard himself condemned with all of Ezekiel's savage ruthlessness, in the name of the most terrifying Judge he could imagine. Small wonder his heart failed him.

Pelatiah's death will, then, be the one point, between the beginning of chapter 8 and the end of chapter 11, where Ezekiel's vision touches reality. This reality, however, is not that of Jerusalem, but of Ezekiel's Babylonian seance—which Ezek. 11:13, like the *-tem* suffix in 8:16, allows us briefly to glimpse.

Ezekiel's mention of Jaazaniah ben Azzur (11:1) raises another problem, which my reconstruction of the seance will help us resolve. What is this man's relation to Jaazaniah ben Shaphan, whom Ezekiel sees among the "elders of the house of Israel" burning incense to the horrid images in the chamber (Ezek. 8:11)? The two have different fathers and therefore obviously cannot be the same. It is true that Jaazaniah was hardly a rare name in Judah at the time of the destruction.[21] Yet it seems

[21] The Book of Jeremiah mentions two Jaazaniahs: the son of the Rechabite Jeremiah (35:3; this is, of course, not the prophet); and the son of the Maacathite (40:8, cf. 2 Kings 25:23), who is probably the same person as the son of Hoshaiah (42:1). (Jer. 43:2, strangely, gives "Azariah"

an odd coincidence that, of the three villains singled out in this one visionary complex, two have the same name.

Walther Zimmerli (1969), following Arnold B. Ehrlich, Johannes Herrmann, and Alfred Bertholet, wants to delete the awkward phrase *weya'azanyahu ben shafan 'omed betokham* ["Jaazaniah ben Shaphan standing in their midst" (Ezek. 8:11)] as a gloss. This is not very helpful, since, as Brownlee (1986) points out, it is hard to see what purpose such a gloss would have served. G. A. Cooke's proposal (1936) that the two Jaazaniahs are the same after all, Azzur having really been the man's grandfather, is also improbable; why should Ezekiel have introduced this gratuitous confusion? Clearly enough, Cooke was troubled by the coincidence and felt pressed to find some connection between the two names.

Let us imagine that Ezekiel's vision followed patterns akin to those of dreams. Let us further imagine that at least some Freudian beliefs about the understanding of dreams are accurate. We will then suppose that a figure "seen" in a dream or a vision may be a "screen" for the person actually intended, whose importance the dreamer's consciousness is not ready to acknowledge. The insignificant "screen" figure and the significant figure lurking behind it may be linked by some superficial or fortuitous resemblance, such as identity or similarity of name.

A woman of Freud's acquaintance, for example, thought she remembered having dreamt of meeting her old family doctor. Freud was able to show that this recollection was a screen for her actual dream—of meeting her former lover, who shared the doctor's name (1941c). Similarly, Newman, Katz, and Rubinstein (1960) found that hypnotized subjects dreamed about "relatively neutral procedures carried out by the hypnotist". But these were screens for "intense feelings about the hypnotist and the hypnotic situation", which the subjects had carried over from their past experiences.

Freud also proposed (1900a, pp. 333–335) that a series of dreams on a given night will often express the same underlying thoughts, and that these thoughts will emerge with increasing

---

as the name of Hoshaiah's son; and the Septuagint has "Azarias" in both 42:1 and 43:2.) Lachish Ostracon I knows yet another Jaazaniah, the son of Tobshillem (Badè, 1933; Fowler, 1988; Ward, 1962). On the significance of the name, see the preceding note.

clarity as the series progresses. The screens, in other words, will gradually fall away; and that which they disguise will begin to declare itself explicitly. Laboratory experiments on dream sequences—which became possible after the discovery, in the 1950s, that sleepers show rapid eye movements (REMs) when they dream—suggest that Freud underestimated the complexity of their thematic development, but that what he had to say about the emergence of latent thoughts from their disguise was essentially correct (Dement & Wolpert, 1958; Fisher, 1965, p. 215; Offenkrantz & Rechtschaffen, 1963; Trosman et al., 1960).

Two examples will make the point clear. William Dement and Edward Wolpert (1958) describe a series of dreams that consistently express the dreamer's rage. At first, its object is a professor; but, as the series unfolds, the professor is replaced by a male acquaintance, then a by female nurse, and finally by the dreamer's mother. The true object of the dreamer's anger, originally concealed, is thus at last made clear. William Offenkrantz and Allan Rechtschaffen (1963) tell of a subject who goes to sleep feeling angry and competitive towards the experimenter. He then dreams of having outwitted an unidentified "rival", with the result that the rival commits suicide. In a later dream, however, the object of this murderous rage appears: the experimenter himself, cast in the role of the dreamer's lowly research assistant. At first, in other words, the dreamer prudently disguises his "rival's" identity. (The experimenter is, after all, a powerful figure who might take reprisals.) Only later does he become bold enough openly to subjugate and humiliate his enemy in his dreams.

Applying these observations to Ezek. 8–11, we are led to the conjecture that Ezekiel went into his trance with considerable repressed hatred against one member of his audience, Jaazaniah ben Azzur. Whether this hatred was entirely unconscious—there is reason to believe that Ezekiel carried it with him from his childhood, and displaced it onto Jaazaniah and the other elders (see above; and Halperin, 1993)[22]—or whether he initially forced

---

[22] "At other times the experimenter would appear as a character in one of the dreams. The subject appeared to utilize the experimental situation as a screen for the projection of transference reactions which were characteristic of his personality" (Trosman, Rechtschaffen, Offenkrantz, & Wolpert, 1960).

it out of his awareness for fear of offending a powerful community leader, we cannot know. In either case, Ezekiel will have used "Jaazaniah ben Shaphan" in an early episode of the vision as a screen for the other, detested, Jaazaniah. Only later, in Ezek. 11:1, was he ready to express his hostility openly.

This does not, of course, mean that Jaazaniah ben Shaphan did not exist. On the contrary, this hypothesis is best served if we suppose he was a prominent man, well known to Ezekiel and his hearers. There is no reason to doubt the widespread view that his father was Shaphan ben Azaliah, the scribe who conveyed the newly found book of the Torah to King Josiah (2 Kings 22:3–20); and that his brothers included the distinguished scribe Gemariah (Jer. 36:9–12), the ambassador Elasah (Ezek. 29:3), and Jeremiah's powerful patron, Ahikam (Ezek. 26:24, cf. 2 Kings 22:12).[23] But we need not wonder at "how far this son had departed from the conduct of Shaphan's family, which remained faithful to Josiah's reform and to Jeremiah" (Zimmerli, 1969). Jaazaniah ben Shaphan may have lived and died the staunchest Yahwist in Jerusalem. He owes his villain's role in Ezek. 8 chiefly to the accident that he had the same name as Ezekiel's *bête noire* Jaazaniah ben Azzur. He therefore could serve as a vehicle for Ezekiel's repressed hostility.

Two other factors, however, may have influenced Jaazaniah ben Shaphan's appearance in Ezekiel chapter 8. We learn from Jer. 29:3 that Elasah ben Shaphan was one of the two men who carried Jeremiah's letter to the exiles. I have shown (Halperin, 1993) that this letter underlies the polemic of Ezek. 11:1–3. Its bearer, and hence Shaphan's entire family, may thus have been at the forefront of Ezekiel's awareness at the time of his vision.

The second factor relates to Ezekiel's unconscious. I have already commented (above, note 21) on the meaning that the name "Jaazaniah" may have had for him. "*Shaphan*", too, is likely to have been significant. The Hebrew word designates a small mammal, declared unclean in Lev. 11:5 and Deut. 14:7, which finds refuge (Ps. 104:18) and a home (Prov. 30:26) in rocky cliffs. From these references, modern scholars have little difficulty identifying it as the Syrian hyrax (Bodenheimer, 1962; McCullough, 1962).

[23] Who was the father of the future governor Gedaliah (2 Kings 25:22, Jer. 40:5).

A small creature, known for insinuating itself into crevices, the hyrax would be an ideal symbolic representation for the penis. (A symbolization of this sort may very well underlie some modern people's fear of mice; Feldman, 1949.) I have argued (Halperin, 1993) that the dreadful chamber in the polluted temple, where the "elders of the house of Israel" burn incense to images of loathsome creatures, is Ezekiel's representation of the female genitals (Broome, 1946); and that his characterization of it as "abominable" reflects his abhorrence of female sexuality. It is not astonishing that a son of "*Shaphan*", a representation of the male genitals, should appear—standing—within this chamber.

Conclusion

The effect of this argument has been to affirm the authenticity of the temple vision of Ezek. 8–11. It is indeed the work of the prophet Ezekiel, it indeed describes a visionary experience of its author, it was indeed spoken and later written down in the context of the Babylonian exile. At the same time, we have found ourselves moved to deny that the vision has any but the most tenuous links with its ostensible setting, the contemporary reality of the Jerusalem temple.

Its real setting, as Ezekiel himself obliquely tells us, is "the chambers of imagination"—namely, his own. It is a dream shared in the very course of dreaming: communicated at first to men whom Ezekiel hated and resembled more than he could admit; then transmitted, through the canon of Hebrew Scripture, to a long succession of uncomprehending generations.

If, as Freud has taught us (1900a, p. 608), dreams are the "*royal road to a knowledge of the unconscious*", Ezekiel's temple vision can serve as our royal road into the psyche of this extraordinary man. It may perhaps also carry us further, into a deeper understanding of the collective psyches of those religious cultures that were eventually to canonize him.

Comments

Martin S. Bergmann

REFLECTIONS OF A PSYCHOANALYST ON DAVID HALPERIN'S "EZEKIEL AND THE ELDERS OF JUDAH: THE WORKING OF A PROPHETIC TRANCE"

A psychoanalyst accustomed to listening to and, if need be, interpreting dreams of his analysands will to begin with have a different feeling about the primitive imagery of Ezekiel than biblical scholars are likely to have. Take, for example, the command to "bake his bread with human excrement". It recalls coprophagia, the childhood impulse that later succumbs to repression, to eat one's own faeces.

If we keep in mind the distinction that Freud made between primary processes that follow laws governing the unconscious and secondary processes that obey logical laws, then the request that the prophet eat faeces will appear less strange, since God communicates with His prophet by primary processes. A secondary-process interpretation would be that the deity wanted to humble the prophet because it granted him the special power to be its spokesman. Such a power could easily lead to a narcissistic over-evaluation. The eating of the faeces then represents an attempt to counteract the narcissistic exultation.

A psychoanalyst will also be less inclined to judge Ezekiel as a sick man than other psychologists or scholars would be. For what, to a psychoanalyst, differentiates Ezekiel from a classical schizophrenic like Daniel Schreber in Freud's famous study (1911c) is the fact that the prophet maintains contact with real elders as well as contact with the ideas and ideals of Judaism current in his time.

It is striking how little psychoanalytic work has been done on the phenomenon of prophecy in Jewish history. We have, to be sure, Jacob Arlow's by now classic paper "The Consecration of the Prophet", but that paper had appeared in 1951. There Ezekiel is only one of the prophets discussed. What impressed Arlow particularly was the powerful wishes for oral incorporation expressed particularly in the command to eat a scroll. Equally impressive to Arlow is the strength of the prophet's penis awe. Arlow writes:

> But finally it is upon the appearance of his loins even downward that the eyes of the prophet focus. When this scoptophilic crescendo reaches its phallic climax, the prophet is completely overwhelmed, falls upon his face and begins to hear the voice of God speaking. [p. 65]
>
> Ezekiel's concentration on God's loins is expressed by the prophet in terms reminiscent of fellatio—impregnation fantasy. The fiery phallus of the vision has been transformed at this point into a roll which tastes like honey. [p. 66]

It was Greenacre (1956) who made the differentiation between penis awe and penis envy. She applied the distinction to women. Those women who primarily compete with men probably have penis envy, while those who feel totally inadequate towards men are likely to suffer from penis awe. Ezekiel retained and transferred to his god the penis awe he must have experienced as a child towards his father.

Arlow also noted the power of the world-destruction fantasy expressed by Ezekiel. Since the 1911 study of Schreber, psychoanalysts have interpreted this fantasy as a projection of a process that the patient, usually schizophrenic, is undergoing. The world is experienced as coming to an end because the patient has withdrawn his libido from the world, and by libido Freud meant love, concern, as well as interest. In Arlow's interpretation, Ezekiel is overwhelmed by the imago of the father. He is therefore under the sway of the negative Oedipus. In Halperin's psychoanalytic interpretation, there is a greater emphasis on the dangers of incestuous wishes. He says:

> I have argued (1993) that the dreadful chamber in the polluted temple, where the "elders of the House of Israel" burn incense to images of loathsome creatures, is Ezekiel's representation of the female genital. [p. 112]

Halperin also interprets the death of Shafan, one of the elders, whose name is usually taken to mean simply rabbit, but, as Halperin shows, it probably represents the Syrian hyrax. The animal insinuates itself into crevices, and Halperin suggests that it therefore stands for the penis. Halperin's psychoanalytic interpretation implies that Ezekiel was functioning on a higher psychosexual level and was suffering from castration anxiety rather than from penis awe.

Of particular interest in the essay under discussion is Halperin's emphasis on Ezekiel's claim to know not only what the elders are doing but also what they are imagining: "They have lifted their idols upon their hearts." Halperin comments:

> these imaginary abominations, whose nature is left entirely vague, merit the most ferocious retribution. [p. 95]

Here, too, the situation is likely to be more familiar to a psychoanalyst than to a biblical scholar, for psychoanalysts operate with the assumption that the superego of the analysand has direct contact with what is still unconscious and in the id. In all cases of melancholia and in many other mental illnesses, the superego punishes the ego not for deeds committed but because the superego has direct access to the unconscious wishes. It is therefore less surprising to us that Ezekiel assumes that he has direct contact with the wishes of the elders and that he is justified in punishing them for these wishes. Ezekiel merely reproduces interpersonally what traditionally goes on intrapsychically. Religions, we know, tend to blur the difference between deeds and wishes, thus magnifying the guilt feelings of their believers, while the psychoanalyst in his daily work continuously reminds his analysands of the difference between acts and wishes.

If, indeed, Ezekiel was the first prophet to demand punishment not only for abominations actually committed but for the wishes to commit them, then he occupies a pivotal position in the history of religion, for guilt over wishes rather than deeds testifies to the fact that aggression has been internalized and a strict superego has been established. Such a severe superego may not be in the interest of the person and may become a source of depression, but it is associated with the internalization of aggression and the establishment of monotheism. Monotheism does not tolerate expression of any aggression towards God. Ezekiel's phrase "Every man in his room of pictures" strikes me as particularly apt. If we assume that in the unconscious, as in dreams, what is real is what is pictured and not what is thought, the private picture room is an excellent metaphorical description for where our fantasies come from.

Both Arlow and Halperin have presented to us the psychological inner world of Ezekiel with little reference to the historical dimension. It seems to me, however, that the effort to separate psychology from history leaves us with an incomplete picture. The phenomenon of prophecy has to be understood within the realm of Jewish history. In my book, *In the Shadow of Moloch* (Bergmann, 1992), I suggested that the backsliding and abominations that the Israelites were accused of by their prophets were nothing else than the religious norms of yesterday. It is believed by many scholars today that YHWH was for a long time a war-like tribal god whose followers succeeded in conquering parts of Canaan. Under ordinary historical conditions, this tribal god should have been forsaken after the wars with Assyria and Babylon had been lost. But at this point an evolutionary miracle happened—a miracle that gave Jewish history its uniqueness. With the aid of prophets who presented themselves as speaking for their god, an entirely new idea was born. The tribal god became a universal god; he was never defeated in battle, he only allowed his people to be defeated because they had sinned against him. To bring about this change, all aggression towards the image of the deity had to be withdrawn. He had to gain in power and become overwhelming. Ezekiel, therefore, expresses the awe before a god that has become internalized.

According to Scholem (1941, p. 7), the history of religion can be divided into sub-parts. The first is the mythological stage, in which men and God mingle freely. As religion develops, God recedes into greater and greater distance. Jewish prophecy operates in a post-mythological stage of religion, but it succeeds in bringing back a direct communication with God, although this communication is restricted to moral demands that this deity makes. The testimony of Ezekiel teaches us that this process of internalization required, at least from some prophets, a sado-masochistic relationship between the deity and the prophet. The sado-masochistic relationship is, however, a transitional phase, leading to an ultimate internalization of the image of the god as requiring continuously moral behaviour.

ESOTERIC MYSTICISM, *MERKAVAH* AND *HEKHALOT*

CHAPTER FOUR

INTRODUCTION

Disclosure and revelation, and the converse, curiosity and study, are features not only of the apocalyptic complex, but of normative Judaism as well. The observant Jew recites twice a day:

> And these matters that I command you today should be placed upon your heart, rehearse them with your children, and speak of them while sitting in your house, when walking on the road, when you lie down and when you arise. And bind them as a sign upon your hand, and they shall become a symbol between your eyes, and write them on the door-posts of your house and on your gates. [Deut. 6:6–9]

On the other hand, certain things are not to be looked at. In Leviticus, chapter 18, we read of the various incestuous and near-incestuous sexual couplings that are forbidden. In each case, the idiom used is: "Do not uncover the nakedness of. . . ." Looking at the pudenda is a prelude to and metaphor for the sexual act.

Regular study of Torah (in its expanded sense, Tanach, Talmud, and commentaries) is essential to religious life and is treated as a form of worship.

None of this is remarkable. In every religion there are some things that the individual is expected to know and other things that he is expected to ignore or to avoid. Nevertheless, ancient ideas of privacy and propriety differed from our own more than we generally acknowledge. We learn, for example, in Berakoth (B.T. 24a) that a woman may recite a blessing while sitting naked, because when a woman sits on the ground neither the genitals nor the buttocks are exposed. A man, therefore, does not have that privilege. Berakoth (B.T. 62a) tells two stories about inappropriate curiosity. The first story is given in two versions. A younger scholar follows an older one into a privy to observe and to "learn" proper conduct there. One of the versions identifies the enquirer as Rabbi Akiba and the other as Ben Azzai, both of whom figure in this essay on inappropriate curiosity. The second story tells us that Rabbi Kahana once hid under Rab's bed to observe his conduct during intercourse. "It is a matter of Torah and I must learn." Yet he knew enough to comment that Rab seemed inexperienced. Rab became aware of Kahana and dismissed him with the comment that his conduct was rude (that is, incompatible with *derekh 'erez*). Shortly after the comment about the naked woman, the text tells us that gazing at a woman's leg, or her hair, or even a handbreadth of exposed flesh, or even listening to her voice is sexually arousing and is therefore incompatible with a prayerful attitude. These anecdotes caution us that our own standards of what is and what is not decorous are culture-bound. For the editors of Berakoth, a naked woman who is seated is not indecorous from a religious point of view; an intruder into a privy or into a bedroom is merely rude, not in violation of religious standards of purity or privacy; woman's hair or voice is an unacceptable sexual distraction.

The mythic continues as an active undercurrent in all religion and recurrently surfaces. In Scripture, the conflict between curiosity and the prohibition against it appears as early as the story of Adam and Eve in the garden. When God prohibits Adam from eating from the tree of knowledge, presumably He was not thinking of prohibiting Adam from learning the multiplication tables (at least not literally). The prohibited knowledge related to matters of instinctual interest, of identity and destiny. The consequence of eating the forbidden fruit is that Adam and Eve became aware of the distinction between good and evil and also of the need to cover their genitals. They became mortal and were exiled from their infantile or perhaps prenatal paradise into the world of reality, of pain and hard work, of thorns and thistles, and of the grave. But since they are to die, the chain of reproduction is initiated so that life may continue, and so Adam "knew" his wife, Eve. The myth tells us that a paradisiac existence is incompatible with a sense of reality, with self-consciousness, and with values. Curiosity is vital for the human but nevertheless its price is the forgoing of immortality.

We encounter the same problem of prohibited curiosity again in Exodus. In chapter 19, in preparation for the theophany on Mt. Sinai, the people are warned against gazing at God lest they perish (Exod. 19:21–24).

In chapter 33 we learn that Moses requested that God let him *know* Him and His ways (using the same word for knowing that is used in the Garden of Eden myth, *yada*). A few verses further down, Moses asks more directly, "Let me see your presence." God permits Moses some degree of proximity and permits him to see his back, but not his face because "no man may see me and live" (Exod. 33:13–23). The Divine Father may not be seen, and especially not his "face". One may be forgiven for suspecting that it is the genital that is off limits.

The first chapter of Ezekiel may be regarded as the transition from myth to mysticism:

> In the thirtieth year, on the fourth day of the fifth month, when I was in the midst of the exile on the river Chebar, the heavens were opened and I saw visions of God. On the fifth of the month—that was the fifth year of the exile of King Jehoiachin—the word of the Lord came to Ezekiel the son of Buzi, the priest, in the land of the Chaldeans, on the river Chebar. And the hand of the Lord came upon him there.
>
> And I looked and here was a stormy wind coming out of the north, a great cloud and a flaming fire, and a radiance surrounded it, and from within, the appearance of hashmal [amber?]—that is, from within the fire. And from within it the image of four creatures, and this was their appearance: they

each resembled a man in appearance. And each had four faces, and each one also had four wings. And as for their legs, the leg was straight, and the foot resembled the foot of a calf, and they gleamed like the appearance of polished brass. And there were human hands under their wings, on each of their four sides, and their faces and their wings were the same for each. Their wings were joined one to another; they (the creatures) did not turn as they traveled, each could proceed straight ahead. And as for the appearance of their faces, each had a human face, and on the right side, each of the four had the face of a lion, and on the left side, each of the four had the face of an ox, and each of the four had the face of an eagle. That, with respect to the faces, and their wings were separated above; two of the wings of each were joined each to its fellow and two covered their bodies. And each individual could proceed ahead; wherever the spirit went, they went; they did not turn as they moved. And with respect to the image of the creatures, their appearance resembled burning embers of fire and the appearance of flames moved among the creatures, and the fire emitted a radiance, and from the fire, lightning [or sparks?] emerged. And the creatures darted up and back so that they appeared like lightning. And as I looked at the creatures, there was a wheel on the ground alongside the four faces of each creature. The appearance of the wheels and their structure resembled tarshish [beryl or chrysolite], and each of the four had the same appearance, and their appearance and structure suggested a wheel within a wheel. On each of their four sides, when the creatures went, the wheels went, and they did not turn when they moved. And as for their rims, they were tall and frightening, and the rims of the four were covered with eyes all around. And when the creatures traveled, the wheels traveled alongside them, and when the creatures were lifted above the earth, the wheels were lifted. Wherever the spirit was inclined to go, they went; there the spirit traveled; and the wheels were lifted alongside them, for the spirit of each of the creatures was in the wheels. When the one went, so did the other and when the one stopped the other did too, and when they were lifted above the ground, the wheels were lifted next to them, for the spirit of the creature was in the wheels.

> And the image of an expanse, resembling the appearance of the awesome crystal, was stretched above the heads of the creatures. And under the expanse their wings were extended each to its neighbor for each creature, and each of the creatures had two covering wings, that is, covering their bodies. And I heard the sound of their wings, like the sound of rushing waters, like the sound of Shaddai, as they moved, the sound of a tumult, like the sound of an army; when they halted, they dropped their wings. And there was a sound above the expanse above their heads; when they halted, they dropped their wings. And above the expanse above their heads, there was the image of a throne resembling sapphire in appearance, and above, upon the image of the throne, an image that resembled a human form. And I saw the gleam of hashmal, like the appearance of fire within a surrounding frame, that extended from what appeared to be its loins upward, and from what appeared to be its loins downward, I saw the appearance of fire surrounded by radiance. Like the appearance of the rainbow that one sees in the clouds on a rainy day, that was the appearance of the surrounding radiance; that was the image of the appearance of the glory of the Lord; I saw it and I fell on my face and then I heard a voice speaking. [Ezek. 1]

I consider this a transitional statement because it provides a mythic view of God which was purported to have been received in what seems to be a mystical trance. I base that view on the last verse of the section and the first two verses of the succeeding chapter:

> And He said to me, "Mortal, stand on your feet and I shall speak to you." And when He spoke to me a spirit entered me and stood me on my feet and I heard what was being spoken to me.

The myth is the specific description of the Deity. Note that the emphasis is displaced here from the image of God to the square animate vehicle in which He arrives. The reader will remember that vehicles appear commonly in apocalyptic fantasies and that the number four occurs with surprising frequency. This structure is not here called a chariot, *merkavah*, but it has become known by that name in the mystical literature that took this material as its basic text. (The earliest surviving use of *merkavah* to refer to Ezekiel's vision is found in Sirach 49:8.) Not only is the structure of the vehicle described, but also the anatomy of the chariot creatures. They modestly cover their bodies with one pair of their four wings.

However two verses from the end, the Deity himself is visualized, but the only detail given relates to the "loins", radiant and aflame. The radiance and the flame draw attention to God's phallus but at the same time obscure it. As we shall see in the fifth essay, *merkavah* and *hekhaloth* mysticism is oriented to the quest to visualize God in His *merkavah* or in His celestial palace. The quest incurs dangers. These and the methods for combating them are detailed in the mystical literature.

Both the quest and danger create a conflict, or rather recreate it. This essay on the "Four who entered the garden" is based upon an anecdote that appears in Tractate Hagigah of the Talmud. Section two of that tractate reads as follows:

> One may not expound the subject of forbidden sexual relations among (as many as) three people (i.e. only one or two); nor the account of creation among (as many as) two; nor the subject of the *merkavah* with even one, unless he is wise and sophisticated in these matters. Everyone who speculates on the following four subjects would be better off if he had not been born: What is above, what is below, what came before, and what will come afterward. Anyone who does not show respect for his Maker would have been better off if he had not been born.

This passage implies that at the time, there was considerable speculation about these matters, that is, mystical quest, and that the authorities who represented normative religion were trying to combat it. The subjects listed were the principal objects of mystical interest: forbidden sexual relations, esoteric cosmogony, and the image of God. It is precisely these subjects that were the object of mystical investigation in all of the subsequent forms of Jewish mysticism. The problems that concerned the rabbinical authorities were that discussing even sexual prohibitions is arousing, that speculation about the origin of the universe threatens one's confidence in the literal account of the creation given in Genesis, and that study of the *merkavah* leads to unseemly preoccupation with God's anatomy. But why do these subjects become so important for the mystic?

The mystical quest is basically for intimacy with God, seeing Him, knowing Him, understanding His position in the universe. Speaking of the sacredness of the Song of Songs, an explicitly erotic poem, Gerson D. Cohen (1991) proposed that: "If love could not be ignored, it could be channelled, reformulated and controlled, and this is precisely what the rabbinic allegory of the Song of Songs attempted to achieve." I would go further and propose that sexuality is used as a vehicle for the mystical pursuit of approach to and union with God, and so are speculations about cosmogony and God's substance and appearance.

Even the image of the austere, remote, immaterial Godhead seems to have given way to a loving, accessible, visible and tangible parent for the *merkavah* and *hekhaloth* mystics, and as an ultimately unknowable, inconceivable *En Sof* or Infinite for the Kabbalists but an Infinite that acts upon the real world and its people through a variety of very familiar and recognizable potencies. As I proposed in the introductory essay, the mystical attitude can be interpreted as a regression to the state of mind of early childhood; the very young child can find comfort and assurance only in physical intimacy with a parent. Nunberg, in an essay on curiosity (1961), related infantile sexual curiosity to three questions: Where do children come from; what is the difference between a boy and a girl; and what are father and mother doing together? These three questions parallel the three concerns of Hagigah. Where do children come from becomes elaborated into the desire to understand origins—and in the case of the mystic, cosmogony. The difference between the boy and girl is reflected, under the influence of phallic primacy, in curiosity about God's physical appearance, focusing indirectly but ultimately and sometimes more directly on His sexual organs. What the parents are doing together is subsequently elaborated into curiosity about sexual behaviour.

Whether these concerns are provided for by universal biological constitution or are acquired during the experiences of early childhood, we cannot know. We do know that they first become manifest in early childhood and are subsequently repressed or sublimated. Under the influence of the mystical quest, they become reactivated and find expression in the various ways that we have mentioned.

Dr Eleanor Galenson adds to the discussion a description of the evolution of curiosity in very young children, in order to complement our hypothetical constructions with hard observational data.

Four entered the garden: normative religion versus illusion

Mortimer Ostow

> Four entered the garden,[1] namely, Ben Azzai, and Ben Zoma, Aher and Rabbi Akiva. Rabbi Akiva said to them: When you arrive at the (place of the) stones of pure marble, don't say, Water, Water! Because it is said: He who speaks falsehood will not stand before my eyes (Ps. 101:7). Ben Azzai looked and died. Scripture says about him: Blessed in the eyes of the Lord is the death of his righteous (Ps. 116:1–5). Ben Zoma looked and was afflicted. Scripture says about him: If you have found honey, eat (only) your fill, because if you become surfeited, you will vomit (Prov. 25:16). Aher cut the shoots. Rabbi Akiva departed in peace.

M. Ostow, "Four Entered the Garden: Normative Religion versus Illusion." In: H. P. Blum, Y. Kramer, Arlene Richards, & Arnold Richards (Eds.), *Fantasy, Myth, and Reality: Essays in Honor of Jacob A. Arlow* (pp. 287–301). New York: International Universities Press, 1988.

[1] The word that I have translated as garden, *Pardes*, presents some problems. It has been used in two senses—namely, a garden or orchard, and also paradise, with which it shares its Greek origin. Scholem (1960) argues that that term is used literally in the first sense in the story but that the garden is a metaphor for paradise. Halperin (1988), on the

This terse and intriguing story appears in chapter 2 (p. 14b) of a section of the *Babylonian Talmud* called Hagigah. The section deals primarily with the celebration of holidays in Temple worship.

The same story, with minor modifications, is given in at least three other places in the Talmudic literature—the *Palestinian* (as distinguished from the *Babylonian*) *Talmud*, Hagigah 77b; Tosefta Hagigah 2:3–4; and *Midrash Rabbah* to Shir Hashirim (Song of Songs) 1:4. A comparison and contrast of these versions would take us too far afield while contributing nothing of interest to my principal thesis.

The four scholars mentioned in the story, all well-known contributors to rabbinic debate, flourished during the first few decades of the second century. The meaning of the story has occupied many competent scholars, and no consensus has been reached. Rowland (1982) interprets the story as "a metaphorical

---

other hand, contends that *Pardes* was used to signify paradise in Jewish apocryphal literature, but in rabbinic usage it referred only to a pleasure garden or park and was used in rabbinic literature to represent metaphorically "the world, the holy land, the people of Israel and the precepts of the Torah". In this story, he argues, it serves as a metaphor for the "chambers of the merkabah".

The word *Apikoros* signifies the arch-heretic in rabbinic literature. In the *Encyclopedia Judaica*, Louis I. Rabinowitz notes that even though the word derives from the name of the Greek philosopher Epicurus, the rabbis ignored that derivation and saw it as derived from the Aramaic word *hefker*, meaning "abandoned". So there seems to have been some objection to acknowledging the association of the word with Epicurus. The term "Epicurean gardens" was used in the classical world to denote groups of disciples of Epicurus in rabbinic times, though we do not know whether that was true in rabbinic circles. It occurred to me therefore to wonder whether the *Pardes* used in our story could have alluded to the Epicurean garden, and, indeed, Henry Albert Fischel, a student of Epicureanism, offers the same suggestion in his book on Rabbinic Literature and Greco-Roman philosophy (1973) and in his article on Epicureanism in the *Encyclopedia Judaica*, buttressed by the citation of several connecting allusions.

Whatever the origin of the term *Pardes*, there is no doubt that in the context of the story it refers to inappropriate merkavah mystical curiosity, as Halperin argues.

description of the consequences resulting from the occupation of four teachers of the early second century in the study of the Scriptures", upon which layers of other meanings have been subsequently imposed (p. 339). Mediaeval Jewish commentators, Hai Gaon and Rashi, for example, understood the story to refer to a vision of mystical ascent to heavenly structures where the *merkavah* or chariot (described in Ezekiel, chapter 1) could be seen, and where one could visualize the seven heavenly palaces or *hekhalot*. Gershom Scholem (1954), the great modern scholar of Jewish mysticism, sees the story as a warning of the dangers of ecstatic ascent to the *hekhalot*. Gruenwald (1980) considers the story one of several mystical speculations regarding ecstatic experiences associated with the illusion of translation to heaven. Halperin (1980) treats the story as one of seven units that together make up what he terms the "mystical collection". The latter conveys the message that "involvement with esoteric matters, is dangerous and normally to be avoided" (p. 104). The collection does not distinguish among the various forms of mysticism. The fullest recent discussion is given by Yehudah Liebes (1990). Howard Eilberg-Schwartz (1994) suggests that the attractive display in the garden was God's phallus, and the dire consequences of gazing at it are caused by homosexual anxiety.

Even though reliable historical data are sparse, if we wish to draw our own conclusions about the story's meaning, we shall have to take a closer look at the few reliable details that we have. Who were the protagonists? Ben Azzai's name is not associated with any particular exploit or point of view. Some of the basic data of his life are obscured by paradox and uncertainty. First, although he taught that failure to observe the commandment to procreate is as grave a violation as shedding blood, he himself did not marry, offering as an explanation the fact that he loved the Torah too much. Second, although the story tells us that his death was caused by his entry into the garden, there is another tradition that holds he was slain in the Hadrianic persecutions (*Lamentations Rabbah* 2:2,4). Third, although he was revered both for his scholarship and for his piety, he was never ordained, so that his name is never preceded by the title Rabbi. In addition, we know that mystical powers were attributed to him (*Song of Songs Rabbah* 1:10), and he argued that God showed the righteous their future glory before death, a belief typical of the mystical tradition (*Bereshith Rabbah* 62:2).

Ben Azzai's failure to marry in an age when marriage and procreation were religious desiderata suggests a disturbance in his sexuality, a disturbance that found some compensation in his mystical endeavours. Among his mystical interests, some stand out especially—namely, his interest in the physical appearance of God and man. He argued that not even the immortal angels were permitted to see the divine glory, and that because it implied the common origin of mankind, Gen. 5:1 was one of the greatest verses of Scripture: "This is the record of Adam's line. When God created man, He made him in the likeness of God; male and female he created them" (Sifra 7:4). Apparently, because Ben Azzai died at an early age, his unexpected death was attributed to his involvement in mystical practice and thought.

In the case of Ben Zoma, we encounter a different problem. The story as given says only that as a result of his looking into the garden, he was "afflicted" [*nifga*]. The affliction is generally understood as a euphemism for mental illness (see Rashi, commentary to B.T. Hagigah 14b). Scholem (1960) calls attention to a variant of the story given in *Lesser Hekhaloth* (a collection of *midrashim* of the *hekhalot* genre), that voices this tradition.

> Ben Azzai beheld the sixth palace and saw the ethereal splendor of the marble plates with which the palace was tessellated and his body could not bear it. He opened his mouth and asked them [apparently the angels standing there]: "What kind of waters are these?" Whereupon he died. Of him it is said: "Precious in the sight of the Lord is the death of his saints." Ben Zoma beheld the splendor of the marble plates and he took them for water and his body could bear it not to ask them, but his mind could not bear it, and he went out of his mind. . . . Rabbi Akiva ascended in peace and descended in peace. [p. 15].

Like Ben Azzai, Ben Zoma never achieved ordination, though his scholarship was proverbial. Of his published comments, some imply a narcissistic orientation, though they explicitly profess reverence for God. Upon seeing a crowd on the Temple mount, he observed that he was fortunate that there were so many people labouring to provide him with food and clothing. He taught that man should appreciate how much God does for him and that the world was created only to be of service to him who fears God and respects His commandments. One of his best-known aphorisms emphasizes paradox.

> Who is a wise man? He that learns from all men. . . . Who is a mighty man? He that subdues his evil impulse. . . . Who is a rich man? He that is content with his portion. . . . Who is an honorable man? He that honors mankind. . . . [Pirke Avoth 4:1].

The story of the four who entered the garden is followed in Hagigah by the following:

> Our Rabbis taught: Once Rabbi Joshua Ben Hanania was standing on a step on the Temple mount, and Ben Zoma saw him and did not stand up before him. So [Rabbi Joshua] said to him: Whence and whither, Ben Zoma? He replied: I was gazing between the upper and lower waters, and there is only a bare three fingers' [breadth] between them, for it is said: And the spirit of God hovered over the face of the waters—like a dove which hovers over her young without touching [them]. Thereupon Rabbi Joshua said to his disciples: Ben Zoma is still outside [15a].

If Rashi's intuition is correct—that is, that Ben Zoma's affliction is mental illness—then Rabbi Joshua's comment may be interpreted as confirmation, that is, "outside" means "out of it", or insane.

But an important question for us is, did he become psychotic, as the story would have it, *because* of his mystical activities, or did his tendency to seek disengagement from the world of reality induce him to attempt the mystical escape? [Fischel (1973) proposes that the latter tale is based upon a Greco-Roman literary genre that ridicules the Sage as absent-minded, impractical, and other-worldly. Ben Zoma's insanity and sudden death, described in other versions of the story, suggests, he adds, that the original tale was revised to constitute a warning against mystical speculation, or against Epicureanism.]

Aher, the name given to Elisha ben Avuya when he became an apostate, means something different, something other, and is intended to be pejorative. The meaning of the statement that "Aher cut the shoots" is no longer evident, and it is variously interpreted. The best scholarship today understands it as a metaphor for his having denied the basic principles of his religion.

Elisha ben Avuya was well known as a learned scholar, and his apostasy was bitterly resented by his former colleagues. The nature of the apostasy is no longer clear, and many suggestions have been made, including his possible defection to the Greek religion, to Gnosticism, to some other Middle Eastern religion, or to atheism. Louis Ginzberg (in *The Jewish Encyclopedia*) suggests that he left the Pharisees to become a Sadducee. The Hagigah text itself tells us that he sang Greek songs and secretly read heretical books. It also suggests that he became a dualist, as the Gnostics were. During his mystical ascent, the text reports, he interpreted what he encountered to mean that there might be two domains, a dualist gnostic conception. It tells us also that he became bitter and resentful. Yet he had friends and supporters, one of whom was his distinguished pupil, Rabbi Meir. They sought to mitigate the general harshness towards him and to find virtue in his impressive scholarship.

The question for us is, did he become an apostate because he engaged in ecstatic mysticism, as the story suggests, or was mysticism attractive to him because he had rejected Pharisaic religion? Certainly nothing in the material that has come down to us excludes the latter possibility.

Rabbi Akiva is generally considered "probably the foremost scholar of his age, patriot and martyr, who exercised a decisive influence in the development of the halakhah" (*Encyclopedia Judaica*). It is surprising to find him listed among the four who entered the garden, as mysticism plays no prominent role in his recorded activities or remarks. The Hagigah text tells us that during his ascent the angels tried to push him away, but God interceded, saying that Akiva was worthy of enjoying His glory. The text of the story tells us that Akiva departed in peace, and the subsequent discussion, that he ascended in peace and descended in peace, thus confirms the interpretation that the story alludes to the mystical ascent to heavenly realms. However, the text misleads us if it implies that no adverse consequences followed from his flirtation with mysticism. For it may well have led to his readiness to support Simon ben Kozeva, called Bar Kokhba ["son of the star"], as the Messiah who would liberate Israel from its oppressors. It was Bar Kokhba's revolt in C.E. 132 that led to the catastrophic slaughter of Jews by Roman troops in the final defeat of 135. Akiva's colleagues did not follow his leadership in this venture. "Grass will grow on the cheeks and the Messiah will still not have come"—this comment is attributed to Rabbi Johanan ben Tortha (*Lamentations Rabbah* 2:2,4). It is interesting that none of the references to Akiva in the literature of that time takes him to task for his misguided messianism.

What do we learn from the story of the four who entered the garden? It seems evident that the narrator or redactor is telling us that engaging in gnostic, mystical exercises poses danger for the individual: losing one's faith in one case; losing one's mind in a second; and losing one's life in a third. Presumably it was observed that among the adepts of gnostic practice a relatively large number of disturbed or deviant individuals was to be found, and it was inferred that the deviance followed from the mystical practice. We can question this inference, of course, and it is not unlikely that involvement in mystical practice simply gave expression to an already present tendency to deviate. Ben Zoma's neglect of a normal gesture of respect—rising when addressed by one's teacher—and his rumination about the approximation of the upper and lower waters were interpreted by some as the consequence of immersion in cosmogonic speculation. But Rabbi Joshua was probably correct when he said that Ben Zoma was "still outside"—that is, psychotic. Involvement in mysticism in the case of Elisha ben Avuya was only one of a number of excursions into heterodoxy, irreligion, and alien cultures and activities. On the basis of the similes attributed to him in chapter 24 of Avoth d'R. Natan, Louis Ginzberg (in *The Jewish Encyclopedia*) infers that in addition to Greek culture and foreign literature, he showed considerable familiarity with wine, horses, and architecture.

The fantasy of flight through the heavens to a place of comfort and protection occurs not only in gnostic theosophy, but also in the recovery component of apocalyptic fantasies and in the dreams of patients in treatment. Such fantasies and dreams occur especially frequently among psychotic patients, borderline patients, and depressed patients. The classical literary apocalypses frequently include accounts of celestial journeys, but they are intended to amplify the revelation rather than to repair the apocalyptic damage.

Clinical evidence has led me to believe (Ostow, 1986) that the gnostic journey represents a translation to comfort in physical intimacy with the mother, or with both parents—that is, a return to the inside of the mother's body, to a seat on her lap, to comfort in parental arms, or between the parents in bed. Idel (1988b) demonstrates that in mystical literature weeping, the usual call for mother's attention and love, facilitates a mystical experience—sometimes, in fact, the visualization of the *Shekhinah*. Being lifted into parental arms finds expression in the experience of ascent. Merkur (1989) cites further instances of weeping, especially as a component of mourning, and proposes that the deliberate invocation of a depressive affect invokes also a corrective experience of elation. The vehicle itself may signify the proverbial claustrum, as does the chamber that the mystic seeks. In our story it is the garden that signifies the *hekhal* or chamber, the goal of the adept in the *hekhalot* literature, and it symbolizes the chambers associated with the mother's body. Here are two dreams reported from the same night by a woman who was troubled by her destructive fantasies and chronic, though fairly well-controlled anger.

> *"I was in the woods. A man at the edge was drawing pictures. I was buying toys for a child. I was there more than a day. The woods became wet, swampy, rainy, warm, and dark. It looked so beautiful in the rain, like a jungle. The trees twisted. There were vines and high bushes. One tree started to reach out like an umbrella, down to the bushes which clung to the tree. It was very beautiful. There were many greens. It was so rich. The water rose halfway up the trunk of the tree. After seven days I left the garden. I felt very inspired by its beauty. I was very sad for the lonely man standing outside the garden. He was a lonely bum. I had to go back to my children.*
>
> *Mother showed me her vagina. She wanted me to make love to her. I said, "No. It's not right." She said, "Come on." I was repelled by it. It was disgusting. The pudenda, the wetness. It was a long rectangle, not sharp at the end, grayish, darkish, and hairy."*

Among her associations to the second dream, she told me that as a child she was unhappy about sleeping with her mother, and that her mother had indeed often exposed her pubes to the child. Here the second dream interprets the first: The garden with its wet foliage represents mother's genitals, to which she unconsciously aspired to return. The seven days may indicate the period required for the creation of the world—that is, the period of intrauterine development. The man at the edge represented her father, who had always resented her intrusion into the parental bed.

I would infer, then, that the gnostic thought and practice that prevailed in Palestine during the two centuries before and the first several centuries of the Common Era attracted individuals who found themselves uncomfortable in the world of reality, and who harboured an unconscious desire to leave it for an illusory haven. Among them I would expect to find psychotics, depressives, and borderlines, as well as those whose external reality was too painful to bear. The various cults and religions that flourished throughout the Middle East at that time attracted such individuals and tempted them to turn their backs on the reality and on the known doctrines of their own tradition in order to find comfort in the proffered illusions. It is hardly surprising, then, that when these individuals gave evidence of clinical decline, the blame was placed on the mystical practice, on the principle of *post hoc propter hoc.*

The reader will have observed that not only was the ascent to the garden thought to pose a threat to the mystic, but danger lurked, too, in the fantasy of the journey. The story of the four who went into the garden includes the warning of Akiva, and the related story adduced by Scholem from the *hekhaloth* literature describes the danger involved in mistaking the shimmering luminescence of the marble stones for water. Why was that dangerous? Perhaps failure to recognize the heavenly luminescence for what it is, interpreting instead the visual experience as that of glittering waters, means that the celestial traveller has not entered completely into the illusion, has not left behind normal reality testing and the categories of logic, as the gnostic journey requires. But there is yet another danger—namely, the opposition of the heavenly host. I have mentioned that Hagigah has it that when Akiva ascended to the divine *hekhal*, the angels attempted to eject him, and that he was saved only by divine intervention. Hostile celestial forces, endangering the human traveller, are reported in the gnostic religions, and in their Jewish counterparts as well. But if the purpose of cultivating the illusion is to achieve peace of mind, why are these intrusive elements permitted to spoil it? One could easily construct an illusion in which the traveller achieves his goal unhindered.

For the solution to this problem, we can turn again to clinical experience. When the depressed patient dreams of finding some relief from danger, the achievement of that relief will always be precluded by some interfering influence—an intruder, an unfavourable change of environment, an insuperable obstacle. It is only when the patient is about to recover from depression, or is recovering, that he succeeds in finding comfort. The celestial antagonists encountered in gnostic fantasies play the part of these interfering agents in such dreams. They symbolize the intrapsychic, self-defeating elements that will not be overcome unless the individual is ready to accept salvation. In gnostic theosophy, salvation is to be achieved by gnosis, special esoteric knowledge. It is a self-fulfilling system. If the traveller succeeds in reaching his goal, he does so because his gnosis was adequate; if he does not, it was inadequate. In psychoanalytic practice, "salvation" is to be achieved by a special knowledge called "insight". The analyst plays the role of the apocalyptic seer who provides the revelation. In the first of the two dreams presented above, "the man at the edge" of the woods "drawing pictures", represents not only the father, but also the psychoanalyst who, taking notes, was not appreciated as having helped in the patient's reunion with her mother and is himself ineligible for admission to the garden. In fact, then, two kinds of danger are said to threaten the gnostic mystic. First, during the ascent he may be not only deterred but actually destroyed by the heavenly host. Second, as human observers attest, individuals attempting the ascent are in danger of succumbing to a personal catastrophe.

But there is yet a third danger, one mentioned neither in gnostic theosophy nor in the rabbinic response to it. This danger is exemplified in the case of Rabbi Akiva, the hero of the story and of his age. Akiva is not known to have been a mystic. I am not aware of a report anywhere in the literature of his involvement in such activity. However, late in life, perhaps in his eighties or nineties, he recognized Simon ben Kozeva as the Messiah and thereby lent his sanction to a catastrophic rebellion against Rome (B.T. Sanhedrin 97b; *Lamentations Rabbah* 2:4). Messianism must be recognized as a component of the apocalyptic vision. It would seem that Akiva's messianism was not caused by his mystical experience, but, rather, that both followed from a readiness to resort to illusion when circumstances justified it.

A third danger, then, is danger not to the individual, but to the community. When individual suffering is brought on by external circumstances so that a large part of the community suffers, even those whose individual disposition does not favour apocalyptic thinking are attracted by it when they encounter it circulating in society, especially when it is sponsored by a charismatic leader. Since most militant apocalyptic thought arises ultimately from self-destructive impulses, millenarian movements almost always end in the defeat of the community, whether in the case of Bar Kokhba, Nazism, or Jonestown. The most serious danger that arises from indulgence in any of the forms of apocalyptic engagement, whether gnostic, mystic, millenarian, messianic, or utopian, is the possibility that an entire community will be seduced and destroyed by it. It was in the aftermath of the Bar Kokhba revolt and its catastrophic defeat that some rabbis denounced active military resistance to the dominant empires, and counselled passive accommodation.

> Rabbi Jose son of Rabbi Hanina . . . said: "What was the purpose of those three adjurations? One, that Israel shall not go up [altogether as if surrounded] by a wall; the second, that whereby the Holy One, blessed be He, adjured Israel that they shall not rebel against the nations of the world; and the third is that whereby the Holy One, blessed be He, adjured the idolaters that they shall not oppress Israel too much." [B.T. Kethuboth 111a].

> Rabbi Jose ben Hanina said: "These are two adjurations, one addressed to Israel and one to the other nations. God adjured Israel not to rebel against the yoke of the governments, and he adjured the governments not to make their yoke too heavy on Israel, for by making this yoke too heavy on Israel they would cause the end to come before it was due. . . ."

> Rabbi Helbo said: "Four adjurations are mentioned here. God adjured Israel that they should not rebel against the governments, that they should not seek to hasten the end, that they should not reveal their mysteries to the other nations, and they should not attempt to go up from the Diaspora by force" [*Songs of Songs Rabbah* 2:7,1].

There follows a discussion of four generations that "tried to hasten the end", that is, force the coming of the Messiah, and one of the four is listed as that of Ben Kozeva.

> What did they do? They assembled and went forth to battle, and many of them were slain. Why was this? Because they did not believe in the Lord and did not trust in His salvation, but anticipated the end and transgressed the adjuration [*Song of Songs Rabbah* 2:7,1].

It was the strategy of the reed rather than of the cedar that these scholars promoted, the strategy that characterized Jewish resistance to oppression for seventeen hundred years and that served reasonably well until the Nazi apocalypse.

The apocalypse pattern attracts and seduces. By promising salvation following destruction, it offers hope in place of despair. How much of the pattern is constitutionally given and how much learned is not evident. One can easily imagine an inherent tendency to reject, detach, and kill, that of itself would generate both anxiety and an automatic recovery response that gives expression to a conscious hope and expectation of rebirth. The sequence of death and rebirth is displayed fairly consistently in response to major shifts in psychic energies. A sharp increase in psychic energy generates the classic *Weltuntergang* fantasy of incipient schizophrenia, which is then followed by delusional rebirth. A decrease in psychic energy generates fantasies and dreams of destruction, but here rebirth usually fails. The stereotypy of apocalyptic fantasies—the regular inclusion of journeys, vehicles, seers, saviours, and antagonists—may be taken as evidence for a constitutional basis for the pattern, but it may also be argued that this stereotypy simply reflects the constants of early infant experience. In any case, the promise of redemption after suffering invites commitment to the illusion.

The tenacity of the apocalyptic vision is remarkable. Its derivatives—mysticism, millenarianism, utopianism, gnosticism, messianism—survive underground for long periods of time, like an infection that has been suppressed but not eradicated, only to spring to life and flourish again when circumstances are propitious. The recent eruption of neo-Nazi apocalyptic groups in farm regions of the United States well exemplifies this tendency.

Given the ubiquity and tenacity of these illusions and the usually disastrous consequences of subscribing to them, at least one deterrent to involvement in the apocalyptic programme, or to acting upon it, must be at work if civilization has not been destroyed. On the individual level, the only one I can see is the function of reality testing, and the sense of reality it confers or withholds. That function, however, is easily overridden in most of us at the level of inference, but in psychotics even at the level of perception. The apocalyptic sequence begins with the abrogation of reality testing and a rejection of the real world, a rejection that permits the rest of the sequence to unfold.

Reality testing can be preempted by the group. What the group believes is real—in politics, in culture, and especially in religion. Since groups readily come to grief when they engage in apocalyptic behaviour, it becomes necessary for them, for their own survival, to discourage it. The problem is that the apocalyptic claims that his revelation supersedes current group beliefs; he becomes a law unto himself. That is why organized religion fears mystics and condemns them as antinomian. The usual response of organized religion to mystical movements is to co-opt them, creating organizational forms whereby the deviation can be controlled. But if organized religion will not co-opt mysticism, for whatever reason (e.g. fear of being contaminated or diluted), it can nevertheless oppose it openly.

That is what we see in the story of the four who entered the garden, and in fact in the whole of chapter 2 of Hagigah. The story is placed there to warn the community that mystical exercises and the induction of trances or states of ecstasy, though often presented as forms of religious experience, are disapproved of as dangerous. Note that they are not denounced as antinomian, though the story of Elisha ben Avuya implies that they invite antinomianism. The reason for the warning is that a number of fairly distinguished rabbis and scholars had become involved in mystical practices and had very carefully dissociated themselves from pagan and Christian gnostics by adhering closely to rabbinic law and values. By excluding anything explicitly antinomian in their teachings, the rabbinic practitioners of throne, chariot, and *hekhalot* mysticism were able to appeal to a broader segment of the community. The injunctions to avoid militancy that were issued after the failure of the Bar Kokhba revolt were intended to deter any further messianic adventures.

Messianism posed a serious problem for the rabbis of that era. The Messiah was anticipated and eagerly awaited by almost all. But since he had not come, there had to be an explanation. A discussion of the problem is to be found in *Babylonian Talmud* Sanhedrin 97b. There Rabbi Samuel bar Nahmani, in the name of Rabbi Jonathan, curses those who "calculate the end"—that is, those who would anticipate the Messiah's advent at a specific time. His reason is that if the Messiah does not come when anticipated, people will lose faith.

To be sure, the rabbis disapproved of both esoteric, mystical speculation and active messianism, but to my knowledge they did not relate the two. This disjunction becomes especially clear in the case of Akiba. In the *Pardes* story he is said to have remained uncorrupted by his mystical experience—but no mention is made of his catastrophic messianism. Is this an omission, or are they refusing to make the connection?

Maimonides, the great scholar and physician of mediaeval Jewry, discussed the advent of the Messiah as an event to be expected, but he saw the messianic world as one free of mystical elements. "Do not assume that in the days of the Messiah any of the laws of nature will be abrogated, or any innovation introduced into creation", he wrote; "The world will follow its usual course. . . . Do not assume that the King Messiah will have to perform signs and wonders [i.e. miracles], create anything new, revive the dead, or do similar things. It is not so." Maimonides is here promoting a tempered messianism, one divorced as much as possible from its apocalyptic matrix. Such a view, tending to preserve the optimism of messianism while discouraging messianic activism, may prevail for limited periods of time, but the very concept of messianism would seem to invite activism.

Regarding the role of Rabbi Akiva, Maimonides takes the position that he

> . . . was a distinguished scholar among the scholars of the Mishnah, yet he was also armor bearer of the King Ben Koziba. He declared that Ben Koziba was the King Messiah; he and all the wise men of his generation believed that he was the messianic king until he was slain for his sins. When he was slain it became known that he was not. Yet the scholars had not asked him for a sign or indication. The general principle is this: this Torah with its statutes and ordinances is valid forever and for all eternity; it is not to be added to or taken away from.

Here Maimonides is clearly opposing messianism while trying to show respect for the messianic allusions of the Bible and the messianic aspirations prevalent among the people (Mishneh Torah, Book of Judges, Chap. 11, para. 3).

I would like to advance the hypothesis that one of the major functions of organized religion is to discourage individual mystical speculation and, more important, to contain apocalyptic and millenarian campaigns at the collective level. Freud spoke of religion as an illusion, but he failed to apprehend that organized religion, by offering an illusion sponsored and controlled by the collectivity, tries to discourage irresponsible and self-defeating mysticism, even though the latter might cloak itself in the terminological trappings of traditional religion. The devastating millenarian movements in history—including, for example, the Nazi apocalypse—have always rejected the discipline and restraints of organized religion, on their own authority overriding these restraints. Despite the traditional antisemitism of most of the organized European churches from the time of the Crusades right through the Holocaust, they attempted much more often than might have been expected to contain the fury of apocalyptic mobs who were attacking Jews (see, for example, Cohn, 1970, pp. 70, 283). And this, I submit, is the lesson that we are taught by the story of the four who entered the garden.

Comments

Eleanor Galenson

DEVELOPMENT AND CURIOSITY IN CHILDHOOD

In the course of human development, children learn to acknowledge certain realities and to distinguish these from fantasy, while at the same time they are permitted to ignore or even deny certain other realities in the interest of maintaining an adequate degree of psychological equilibrium. Despite the infinite number of individual variations in the psychological processes through which these tasks are accomplished, infant researchers have been able to identify consistencies and commonalities whereby the sense of oneself as an individual with wholeness and continuity over time is required, along with the reciprocally acquired sense of the other, usually the primary caretaker.

We know that recognition of the psychological sense of self as distant from the other is achieved in most infants during the second half of the first year of life (Mahler, Pine, & Bergman, 1975). While this recognition results in a disequilibrium that involves every aspect of the developing personality, it is particularly in regard to loving and hating feelings that psychological instability is evident. This instability is reflected in a variety of behavioural sequences. The infant now both loves and hates the other, just as he loves and hates himself—an unstable psychological state that appears to be served effectively in a remarkable new developmental step. Two different channels are now utilized, activated by and ultimately providing discharge pathways for these two opposing psychological views of the other and of the self. The infant's attachment to the other and his sense of his own "oneness" are preserved temporarily. Ultimately, the solution lies, of course, in a synthesis of the loving and the hating self, of the hated other with the loved other.

The temporary, normal splitting or primary ambivalence of the second year is thus dynamically related to the emergence of anal and early genital zone arousal. The anal zone serves as a channel for the discharge of aggression by virtue of its structural capacities for retention and expulsion. The genital zone has been gradually prepared during the first year as the site of pleasurable sensations, along with the closeness and warmth experienced passively in the rest of the body during various maternal nurturing interchanges. A similar type of pleasure is now actively produced by the child himself at the genital zone, again by virtue of its structural properties—namely, the capacity for venous engorgement in response to psychological stimulation and an extraordinary degree of tactile sensitivity. As with all other sensate zones that influence psychological development, the anal and genital zones gradually begin to serve as bodily nuclei to which psychological representation of feelings are attached, the predominantly loving ones to the genital area and the predominantly hating ones to the anal area.

The psychological capacity to distinguish self from others develops only very gradually and is facilitated by the simultaneous unfolding of a variety of biological and psychological functions during the first year. Among the various attributes of the infant is the tendency to search for a repetition of somatic and psychological experiences that have afforded an appropriate type and degree of stimulation. Oral experience is particularly illustrative of this attribute. Having sucked on finger or milk, the infant seeks to repeat the experience in a variety of ways. Indeed, he/she expands the use of his mouth to explore eventually the body and any other animate or inanimate object within his or her reach. One might consider this search for repetition as a bedrock aspect of curiosity, since it helps to amass a variety of experiences that eventually inform the infant of the many similarities and differences in the objects he has encountered. Ordinarily, the experiences are sorted out and identified as belonging to different groups, some producing subsequent sensations in one's body while others do not. Eventually the illusion that others have the same reaction that we have to an experience has to give way to the reality of a separate other, although we never abandon the tendency to return to this illusion during times of stress, in our fantasies, and also in everyday life when we assume that others think and feel as we do without having the evidence to support this view.

By the end of the first year, then, a critical level of complex psychological capacities allows, or perhaps forces, the infant more or less to acknowledge the existence of another who is not himself, and to acknowledge his now often conflicting affects towards both of them. Behavioural evidence of the emergence of two major pathways for discharge of conflicting affects has not been difficult to obtain.

Sometime between the 12th and 14th months, both boys and girls begin to be aware of their anal functioning (Galenson & Roiphe, 1971, 1974, 1976, 1980; Roiphe & Galenson, 1981). Ego reflections of this new level of organization include behavioural evidence of curiosity about their own anal zone and its products, followed by anal curiosity regarding other people, animals, dolls, etc. Many play sequences in infants of this age replicate anal structural characteristics, and the anal drive-connected affects of directed aggression and ambivalence emerge.

Pre-oedipal genitality begins to appear, along with urinary awareness, some time between 14 and 16 months. Attention to the urinary stream, attempts to control it, curiosity about this area and function in other children and in adults, and games that derive from and reflect the urinary interest are readily observable in infants of both sexes at this time. Early genitality is reflected in increased intentional genital self-manipulation and curiosity expressed verbally and behaviourally about the genital anatomy of other children and adults, of dolls, and of animals (both animate and inanimate).

Although parental responses to this burgeoning curiosity differ, of course, almost all the infants observed in the study cited above were allowed to witness the mother's toileting, and most of them were also admitted to the bathroom by the fathers as well during the first two or three months of the infants' newly emergent curiosity. Many of the fathers soon banished their female children from observing their toileting.

As the infants begin to acknowledge the genital and urinary differences between the sexes, the subsequent developmental direction of the boys and girls begin to diverge. Boys begin to avoid exposure to the mother's toileting and tend to accompany the father instead. They direct their attention to body protuberances (breasts, nipples, umbilicus), are concerned about body injury, and again become anxious about separation from the mother. The increase in their general motor activity at this time may be another avenue for expression of their heightened preoedipal castration anxiety.

Infant girls react to their appreciation of the genito–urinary differences they have observed with heightened hostile ambivalence towards the mother, a large variety of exploratory play with dolls and toy animals, a new type of erotic flirtation with the father, various body damage concerns, depressed mood states, and other evidence of their underlying castration reaction.

The reaction of parents to the infant's genital interests and behaviours appears to vary a great deal. However, most parents tend to "forget" what they have witnessed until reminded of it by seeing it duplicated by another young child. Repression of the memory of this early sexuality seems to be equally profound in both the parents and their children.

It is of great interest and importance that the so-called disorders of gender identity are far more common in boys than in girls, and that they begin to emerge towards the end of the second year. It is likely that this disorder has its origins in traumatic experiences during the first year of life, if these experiences have interfered with the developing mother–child relationship. In regard to the preponderance of the gender disorder in boys, it is thought that the boy's recognition of the genital anatomical difference requires that he disengage from the mother if he is to retain his phallic identity. However, if the relationship with the mother is an unstable one, such a boy needs to remain closely attached to her in an attempt to avoid excessive anxiety brought on by separation.

The early genital phase may be viewed as a "psychic organizer" in the average child in that the psychological system is restructured on a higher level of complexity. Through self-induced genital stimulation, the infant can now *actively* achieve the pleasure previously derived from the mother's ministrations—a shift in the passive–active balance that aids in consolidating differentiation of self from object. While masturbation and its accompanying fantasy state provide a feeling of closeness to the mother, they simultaneously enhance differentiation from her, specifically around the new supremacy of genitality. Masturbation and its fantasies also provide something equivalent to trial action, offering specific satisfaction at the genital level and facilitating repression of regressive pre-phallic fantasies of merging with the non-sexual mother of early infancy.

The pathway to the oedipal phase

Mahler, Pine, and Bergman (1975) have emphasized that the period of the rapprochement crisis, at the close of the second year, is more troubled for the girl than for the boy. Children's recognition of the sexual difference probably accounts in part for this difference in response. In girls, the heightening of the aggressive aspect of ambivalence to the mother that results from recognition of the genital anatomical difference leads to a loosening of the tie to the mother and an increasingly erotic turn to the father. This provides a developmental precondition for the future positive–oedipal constellation. Those girls who develop severe castration reactions at this time have experienced difficulties with the mother during their first year. The hostile ambivalence to the mother becomes very intense, the maternal attachment is heightened, and the turn to the father does not occur.

Overtly, the boy is far less disturbed by the discovery of the genital difference. In fact, however, he defends himself against castration anxiety by more profound denial and displacement—both of which may affect development in other areas as well. The father's availability at this time plays a crucial role in supporting the boy's gradual distancing from his mother and the increasingly stable sense of his phallic identity.

While soft stuffed animals are used for various kinds of self-comforting during the first and second years, interest in dolls has emerged by the end of the second year in most girls and increases in intensity and complexity from that time until the 6th or 7th year. Early semi-symbolic doll play seems to replicate the little girl's experience with her own mother—repeating with her doll the same care-taking that she herself has received. It is difficult to distinguish this early identification with the mother's nurturing activities from the more advanced doll play in which the doll represents the little girl's wished-for baby of her own. Most 3- to 3½-year-old girls have begun to pretend that they have a baby inside their abdomens, particularly if they have had the opportunity to observe a pregnant woman. And this is followed by curiosity as to how the father's "seed" gets into the mother's stomach and how the body then emerges.

While doll play is desultory at best in boys, they, too, are keenly aware of pregnant women beginning at about 3 to 3½ years of age, and they develop curiosity about birth and impregnation within the next six to eight months, although they may indicate their curiosity by action rather than words.

During the third and fourth years, both sexes continue to acquire a sense of sexual identity. Exhibitionism and scoptophilia are pronounced components in both sexes, with a gradual divergence between girls and boys becoming evident in regard to drive-derivative fantasies, sexual identification, and object relations. Sexual wishes and fantasies are still in a one-to-one relationship. For the boy, castration anxiety of this earlier period differs from oedipal castration anxiety, while the penis becomes a highly valued body part and the main source of narcissistic gratification. The boy may fear its loss at the hands of envious females or as punishment by his father, and he may even fear that damage may come to him through masturbation, but he does not anticipate its loss as punishment for his wish to banish or castrate his father. In the girl, the wish for a penis may build on earlier wishes she has had for other objects she did not possess; these yearnings are intensified by the discovery of the genital difference. Penis envy with lowering of her self-esteem may interfere with the development of her feminine identification.

Oedipal-phase development

The child's dyadic relationship slowly merges into the oedipal triadic relationship with the parents by the end of the fourth year, ushering in a severely conflictual situation for children of both sexes. If identification with the parent of the same sex has been proceeding well, this identification now serves as a stabilizing force, facilitating the temporary surrender of incestuous wishes and the modulation of hostile aggressive wishes towards the parent of the same sex. Sublimation of the sexual and aggressive drive derivatives can now proceed, with curiosity directed towards other areas. A significant landmark during latency is the gradual emergence of a scientific approach to learning and thinking. The why and wherefore of things become very important: concepts of the world and people begin to expand, and the development of reasoning steadily advances. Curiosity about sexuality gives way, under reasonably adequate psychological conditions, to curiosity about the wider aspects of the world, a sublimation of a portion of sexual as well as aggressive wishes that continues into adult life unless inhibitions arise because of psychological conflicts that were insufficiently resolved during the pre-oedipal and oedipal periods.

CHAPTER FIVE

INTRODUCTION

Chapter four dealt with revived childhood wishes to approach, to behold, and ultimately to be embraced by and to unite with a parent figure. The wish and the anxiety that the wish engenders are expressed in the account of the dangerous fascination of the mystical garden, the *pardes*.

But the chariot, the throne, and the garden are obviously claustrum symbols—symbols of mother's body, the literal Garden of Eden, which attracts us all when we regress. Claustrophilia and claustrophobia become the organizing principles that evoke such fantasies.

This chapter describes variants of such fantasies, variations of a basic pattern in which the individual encounters or hopes to encounter father or father's penis inside mother's body. When one is sensitized to these patterns, one can find them surprisingly frequently in the fantasies and dreams that patients report. The *merkavah* and *hekhaloth* images form a direct link between apocalyptic and mystical ideas and drives on the one hand, and material of clinical significance, namely, symptoms, fantasies, and dreams on the other.

The psychodynamics of *merkavah* mysticism

Mortimer Ostow

Merkavah mysticism prevailed as the dominant form of Jewish mysticism for about a thousand years, starting a few centuries before the Common Era and enduring to close to the end of the first millennium, when it overlapped with and was succeeded by Kabbalah, which, in turn, was gradually replaced by Hasidism starting in the eighteenth century. (A fascinating, probably complete and searching analysis of *merkavah* materials is given by Halperin in *The Faces of the Chariot*, 1988a.)

Merkavah mysticism takes its name from the throne-chariot described in the first chapter of Ezekiel. A kind of divine throne is also referred to in a number of early apocalypses and in the Book of Revelation. (The word "*merkavah*" means "chariot".) The Ezekiel material is given in the introduction to chapter four. The four creatures with their wheels constitute the chariot, and the throne is carried on a platform above them. As noted above, the term "*merkavah*" does not appear there

I should like to thank Dr Jacob A. Arlow for his generous assistance in organizing this material for presentation.

or elsewhere in the Jewish canon with respect to the vision of Ezekiel. (The earliest surviving use of *merkavah* to refer to Ezekiel's vision appears in Sirach 49:8.) Please note the many references to fire, gleam, crystalline substance, amber and sapphire, radiance and the rainbow; the fact that what is described is both a vehicle and a seat; and that there are four creatures, four faces to each, four complex wheels, and four sets of wings. The image is awesome and frightening, and the prophet collapses.

The first five verses of chapter 6 of the Book of Isaiah contains a throne vision, which includes the familiar doxology, "*Kadosh, kadosh, kadosh*" [Holy, holy, holy], which we find in the *Kedushah* of the liturgy and which is repeated over and over in the *Hekhaloth* texts, which we discuss below.

> In the year of the death of the king Uzziah, I saw the Lord sitting on a high and lofty throne, and his skirts filled the chamber. And seraphs were standing in attendance, six wings, six wings to each. With two each covers his face, with two he covers his legs and with two he flies. And each calls to the other and says "Holy, holy, holy. The Lord of hosts. The earth is filled with His glory." And the doorposts were moved at the sound of Him who called and the building was filled with smoke and I said, "Woe is me because I am undone. For I am a man of unclean lips and I reside among a people of unclean lips. For my eyes have seen the king, the Lord of hosts." [Isa. 6:1–4]

A similar vision is found in Revelation:

> After this I looked, and, behold, a door was opened in heaven: and the first voice which I heard was as it were of a trumpet talking with me; which said, Come up hither, and I will show thee things which must be hereafter. And immediately I was in the Spirit: and, behold, a throne was set in heaven, and one sat on the throne. And He that sat was to look upon like a jasper and a sardine stone: and there was a rainbow round about the throne, in sight like unto an emerald. And round about the throne were four and twenty seats: and upon the seats I saw four and twenty elders sitting, clothed in white raiment; and they had on their heads crowns of gold. And out of the throne proceeded lightnings and thunderings and voices: and there were seven lamps of

> fire burning before the throne, which are the seven Spirits of God. And before the throne there was a sea of glass like unto crystal: and in the midst of the throne, and round about the throne, were four beasts full of eyes before and behind. And the first beast was like a lion, and the second beast like a calf, and the third beast had a face as a man, and the fourth beast was like a flying eagle. And the four beasts had each of them six wings about him; and they were full of eyes within: and they rest not day and night, saying, Holy, holy, holy, Lord God Almighty, Which was, and is, and is to come. And when those beasts give glory and honor and thanks to Him that sat on the throne, who liveth for ever and ever, the four and twenty elders fall down before Him that sat on the throne, and worship Him that liveth for ever and ever, and cast their crowns before the throne, saying, Thou art worthy, O Lord, to receive glory and honor and power: for Thou hast created all things, and for Thy pleasure they are and were created. [Rev. 4]

If we examine all of the references in the Jewish Bible to *merkavah*-type material, we find the following composite image: God is sitting on a throne; He has the appearance of a man (Ezekiel) and particularly that of an old, white-haired man (Daniel); God is sitting in a palace (2 Kings, Isaiah, and Daniel); fire occupies an important position in the vision (Ezekiel, Daniel, and indirectly also Isaiah); God is accompanied by angels who minister to Him (2 Kings, Isaiah, Ezekiel, and Daniel); the angels recite hymns (Isaiah) (see Gruenwald, 1980, p. 31).

We meet the term "*merkavah*" applied to this type of theophany in various Talmudic and other rabbinic sources (Tosefta Hagigah 2:1–7; Mishnah Hagigah 2:1; *Babylonian Talmud* Hagigah 11b–16a; *Palestinian Talmud* Hagigah 77a–d). The sources speak of Ma'aseh *Merkavah*—literally, "the account of the *merkavah*", referring either to the text itself, to the narrative, or to mystical ideas associated with it. They associate it with *Ma'aseh B'reshith*—that is, cosmogony—and also with the laws delineating sexual prohibitions, none of which may be taught in public, but only to very limited groups of scholars, in the case of *merkavah* mysticism to (or by) only one person, and then only in hints. They provide anecdotal commentary about both laudable and improper involvement in this mystical doctrine. On the other hand, we note that the Biblical and apocalyptic visions of God were not only not restricted, but actively publicized. Why the difference? In the Bible and apocalypses, the revelations were employed in order to lend authority and force to the moral and religious message that the writer wished to transmit. The rabbinic literature, on the other hand, seems to imply that a mystical practice intended to achieve visualization of the Godhead, accompanied by no moral or socially responsible message, was dangerous both to the individual and to the community. Individual mystical experience can also be used to circumvent and to supersede normative religion. From rabbinic sources, it becomes evident that interest or engaging in mystical praxis was common, that study of it was considered dangerous, and that though it was important to transmit, that transmission had to be regulated stringently.

At some point the *merkavah* fantasy became associated with and gradually gave way to a similar one. It emphasized methods to ascend through the various heavens to the *hekhaloth*, the chambers, the halls or palaces where ultimately God could be seen sitting on His throne. Seeing and approaching God were the declared aims. Achieving this confrontation with God was an ordeal: one prepared for it by prolonged fasting, restriction of activity, assuming deferential postures or the use of ritual baths, or a combination of these. Gatekeepers at the various *hekhaloth* might not only prevent the entry of the petitioner, but without much provocation might kill him. The texts therefore were a combination of descriptions of the appearance of God, methods to achieve the ascent, a technical manual, and prayers, hymns, and incantations and other apotropaic manoeuvres intended to avoid danger and to assure a successful ascent. [Martha Himmelfarb (1993, pp. 108f.) accepts arguments by Halperin (1984) and Schäfer (1992, pp. 150ff.) that find the ascent component of the *hekhalot* literature of less than primary significance. What they mean is that the texts were not meant to be practical manuals of instruction on how to achieve mystical ascent, but rather texts for study and ritual repetition.]

These mystical texts, while spiritual, do seem to reflect a considerable ambivalence in that they speak of seeing, looking at, or approaching God, all prohibited activities in both Biblical and Talmudic Judaism. The rebelliousness implied in the various ascent texts is dealt with by the description of dangers and hazards that await the mystic. Interestingly, the post-scriptural Jewish mystical writings [*midrashim*] come not from heretics or rebels, but from within the rabbinic establishment itself. These presumptuous fantasies seem to express impatience with the distance between God and man in classical Judaism and eagerness for immediate divine comfort, divine knowledge, and divine power. Halperin (1988a, pp. 319ff., 444; 1988b) documents a rebellious theme in some of these texts and infers that it reflects the eternal generational conflict between youth and age. Schäfer (1992, p. 165) prefers to see the *hekhalot* material as the effort to establish a liturgical communion of the *yored merkavah*, the *merkavah* adept, as emissary of Israel, with God.

The texts also describe the angels singing hymns, the very same hymns that the human traveller is advised to sing. The hymns are given *in extenso.* They consist mostly of repetitive hyperbolic praise of God with almost no ideology, morality, or reference to individual spiritual concerns. I shall give here a few samples of this material, but brief samples cannot convey the impression created by the prolixity, the repetitiousness, and the interesting structure that itself conveys feelings of progression and ascent (see Janowitz, 1989). The *Hekhaloth Rabbati*, generally translated as *The Greater Hekhaloth*, a major source, starts with a verse that introduces the extensive text that follows.

Rabbi Ishmael said:

> What are the incantations that should be recited by one who wishes to glimpse the merkavah, to descend (i.e. to the merkavah) in peace and to ascend in peace? It is desirable to obligate him, to lead him and to bring him to the chambers of the palace of *aravot* (a name of one of the heavens), to stand him to the right of His throne of glory twice, so that he may stand next to the Lord, God of Israel to see what one does before His throne of glory, and to know everything that is destined to happen in the world. [Jellinek, 1:1]

Here is a classic hymn from the same source. It accents the role of unison singing and worship, it calls attention to the role of fire, which appears in many *merkavah* texts, and it illustrates the hyperbole that characterizes them.

From the praise and song of each day,
From the jubilation and exultation of each hour,
And from the utterances that proceed out of the mouth of
the holy ones,
And from the melody which wells out of the mouth of the
servants,
Mountains of fire and hills of flame
Are piled up and hidden and poured out each day.

[Scholem, 1960, p. 21][1]

This and all subsequent hymns are followed by the Trishagion:

Kadosh, Kadosh, Kadosh,

that is,

Holy, Holy, Holy is the Lord of Sabaoth.[2]
The whole earth is filled with His glory.

That refrain, taken from Isaiah, chapter 6, is repeated many times throughout the *Hekhaloth* texts. In fact, a description of the celestial Kedushah (i.e. the liturgical sanctification) follows. Note again the hyperbole, the reference to fire, the unison singing, and the fact that God uncovers his face in response.

> The Holy Living Creatures do strengthen and hallow and purify themselves, and each one has bound upon its head a thousand thousands of thousands of crowns of luminaries of divers sorts, and they are clothed in clothing of fire and wrapped in a garment of flame and cover their faces with lightning. And the Holy One, Blessed be He, uncovers His face. And why do the Holy Living Creatures and the Ophanim of majesty and the Cherubim of splendor hallow and purify and clothe and wrap and adorn themselves yet more? Because the Merkabah is above them and the throne of glory upon their heads and the Shekhinah over them and rivers of fire pass between them. Accordingly do they strengthen themselves and make themselves splendid and

---

[1]This and other translations from Scholem, 1960, were done by Judah Goldin.

[2]*Sabaoth* is a Hebrew word, usually translated as "hosts" (see the selection from Isa. 6, translated above). It may refer either to the heavenly retinue or to stars. Its precise significance is obscure, since it is used in different ways.

> purify themselves in fire seventy times and do all of them stand in cleanliness and holiness and sing songs and hymns, praise and rejoicing and applause, with one voice, with one utterance, with one mind, and with one melody. [Scholem, 1960, p. 29]
>
> Rabbi Ishmael said, this is what Rabbi Nehunya ben Hakanah said: "In the seven hekhaloth (palaces) Tutrasi'i (probably a reference to the Tetragrammaton, the four-letter name of God, YHVH) the Lord God of Israel sits in one chamber within another, and at the entrance of each palace, eight guards stand, four on each side of the door." [Jellinek, 15:1]

The guards are fierce, and unless the mystic appeases them by his piety or by exhibiting appropriate seals, they may drive him from heaven or viciously attack him.

The fierce gatekeepers and their equally fierce horses that threaten the presumptuous mystic are described in *Hekhaloth Rabbati* as follows:

> . . . angry and war-like, strong, harsh, fearful, terrific, taller than mountains and sharper than peaks. Their bows are strung and stand before them; their swords are sharpened and in their hands. Lightnings flow and issue forth from the balls of their eyes, and balls of fire from their nostrils, and torches of fiery coals from their mouths. They are equipped with helmets and with coats of mail, and javelins and spears are hung upon their thews . . . the horses upon which they ride stand beside mangers of fire full of coals of juniper and eat fiery coals from the mangers [taking] a measure of forty bushels of coals in one mouthful. [Scholem, 1960, pp. 31f.]

There are no explicit sexual images in the material to my knowledge, but in a literature so concerned with spying out secrets, inevitably one runs into a number of images that strongly suggest sexual curiosity. If we look back to Ezekiel 1, we find (1:27): "And I saw the gleam of hashmal, like the appearance of fire within a surrounding frame, that extended from what appeared to be its loins upward, and from what appeared to be its loins downward, I saw the appearance of fire surrounded by radiance." It would be difficult to deny that the allusion is to the phallus. Eilberg-Schwartz (1994, pp. 181ff.)

draws the same conclusion, and he attributes a homoerotic component to Ezekiel's visualizing God's phallus.

Fire is a powerful if ambiguous symbol. Light usually promises rebirth—for example, the light at the end of the tunnel. It can be threatening or destructive, as, for example, sunshine in the desert. Flames can warm, or they can harm. Fire that contains these potencies symbolizes power. It is attractive but dangerous; for example, the fire and lightning of the theophany on the occasion of the revelation at Mt. Sinai. Therefore it occurs commonly in the dreams and fantasies that accompany the members of the apocalyptic complex, which deal with destruction and rebirth in close proximity. We know that the father's phallus is a source of fascination for the child (see Galenson, chapter four) but also of danger. In Ezekiel's *merkavah* images, the fire hides the phallus itself, but symbolizes both its attractiveness and its dangerousness.

Intense visual sensations, lights of various colours and shapes are described by users of hallucinogenic drugs. Apparently the mystical state of mind, whether induced by psychological preparation or by hallucinogenic substances, favours intense visual experience.

Arlow (1951), in an early and important essay on the mystical experiences that accompany the consecration of the Biblical prophets, establishes from the texts that not only are the prophets confronted by the appearance of God, but the confrontation is accompanied by oral incorporation of His phallus, by means of which the prophet acquires His power of prophecy and His authority as spokesman for God. The mystic who would ascend to the *merkavah* or the *hekhaloth* also hopes to see God plainly, presumably expecting that the vision will not only give him comfort, but also, by a process of oral incorporation, lend him some of the divine potency and knowledge.

David J. Halperin (1987) argues that the eyes of the "holy hayyot" (the creatures of Ezek. 1) symbolize the female genital in the following verse in *Hekhalot Rabbati*:

> Each one of the eyes of the holy *hayyot* is split open, the size of a large winnower's (?) sieve, and their eyes look as if *they race like lightnings*. Besides them, there are the eyes of the mighty cherubim and of the *'ofannim* of the Shekhinah,

> which look like torches and flaming coals. [The words in italics appear in Ezek. 1.]

His argument, involving comparison with other verses using a similar metaphor, seems to me persuasive. Presumably the same argument would apply to the eyes that covered the rims of the wheels of Ezekiel's chariot. (In dreams, eyes and what they see can symbolize each other.)

A primal scene is suggested by the following anecdote given in the *merkavah* unit of Hagigah (BT, 14b).

> Now when these things were told to Rabbi Joshua, he and Rabbi Jose the priest were going on a journey. They said, Let us also expound the "Work of the Chariot" (Ma'aseh Merkavah); so Rabbi Joshua began an exposition. Now that day was the summer solstice; (nevertheless) the heavens became overcast with clouds and a kind of rainbow appeared in the cloud, and the ministering angels assembled and came to listen like people who assemble and come to watch the entertainments of a bridegroom and bride.

[Halperin sees a confirmation for the suggestion that BT Hagigah describes a primal scene, in the presence of the *rainbow in the cloud.* BT Sanhedrin 92a says, *kol hammistakkel be'ervah qashto nin'eret,* which presumably means something like, "Whoever gazes at genitalia [female?], his bow [= penis] is impaired" (see Rashi, commentary on BT Sanhedrin 92a; and Jastrow, 1950, s.v. *n'r*). The formation is remarkably similar to that of BT Hagigah 16a, *kol hammistakkel bisheloshah devarim 'enav kehot baqqeshet uvannasi' uvakkohanim,* "Whoever gazes at three things, his eyes grow dim: the bow, the prince, and the priests". In context, the "bow" obviously means the rainbow. But, especially in view of the Sanhedrin passage, it seems reasonable to postulate a latent allusion to the penis: looking at (your father's?) penis is punished with blindness.]

One of the more unusual texts of the *hekhaloth* material is called "*Shiur Qomah*"—literally, "the measure of the body". It is a theurgic text, the recitation of which, it was hoped, would obtain for the mystic gratification of many of his desires. Whereas the other *hekhaloth* texts idealize God for His many virtues as well as His grandeur, power, and knowledge, this aggrandizes His literal size, here given in cosmic terms.

> R. Aqiba said: I give testimony that Metatron said to me, [Metatron, who is] the great prince of testimony, our lord and master, who exalts our blood and who saves us and redeems us from every evil thing. From the place of the seat of His glory and up [is a distance of] 1,180,000,000 parasangs. From His glorious seat and down [is a distance of] 1,180,000,000 parasangs. His height is 2,300,000,000 parasangs. From the right arm [across] until the left arm is 770,000,000 parasangs. And from the right eyeball until the left eyeball [is a distance of] 300,000,000 parasangs. The skull of His head is 3,000,000,003 and a third parasangs. The crown on His head is 600,000, corresponding to the 600,000 Israelite minions. Thus He is called the great, mighty and awesome God *kaliote* [*klyvtyh*]; *sazioyte* [*szyvtyh*]; *haqtas* [*hqts*]; *ba'avur* [*b'bvr*]; *masos* [*msvs*].[3] Blessed be He and blessed be the name of the glory of His kingdom forever. [Cohen, 1982, pp. 440f.]

A parasang is a Persian mile, about three-quarters of a modern mile, but the author himself defines it as a truly infinite measure (Cohen, 1982, p. 468).

What is especially bold is attributing to God literal human organs. Cohen (1982, pp. 464, 471) reads allusions to God's penis in the text.

Let us summarize the features that characterize *merkavah* texts and *hekhaloth* variants. Primarily, the texts deal with the attempt to visualize and to approach a divine being, specifically the Jewish God in all of the instances that I have mentioned. The Deity is idealized and adored, and the mystic who aspires to the *merkavah* will often abase himself. The affect implied is awe and fear. The Deity is usually to be found, if not at the top of a mountain, then on a throne, in a chariot, in magnificent chambers within magnificent palaces, on an elevated place, one of the postulated heavens, in these texts usually the seventh.

The number four occurs with surprising regularity in these texts. The *merkavah* in Ezekiel, is a four-sided structure made up of four creatures, each of which has four faces and four wings. In the Daniel and Revelation apocalypses, different sets of

---

[3] If these terms have meanings, we do not know them. Presumably they are intended as names or qualities of God (M.O.).

four beasts or beings are described. The chamber and palace structures may be presumed to be quadrangular.

The Deity is attended by enormous retinues of angels, many of whom are referred to by name, by function, by appearance, by rank, or by origin.

The issue of danger looms importantly. In the apocalyptic texts, the visionary is involuntarily transported to the locus of his meeting with the Deity. In the prophetic visions, the prophet is awed and terrified but is then reassured. The rabbinic texts emphasize the danger that arises from the spread of *merkavah* mystical interest and practice, and strictly limit its dissemination. The *pardes* text (the garden text of the previous essay) emphasizes danger. The *hekhaloth* texts all emphasize the mortal danger that awaits the mystic who attempts the ascent (or descent—paradoxically both metaphors are used, apparently indiscriminately) to the *merkavah*, improperly prepared. Presumably, the preparation involves trance-promoting manoeuvres for the cultivation of a properly self-effacing frame of mind. Much of the danger is attributed to the hostility of the heavenly host, the fierce gatekeepers described above, and other envious angels. To offset the danger of the ascent, apotropaic manoeuvres are recommended; the chief of these is the recitation of formulas, the singing of hymns, and the recitation of incantations embodied in the text. The effect intended is extravagant self-effacement and self-abasement. Other forms of magic are described—the presentation of seals, the use of names for conjuring, especially the many names given for God. Although the danger is attributed to the heavenly hosts, jealous of their prerogatives and primacy, one must infer that it is the presumptuousness of the ascent to forbidden regions and of engaging in a forbidden looking that creates the danger of punishment.

The heavenly retinue is described in hyperbolic numbers and power. They attend the Deity in every possible way. When not otherwise engaged, they spend their time singing hymns of praise, some of which are identical with portions of synagogue liturgy already established, and others that were subsequently incorporated into it. While the texts emphasize the harmony of this music and the synchrony of their actions, there are a number of references to rivalry among them and towards the human aspirant to the *merkavah*.

The issue of secrecy is emphasized. The visions in the biblical passages and the apocalypses are announced publicly in the hope that they will lend authority and cogency to the message of the prophet or the promoter of the apocalypse. (Nevertheless, many apocalypses use a fictional secrecy to enhance their allure.) The rabbinic authorities prohibited the public discussion of this type of mysticism except under the most protected circumstances, implying that violation of the prohibition incurs great danger, presumably for the individual as well as for the community where such indiscretion occurs. For the *merkavah* mystics, the texts are meant to instruct the would-be seeker of the mystical experience, but the danger is attributed to the attempted ascent if it is not properly prepared and performed, using manoeuvres intended to induce the appropriately self-effacing attitudes.

The *merkavah* vision is attained in a state of altered consciousness, described or implied by the prophets, apocalypticists, rabbis and mystics. The term "trance" would seem to apply to most instances. (The psychology of the trance state is discussed in chapter one.) These trances were imposed upon the prophets and apocalypticists, occurred spontaneously during the studies of the rabbis, and were induced by serious effort among the *merkavah* mystics.

We are now in a position to study the psychodynamic implications of these visions and fantasies. Halperin (1988a and 1988b) suggests that the ascension of the *merkavah* adept to the divine realms can be construed as an oedipal invasion. One finds few if any obvious current clinical homologues of the *merkavah* or *hekhaloth* mystical dynamics—that is, symptoms or fantasies. They do occur in the hallucinations and delusions of schizophrenics, but usually the material there is so florid that the specifics of this pattern are easily lost.[4]

[4] In the best-known instance of schizophrenic psychosis in psychoanalytic literature, the Schreber case, one easily recognizes the central features of the hekhaloth fantasy. Daniel Paul Schreber, a nineteenth-century German jurist, described his experiences in a number of episodes of psychosis, in his *Memoirs*. Freud (1911c) analysed these memoirs and gave us our first understanding of the dynamics of schizophrenic psychosis. (For an extensive discussion of Schreber, his background, and his illness, see Lothane, 1992.) In Schreber's delusions and hallucinations

The dream world, on the other hand, is not limited by what is culturally acceptable, and here we shall have no difficulty in recognizing clear representations of the same Gestalt that we encounter in *merkavah* mysticism.

In *The Interpretation of Dreams*, Freud (1900a, pp. 209ff.) reports his own dreams, including the following:

> A crowd of people, a meeting of students.—A count (Thun or Taaffe) was speaking. . . . It was as though I was in the Aula (the great ceremonial hall of the University); the entrances were cordoned off and we had to escape. I made my way through a series of beautifully furnished rooms, evidently ministerial or public apartments, with furniture upholstered in a colour between brown and violet; at last I came to a corridor, in which a housekeeper was sitting, an elderly stout woman. I avoided speaking to her, but she evidently thought I had a right to pass, for she asked whether she should accompany me with the lamp. I indicated to her, by word or gesture, that she was to stop on the staircase; and I felt I was being very cunning in thus avoiding inspection at the exit. I got downstairs and found a narrow and steep ascending path, along which I went. . . .
>
> I wondered whether to go to Krems or Znaim, but reflected that the Court would be in residence there, so I decided in favour of Graz, or some such place. I was now sitting in the compartment, which was like a carriage on the Stadtbahn [the suburban railway]; and in my buttonhole I had a peculiar plaited, long-shaped object, and beside it some violet-brown violets made of a stiff material. This greatly struck people. [At this point the scene broke off.]
>
> Once more I was in front of the station, but this time in the company of an elderly gentleman. I thought of a plan for remaining unrecognized; and then saw that this plan had already been put into effect. It was as though thinking and experiencing were one and the same thing. He appeared to

---

the divine figure is presented either as the God common to the writer and his audience, or as his doctor, Flechsig, or the sun. We find a celestial host of subordinated, supernatural creatures, the miracled birds, Schreber's attempts to gaze at the sun, the symbol of the fiery divine figure. We find also a concern with enclosures, the "fore-courts of Heaven". (This material is discussed in greater detail in chapter two.)

be blind, at all events with one eye, and I handed him a male glass urinal (which we had to buy or had bought in town). So I was a sick-nurse and had to give him the urinal because he was blind. If the ticket-collector were to see us like that, he would be certain to let us get away without noticing us. Here the man's attitude and his micturating penis appeared in plastic form. [This was the point at which I awoke, feeling a need to micturate.]

We encounter here features familiar to us now from our *merkavah* discussion: a crowd surrounding the distinguished central figure, the Count, and later the "elderly gentleman" whose penis is visualized; a series of beautifully furnished quadrangular rooms and apartments that had to be traversed, presided over by a woman seated in a corridor; a need to escape via exits, using passes; a royal court; a quadrangular vehicle, the railroad carriage. Here, however, the attitude is quite the opposite of that characteristic of *merkavah* mysticism. The dreamer is leaving rather than arriving. He descends the stairs, although he later ascends. Freud, the dreamer, refuses to defer to the authority and expresses contempt both explicitly and implicitly, presuming to enter apartments where he was not welcome. The associations lead to a discussion of his inclination to rebel against authority. We recognize there not only his political liberalism, but also his professional courageous independence. Ultimately the dream portrays Freud's ambivalence towards his beloved father.

In the following dream we shall recognize some of the features that are found in the *hekhaloth* materials. It was reported by a man who had been depressed for years, but was now in partial remission with the assistance of medication. The story of his life is one of repeated perverse rebellion, followed by downfall.

"I was in Brooklyn on Eastern Parkway driving past the headquarters of the Lubavitch Rebbe. I was sitting in a room with Hasidim. They said, 'This time it really happened.'—'No, it couldn't.' What were they talking about? I walked out. They were all talking. It turned out that the Rebbe had died and these people believed that he was directly related to God. A number of times he'd been sick, but hadn't died. Now he had

died. If he had had divine protection he should not have died. They paraded him around on a chair. He would ascend to heaven in a fire. They put me in a chair, which I thought was strange. They were rocking me back and forth. I fell off the chair. There was a fire. I fell into it."

There is a room in a headquarters. The Lubavitch Rebbe is presented as a charismatic, religious figure. We find a *merkavah*, the chair in which the Rebbe would be translated into heaven. The patient associates to the Jewish wedding custom of elevating bride and groom on chairs carried by the more vigorous guests. Occupying the chair represents an oedipal violation of the father's privilege. The dreamer specifies a host of ministering subordinates, the Hasidim, who, like the hostile angels of the *hekhaloth*, throw the dreamer down to his fiery death. Fire both accompanies the ascent to heaven and awaits the traveller who is ejected. Clearly, the intent of the dream is Promethean, to ascend to divine heights and to displace the father god. For that, the dreamer is punished.

Here is the dream of a woman who came for treatment of hysterical blindness. In her mid-forties, after her children had grown, she had gone back to work in the same business in which her father had been engaged. She had loved him very much as a child, but, as she remembered, her mother had come between them and prevented any significant exchange of affection. He had died a number of years ago.

"I was in my father's bedroom. We were talking about business. He was familiar with the issues that concerned me. I asked, 'How did you know?' I marvelled about how smart he was. He worked hard and was familiar with the background material. There was someone else in the room, not my mother. I was thrilled because I was able to talk to my father about business. He was very young and strong, very vital. I enjoyed listening to his usually loud voice, forceful, smiling. I was very happy, perhaps 23 or 25. He told me what to do, but I wasn't sure I could do it. I could work for him. I was a little frightened that I wouldn't do a good job. Perhaps that was not such a good idea."

He became impatient. I was back in the bedroom. It was very dim. I tried to see him, but I couldn't see him so clearly. He put on his shoes. He was getting dressed. I kept saying, 'How did you know that that's the right thing to do?'"

In the dream, the patient realizes her wish for reunion with her father, now dead, to see him and to hear him, and she aspires to identify with him. She idealizes him, which she tends to do in waking life. Her mother was there ("not my mother"), but does not interfere, though her influence is felt. In childhood, the mother had kept father and daughter apart. The patient feared that she would not be able to please her father. Her desire to see was frustrated; there was not enough light. In fact, she was very angry with her male employer, whom she (probably correctly) considered stupid. When she was a child, it was her brother's intelligence that was celebrated by her mother. She was left feeling stupid, as her employer made her feel currently. The dream expresses her transference desire to know and see more of her father and analyst, to identify with them, and to win their admiration and love for her. The *hekhalot* mystical dynamic here consists of attempting to combat her employer's depressing disparagement of her by reminding herself of her love for her psychoanalyst and the hope that he valued her, and her tremendous admiration for her father, as well as her effort to see his body, as she had watched him dress every morning in the bedroom when she was a child, and to watch him shave in the bathroom. She hoped for revelations from her father and her analyst. Like the *merkavah* and *hekhalot* mystics, frustrated and distressed by the reality of daily life, she recreated in her dream her earliest gratifying, exciting, and inspiring experiences, visualizing her impressive, beloved, and loving father in an intimate and implicitly sexual context.

This is the dream of a married woman of 37. She had been writing stories about her mother, focusing on their anger with one another.

"I was looking for an apartment. There was a Hispanic woman with me, perhaps a housekeeper. There was a baby or a child and also another woman. The apartment was too small. I required a larger apartment.

> *I was on a boat in very deep water. It was a clear blue day. The sides of the boat were open. There were a large number of sailboats in the water. People and porpoises were there, and the porpoises could be seen jumping up."*

Just before telling me that dream, the patient told me of a dream that she had had in the past:

> *"I saw the Taj Mahal. It was sitting on a small island alone in the distance. It was illuminated only by its own power. There was a woman banging on the door and screaming to get in.*
>
> *There were a number of people in the water. It was very deep. They held onto the edge as if the edge of a pool. They couldn't swim to the island. They were afraid to try because they might not make it. I talked to them about it and decided to take a chance and swim there myself. When I got close, I could see the figure of the woman banging on the door."*

The porpoise, she told me, was a friendly animal whose presence protects one against the presence of sharks in the water, because porpoises drive sharks away. They are like humans, and their presence is reassuring.

One is reminded of an episode in the Apocalypse of Zephania in which the visionary is transported to paradise in a boat with thousands of angels. "I, myself, put on an angelic garment. . . . I, myself, prayed together with them, I knew their language, which they spoke with me" (Charlesworth, 1983, p. 514).

This woman's mother had died in 1986 of cancer, which she had had for about seven years. Early in the course of her illness, she had come to New York and had lived with the patient for a year, helping with the care of the patient's daughter.

The Taj Mahal dream followed shortly upon her mother's death. The hekhal here is the Taj Mahal (which is a mausoleum) "illuminated only by its own power"; in the more recent dream, the hekhal is the apartment. In both dreams, there is a quest for admission, the woman banging on the door of the Taj Mahal and screaming to get in and the dreamer seeking a larger apartment. There were a number of people in the water, in danger. She remembered that when her father took her and her younger sister swimming, she would ask her father, if the float were to tip over, whom would he save, her or her sister. He said that he would rescue the sister because she, the patient, could look after herself. Apart from the people, there were the porpoises in the water, friendly and protective. There is a vehicle, the boat. Here again we see a hekhal, but without a central male figure. Clearly it represents the mother. The dream had occurred on the night of a wedding anniversary, celebrated with an episode of sexual intercourse, which did not occur that frequently. Her husband was a wealthy man; it was by virtue of his financial assistance that she was able to look after her mother in the latter's final days. The man was merely an enabler in her quest to return to her mother.

The person designated in chapter one as C, the man who described a spiritual experience at Machu Picchu, some weeks thereafter reported the following dream:

> *"I was in the old Madison Square Garden with my brother and another man. One walked upstairs several flights up, and on each level there were squash courts, as if the building were a giant amusement park. I lost track of my brother. I met Sally. Other people were milling about, engaged in what might have been after-game conversation. Our heads were very close, on either side of a large chair. I was kneeling on the chair, and she was standing behind it. Our lips were moving together to kiss. At the last moment she pulled away. We were both embarrassed and apologized. She asked why I want to kiss her. I said I wasn't sure, it was a feeling between us. She agreed.*
>
> *We were separated in the crowd. I walked down a long, narrow staircase. I took a taxi to go to my street. But the streets came off at irregular angles, as though they were zigzagging through a brick building. I saw a place that resembled a Roman square—but without trees, only grass. At the far end there was an obelisk—but short and square. There was a building that I associated with Mussolini.*
>
> *I went home, and my parents asked where I had been. My friend said, 'You live at home with your parents? That must be difficult.'"*

I shall ignore the associations and references that relate to individual and personal matters and highlight the archetypes relevant to our discussion.

In this man's subsequent dreams, vehicles and vehicular travel were emphasized. In one instance the dreamer saw himself *lying on a hospital gurney.* In a second, he *steadied a baby who was seated on a flat-bed railroad car that travelled to meet his mother.*

Although C had never heard of Jewish mysticism and was barely aware of any mystical systems, in his description of a building with several levels on each of which squash *courts* could be found he replicates images of the classical *hekhalot* of which we have spoken. (Schreber also speaks of the *fore-courts* of heaven.) The building was located in Madison Square *Garden.* We noted in chapter four that the garden serves as a symbol of mystical wisdom and enlightenment, and also as a symbol of mother's genitals or her womb—that part of her body that encloses, feeds, and protects the infant. Pursuing the symbolic imagery, the people milling about can easily be interpreted as equivalent to the hosts of angels inhabiting the courts and waiting upon God. The dreamer finds himself in a "large chair", equivalent to the throne of *hekhalot* imagery. I see the throne as a symbol for mother or mother's lap. Here the dreamer is about to "kiss" mother, but at the last moment the kiss is averted. They both agreed that "there was a feeling between us". The incestuous coupling is prevented. Kneeling, he said, must have religious overtones.

The next segment of the dream translates the divine chamber imagery to more transparent anatomic imagery. The dreamer descends from the *hekhalot* and finds himself in a kind of labyrinth—often a symbol for mother's body. He arrives by taxi at a square. The reader will recall that in chapter two I suggested that moving vehicles and quadrangular spaces generally represent the mother's body. Grass is a well-known symbol for pubic hair. The short, square obelisk probably represents the clitoris, the stunted penis. The building reminded him of a church. The zigzag streets reminded him of the ruins of Machu Picchu that had moved him so profoundly a few weeks previously.

The final segment interprets the first two—namely, "You live at home with your parents?"

This dream seems to demonstrate the equivalence of the *hekhalot* fantasy image with the fantasy of mother's body—in the sense that they both serve as chambers in which the infant looks for comfort, food, pleasure, and protection but in which he may encounter opposition from siblings (the angels) and from father (the male God) who is ensconced there. In these dreams, the latter appears only implicitly in the plural, parents, and also implicitly by the prevention of the illicit kiss on the divine throne.

What does the pattern of *merkavah* mysticism look like when it functions as the organizing principle of an individual's life? A woman in her middle fifties came for help around the experience of having been abandoned by her second husband, whom she described as "the most vital, creative man" she had ever met. She had grown up in a Catholic family, and as a child she had found gratification and happiness in the church—an escape from home. She was anxious at school, but "awed by intelligence" and, in fantasy, hoped that having been liberated from a castle by a knight, she would be permitted to indulge in a sexual life. We see here a wish to marry an idealized man, religious orientation in childhood, a sense of awe in the presence of intelligence, and a fantasy of sexual experience associated with being liberated by a male saviour from a female claustrum. One of her most exciting experiences, she recalls, was personally meeting a man who had really loomed large in world history. The patient's sexual interest focused on men who were what might be called heroic figures in the classical sense.

On one occasion she visited the Middle East and climbed Mount Sinai at night, accompanied only by two Bedouin youths. She was excited at the top by "the most beautiful thing I had ever seen, the sunrise over the desert". At the top of the mountain she had a sense of "extraordinary alienation from earth". She thought that the desert was so hostile, arid, and rocky that she could understand why this was the scene of the revelation of the Law to Moses. The road leading up Mount Sinai looked golden and reminded her of the yellow brick road that Dorothy followed in *The Wizard of Oz*. She prayed as she climbed, though she ordinarily eschews ritual. She felt "wonderful" for days afterward. She told me of other hazardous trips she had taken and was surprised at "how intensely one can feel the quiet between episodes of danger". She had had moments of "spiritual exaltation". She was fascinated by men who had courageously faced danger and survived. Alongside this appreciation of physical courage, she was impressed by wisdom and yearned for ultimate understanding. When, in the course of her treatment, she met another man of heroic stature who was ready to start an affair with her, she saw that as more than a coincidence. She implied that she believed that it had been supernaturally determined.

> "I deeply believe in intelligences at work that go beyond what we can appreciate. It has given me the ability to bear my burdens."

This woman was able to achieve a mystical experience at the top of Mt. Sinai and the sense of a revelation after, and perhaps by means of, exposing herself to danger. She did not see an image of the Deity sitting on his throne at the top of the mountain, but I infer that she felt as though the sunrise that so impressed her symbolized that. In his discussion of the Schreber case, Freud (1911c) interprets the image of the sun as a father symbol. The awe that accompanied the mountain-top view, and the euphoria that followed it strongly suggest that the mystical experience consisted of a fantasy of visualization of or union with God, the all-powerful father figure. She deeply felt the profound relationship among danger, the illusion of rebirth that escape encourages, and the revelation that passes for wisdom. She obtained knowledge by contact with her heroic men, men larger than life. When I asked her what images of heroic stature had she encountered in childhood, she replied, "the large image of Christ on the large cross in church". Then she said that she had never really been impressed by Christ and all of his suffering, but by God the Father who is never graphically represented in church.

This woman is not a declared mystic, but she seeks exalting experiences in the form of revelations, both visual and cognitive, by exposing herself to danger and attaching herself to courageous men who themselves brave danger and acquire wisdom. Large religious images have impressed her, and the spiritual high point of her life was attained by the climb up Mount Sinai, to participate in the theophany that Moses had achieved. In the real world, her criteria for selecting a husband brought her men who were pathologically narcissistic and unable to give her the love that she craved and that could not be replaced by a revelation. And her continuing search for illusion left her real life, not unsuccessful, but to her, meaningless and unrewarding. (Her comments about Christ on the cross suggest the possibility that that is a striking example of the Deity in his throne chariot, but in this case a particularly hostile throne chariot that torments and kills its occupant.)

A note about heights: In the ancient world, the holy places were the heights. God or the gods were usually visualized as residing on the top of a holy mountain, such as Mt. Olympus, Mt. Sinai. This location reproduces the child's experience of the parent's face and arms as above him, and he longs to be lifted up by their arms. When the gods are not visualized on an accessible mountain, they are visualized in heaven. The *merkavah*, Ezekiel's chariot, is visualized in the heavens. At some point the gods are domesticated by being brought into a building, a temple, a hekhal. Often the two concepts are combined. The mystic ascends through the various heavens—usually seven—to the court in which the god is to be found. A similar combination occurs in the last dream reported: the dreamer ascends inside a building to the court at the top level. In general, in the early *merkavah* materials, ascent is emphasized. In the *hekhalot* materials, it is the chamber, the interior, that becomes salient.

My aim in presenting these dreams is to show that despite wide differences in material and social circumstances, the basic structure of the *merkavah* and *hekhalot* mystics is reproduced with amazing precision in the dreams and fantasies of moderns, whether Europeans or Americans. In both we find: a central authority, a parental figure, residing within a quadrangular chamber, a room or a space called a court or a garden; the figure is often seen on a chair, throne, or other seat; the subject strives to see him and approach him, not daring to hope to touch him; occasionally the genital is explicitly the object of interest; the subject encounters obstacles—whether inanimate barriers or hostile creatures—in his quest; occasionally the latter are controlled by benign friendly creatures; often crowds are encountered, angels in the mystical images and other humans in the dream; often vehicles convey the subject to his goal. The scholar of Jewish mysticism will search for the determinants of the details of these images in the natural environment and in the artefacts of the authors of the images. The psychoanalyst, acknowledging the relevance of these realia, will try to explain why these specific items were selected by referring to the universal unconscious fantasies of mankind, which are based upon childhood experience and fantasy.

The pattern is simple. The individual aspirant cultivates the illusion that he will approach or unite with a paternal figure who is ensconced in a maternal claustrum. The desired elevating experience may be limited to seeing God, or it may proceed to approaching Him. In *merkavah* mystical texts, we do not encounter any attempt to unite with or supplant Him. The retreat to mystical experience is usually precipitated by a stress, chronic or acute, and itself constitutes a regression. The mystic rejects, retreats from, or mentally destroys the real world and achieves rebirth by regressing to illusion, the illusion of revisiting an early, probably historical state, namely, participating in powerful intimacy with parents, such as being in bed with them.

The basic *merkavah* fantasy may be replaced by any of a number of variants. First, the most primitive variant suggested is the infant's wish to return to the safe, maternal claustrum.[5] That claustrum is symbolized by a container of whatever form.

As we observed above, one quality that occurs with surprising frequency is rectangularity, sometimes symbolized by the number four. Rectangularity and the number four are encountered in both the mystical texts and clinically encountered dreams. Since four also symbolizes the four basic directions of space, it can sometimes refer to the entire cosmos—the converse of the claustrum. The *merkavah* in Ezekiel is a four-sided structure incorporating four creatures, each of which has four faces and four wings. In the Daniel and Revelation apocalypses, different sets of four beasts or beings are described. The chamber and palace structures may be presumed to be quadrangular. The prophecies of both Isaiah and Ezekiel at other points refer to the four compass points.

---

[5] Lewin, in his classic paper, "The Body as Phallus" (1973), rings changes on this symbolic equation. He demonstrates its pregenital roots and an associated "post-phallic reorganization of the libidinal components". He also considers the possible combinations of respective owners of the body and the phallus.

I believe that the number four symbolizes the maternal claustrum. Rectangularity may symbolize either the claustrum itself or the vehicle that transports the dreamer to the claustrum. Jung (1958) discusses the quaternity at length—but as a Christian symbol. He sees it as a modification of the Trinity by the addition of a fourth element, which might be the female, the devil, or the unconscious. The quaternity, he says, "issues from" the *anima*, a feminine figure who becomes the *matrix* of the quaternity, or *Mater Dei.*

In a second variant of the fundamental pattern, access to the claustrum is impeded by obstacles or by dangerous creatures who serve as its guardians. Chasseguet-Smirgel, in an essay entitled "The Archaic Matrix of the Oedipus Complex" (1986), proposes that:

> There exists a primary desire to discover a universe without obstacles, without roughness or differences, entirely smooth, identified with the mother's belly stripped of its contents, an interior to which one has free access.

Following Melanie Klein, she interprets the obstacles usually encountered in the return trip to the maternal claustrum as the father's penis, other children, and the faeces in the mother's body. Although closed doors, snow, heights, and other barriers impede the traveller in some clinical instances, I find that in most fantasies and dreams it is hostile creatures that bar the way, fierce and frightening enemies, numbers of children, or unfriendly animals. Chasseguet-Smirgel proposes that the obstacles represent reality—the reality that dictates that, having left the maternal protective envelope, the child cannot possibly find its way back. In many instances, the individual is not only impeded, blocked, challenged, or threatened, but actually destroyed, as, for example, in the "Four Entered the Garden" text and in the second dream. Accordingly, we must emphasize not merely the impossibility of returning, but actually that the attempt to return is hazardous.

I infer the existence of an affect-regulating system that automatically acts to oppose an impulse of excessive strength, in fact, to activate an opposite tendency. Too strong a desire to move towards one goal, or too presumptuous a move, either in reality or fantasy, automatically elicits an equally vigorous tendency to move towards its opposite. One sees in many dreams a series of automatic, reciprocal, overcompensating corrections. In the second dream, we find one such overcompensating correction: the Promethean replacement of the father in the throne–chariot results in the dreamer's literal downfall.

That the maternal, uterine claustrum is imagined to be the site within which rivals were encountered in the past was established by Arlow (1960, 1972). In accordance with this fantasy, some of his patients presented clinically with claustrophobic or claustrophilic symptoms.

Both texts and dreams speak of the creatures that either facilitate or oppose the mystical quest. They may be adults, children, animals, or angels, sometimes chimeras—friendly or unfriendly—such as the chimeras of Ezekiel's chariot. The images might arise from a fragmentation and distortion of actual parental or sibling images, such as are encountered in delirium. In chapter two, I observed that perception is basically modular. Whole percepts consist of a construction of elementary components. However, in pathology or other unusual circumstances the integration may go awry so that unreasonable connections are made or unrealistic composites imagined. These creatures may also represent the earliest form of society into which the child must enter in latency as he prepares to leave his parents. This feature of the *merkavah* fantasy permits the expression of either mystical identification or rivalry with siblings.

The third major variant that we must consider is the aspiration to encounter the father within the maternal claustrum. In the *merkavah* and *hekhaloth* texts, the maternal claustrum is symbolized by the throne on which he sits, or the *hekhal* or chamber in which he is found. In *Hekhaloth Rabbati* (3:2), the throne bows to God and begs Him to be seated on it, reassuring Him that He does not rest too heavily upon it (her). At another point (24:1), the throne joins in singing hymns to God. Gershom Scholem (1962) quotes a parable from the book *Bahir*, a very early Kabbalistic text:

> He said: the thing is like a king who had a throne. Sometimes he took it in his arms, sometimes he put it on his head. They asked him: why? Because it was beautiful and it saddened him to sit upon it. They asked him: and where does he put it on his head? He said: in the open letter *mem*, as it is written:

> [Ps. 85:12] "Truth springs up from the earth; justice looks down from heaven." The open *mem* is . . . a symbol of the feminine. [p. 60]

A child of eight reported the following dream:

> *"I saw a crocodile or alligator, and I was in a small sort of cabin. The crocodile stuck his head between the bars, and that looked funny. And the crocodile kept on moving from side to side, and I kept on jumping from side to side too. And finally he got me. And instead of biting a chunk out of me, a sort of tooth stuck in me. And I tried to pull it out, and I did not succeed. Then we went to supper,* and then I woke up."

The child has taken refuge in the maternal claustrum, but she is still not safe from the father's aggressive intrusion (though the outcome is not altogether unhappy).

Encountering father within the maternal claustrum may represent either of two organizing fantasies—namely, being confronted with a primal scene or wishing to be loved by both without the stress of rivalry, as the child feels when he is in bed between both parents.

One may approach the royal father out of love and a yearning to be transformed, invigorated, reborn by the approach or contact with him. On the other hand, one may approach him in an arrogant, defiant way, with the Promethean intention of looking at what one should not look at, or deposing and superseding him (cf. Freud's "Count Thun" dream). In the latter case, the danger of destruction lends itself to interpretation as punishment. The oedipal fantasy in this context may be considered a variant of the Promethean. It is to signal (and effect) deference in the approach that the *hekhaloth* texts prescribe hymns and liturgies idealizing the deity and effacing the self.

We must take note of the fact that in almost all *merkavah*- and *hekhaloth*-type dreams the dreamer encounters resistance to his quest. He fails to arrive at his destination. Or his path is obstructed. Or he encounters hazards such as unstable bridges, rivers difficult to cross, insecure high places. Or hostile forces attack him or bar the way. Or he encounters dangerous animals. Or the claustrum itself ejects him. As an adult, the eight-year-old child reported also the following dream:

> *"I was in the desert. It was strange. There was a whirlwind around a hole in the desert, an oasis, a sinkhole, or a pit in the sand or quicksand. I looked at it. There were animals around it, desert animals, strange and interesting. A woman had painted a picture of it. She said, 'It's a real scene.' She was an older woman. The animals weren't real. They looked rather like animal-like jewellery."*

In the childhood dream, the crocodile threatened her and bit her. In this dream, the oasis was simultaneously a quicksand and was surrounded by "desert animals". She was threatened with being consumed by the mother, whom she rejoined. As I observed above, in the *hekhaloth* texts themselves, the individual who ascends encounters murderous guards, gatekeepers, and angels who behave more like demons than angels. In fact, the prototypic *merkavah* vision of Ezekiel starts with a dangerous windstorm, as does this dream.

I find it of some interest that each of the dangers appears also in classic phobias—that is, fears of travelling, of high places, of bridges, of water, of animals, of closed spaces, of open spaces. That fact encourages the speculation that classic phobias represent one aspect of a prevailing use of a *merkavah* or *hekhaloth* fantasy as a means of resolving anxiety. The patients whose dreams I have reported, and others who present similar dreams, do not present primarily as phobics. Usually their complaints indicate some disorder of affect regulation. But almost all acknowledge some phobic concerns.

Why does danger inhere in these dreams and fantasies? One might propose an oedipal explanation, or an appeal to the Promethean paradigm, which would require punishment for presumption. It is also possible that the anxiety that appears in these experiences is merely the same anxiety that the dreamer is trying to escape by seeking out the safety and gratification of the claustrum, and that now pursues him. It is this anxiety that denies him the comfort and refuge that he seeks.

The singing, and especially the unison singing attributed to the angelic hosts, emphasizes the mutual bonding function of singing for mother and infant.

The declared purpose of the apocalypse is to reveal a secret, to convey some unknown but magically portentous and potent information. In some of the clinical material (for example, the third dream) and the mystical texts, meaningful revelations play an important role. The purpose of the ascent is to see God, the ultimate mystery. To make one's way there one must know the proper hymns and incantations. The concluding section of the *Hekhaloth Rabbati*, known as the Sar-Torah section, starting with chapter 27, guarantees the practitioner the capacity to master sacred learning. Secrecy, esotericism, is used in opposite ways in religious material we are considering. It is a guarantee of potency and relevance in the prophetic and *hekhaloth* texts, but it is used to restrict transmission and diffusion in the Talmudic texts. In Kabbalistic circles, we encounter controversies between those encouraging popular diffusion and those demanding esotericism.

If my thesis that *merkavah* mysticism is based upon an organizing fantasy that prevails broadly in the population is valid, then we must seriously consider the likelihood that all mystical systems are similarly based upon widely prevailing organizing fantasies. That inference remains to be validated.

We must also consider the resemblance between the circumstances of psychoanalytic therapy and the fantasies of *merkavah* mysticism. In the therapeutic chamber, there is a charismatic authority figure, enthroned within a protective claustrum. I remember an incident that occurred during the student riots of 1968. A patient who was a faculty member of a local university came to my office for his session after a particularly difficult day, lay down on the couch, and said, "It's nice to get back to the ivory tower". Negative affects are generated either by excessive frustration of this attachment—as, for example, by the therapist's vacation—or by excessive gratification, which leads to corrective fears. Uncovering secrets relating to the patient's past or to his fate, as well as to the private life of the analyst, is a major quest of the patient. Under such circumstances, the therapy or analysis becomes protective and gratifying by virtue of the experience itself, above and beyond the validity of the interpretations.

Individuals for whom the *merkavah* fantasy plays an organizing role are inclined to form strong idealizing attachments and to react against them equally strongly. Sometimes one, sometimes the other sentiment prevails, and sometimes they alternate.

Summary

Merkavah mysticism refers to a mystical system that prevailed in the Jewish community for about a thousand years, basing itself upon the chariot and throne visions of the prophets and finding expression subsequently in apocalyptic texts, rabbinic discussions, and *hekhaloth* incantations, prayers, and hymns.

The basic fantasy is that of an aspirant hoping to enter into a claustrum to achieve sight of and physical closeness to a male deity seated within it. Vehicles play a part in the movement towards the desired goal, as well as in the image of the claustrum itself.

Similar images—archetypes perhaps—are encountered in the illusions of the delirious, in the hallucinations of the psychotic, and in the dreams of the normal. We infer that a commonly encountered archaic and unconscious organizing psychodynamic fantasy determines the basic patterns of the formulations of *merkavah* mysticism.

In the underlying wish fantasy, the individual seeks to repeat childhood experience or fantasies of participating in parental intimacy.

Individuals who favour this fantasy often describe phobic aversions and tend to form idealizing attachments and ambivalently to rebel against them.

The psychotherapeutic and analytic situation can be seen by such patients as a gratification of the archetypal wish of the *merkavah* mystical aspiration.

Are all mystical systems based upon widely prevailing, unconscious organizing fantasies?

METHODOLOGY

CHAPTER SIX

Methodological reflections on psychoanalysis and Judaic studies: a response to Mortimer Ostow

David J. Halperin

While doing research at the Hebrew University in Jerusalem in the summer of 1989, I had lunch one day with a distinguished Bible scholar whom I had known for some fifteen years. He asked me what I was working on. I told him I was engaged in a study of the prophet Ezekiel from a psychoanalytic perspective. I sketched for him some of the perspectives on Ezekiel that were emerging from this study (which was published some four years later [Halperin, 1993]). As I spoke, I noticed his eyes begin to glaze over. When I finished, he changed the subject. He obviously found what I said unconvincing and perhaps also uninteresting; yet he offered no criticism whatsoever.

I understood the man's response. He did not mean to disparage what I was doing, and certainly not to express personal disrespect for me. But I was advancing proposals for understanding the Bible that were so alien to his universe of discourse that he had no way to respond. Modern critical Bible scholarship, to which he owed his allegiance, simply does not allow certain questions on its agenda; and there is no way to respond when someone decides to raise them, except to say that they are the wrong questions. To quote the pronouncement of one modern Biblicist: ". . . we must prescind from psychology at the distance of millennia" (Heider, 1985, p. 407).

The reaction has a certain legitimacy. The common project of scholarship, like our individual projects, is unlikely to progress unless scholars are prepared to focus their energies upon an agreed-upon set of issues and leave others outside their purview. Yet it can also be tragically limiting.

It is reasonable to insist that a text, ancient or modern, is not a transparent window into the soul of another human being, but a literary creation that is apt to follow quite non-psychological laws of its own. It is reasonable, too, that we recall that "the past is a different country, they do things differently there",[1] and that an ancient prophet or mystic is apt to have been very different from a twentieth-century analysand. And yet books do not come into being by spontaneous generation. They are written by members of the species *Homo sapiens*, who may be assumed a priori to have certain fundamental identities—constituting the now unfashionable term "human nature"—with other members of the species. To refuse to ask psychological, or even psychoanalytic, questions of these texts is to limit our ability to answer those questions that the historians and textual scholars are willing to declare legitimate. It also has the graver effect of silencing the ancients: of refusing the vital testimony they can give on the great questions of who we humans are, why we act as we do, and how we may wisely direct our short and often painful lives.

* * *

It is a great pity, in my judgement, that most professional historians and textual scholars in the field of Judaica are likely to respond to Mortimer Ostow's thoughtful and stimulating papers very much as my Biblicist friend did to my ideas: with a polite and embarrassed silence, and with some relief if the subject can be changed. It will be a great achievement if psychoanalytic thinkers and Judaica scholars, working together with good will and willingness to hear one another, can bridge the gap that must provoke such a response.

---

[1]This is my recollection of the opening lines of the 1971 film *The Go-Between*.

Let us consider how a more-or-less conventional Judaica scholar—whom we shall assume to be a woman—might respond to Ostow's chapter on the Four who entered the garden.

She will begin by noting that Ostow, although plainly aware of a wide range of rabbinic sources concerning the four ancient rabbis of whom his paper treats, seems to take no interest in what these sources are, when they were written, or how they relate to each other and to the historical individuals they purport to describe. This apparent lack of interest will certainly distress her—so keenly, perhaps, that she will stop reading his paper near the beginning.

For questions of this sort are the very essence of her scholarship. She is acutely aware that we have no Jewish texts of the period of the Mishnah and Talmud that even purport to be written by any of the creative figures of this period. What we have is anonymous compilations, usually very difficult to date, which contain a myriad of individual utterances normally *attributed* to one rabbi or another; plus a number of stories (normally themselves anonymous) about these rabbis. No generally accepted method exists for determining the truthfulness of these stories (which are often filled with fanciful details), or the accuracy of the attribution of such-and-such an utterance to Rabbi X (especially since a parallel text may very well attribute the same utterance to Rabbi Y or Rabbi Z, or perhaps vary the wording of the utterance in some crucial way). Our only access to the public and private agendas of the rabbis themselves is via an uncertain number of anonymous authors and compilers, who unquestionably had public and private agendas of their own.

Let me repeat: there is no acknowledged method for making this transition. The approach that may strike the reader as obvious—why don't we compile all the utterances attributed in the rabbinic literature to Rabbi X and let a portrait emerge that differentiates him from the other rabbis?—has so far produced results so unimpressive as to call into question the legitimacy of the approach. A non-specialist writer, therefore, cannot appeal to any consensus of specialists on the biography of this or that rabbi, since no consensus on legitimate method, far less legitimate results, has yet appeared.

What, for example, do we know of Elisha ben Avuya, the heretic and apostate among the Four? We have the *baraita* itself of the Four who entered the garden, quoted with variations in a number of later sources. (A "*baraita*" is an utterance or story attributed to the earliest stratum of rabbinic literature, called the *Tannaitic*, whose last spokesmen lived early in the third century AD) Two of these sources, the *Palestinian* and *Babylonian Talmuds*, attach to this *baraita* a dossier of colourful stories about Elisha (PT Hagigah 2:1, 77b–c; BT Hagigah 15a–b), plus a few seemingly isolated comments whose original context is unclear.

Some of our most important bits of data, or pseudo-data, derive from these remarks. *What was Aher's* [= Elisha's] *case?* asks the *Babylonian Talmud* at one point. And it goes on to reply: *Greek song poured ceaselessly from his mouth. They* [= who?] *said of Aher that whenever he stood up in the study house, many heretical books fell from his lap.* The question is couched in the phraseology we associate with the editorial layers of the *Babylonian Talmud*, which was compiled in the sixth century AD The first sentence of the answer is in Aramaic, the second in Hebrew. No name is attached to either part of the answer, nor is it clear how the two parts relate to one another. Did one or both of them exist, in oral or written form, prior to the formation of the context in which they now appear? Or were they fabricated by some editor of the Talmud, perhaps four hundred years after Elisha ben Avuya's death? There seems no way to answer this question.

A few utterances outside these Talmudic passages are attributed to Elisha. A passage preserved in the central Tannaitic text, the Mishnah, represents him as comparing one who learns as a child to *ink written on new paper*, while one who learns as an old man is like *ink written on paper that has been blotted out* (Avot 4:20; tr. Goldin, 1955). A text of uncertain date, *The Fathers According to Rabbi Nathan*, quotes a series of sayings in which Elisha praises the combination of study and good deeds but deplores the ill effects of study unmixed with good deeds. For example: *one in whom there are no good works, though he has studied much Torah, to what may he be likened? To a horse that has no bridle: when one mounts it, it throws him off headlong* (chapter 24; tr. Goldin, 1955). How appropriate for a learned heretic! we think; and are therefore disposed to treat the attribution as authentic. But wait a moment: perhaps the same thought had occurred to the compiler of *The Fathers According to Rabbi Nathan*, who therefore decided to attach Elisha's name to what had been a string of anonymous proverbs? The problem of the relation between the literary image of an individual and the *utterances* that are attributed to that individual is a very difficult one. It is possible, of course, that their nexus lies in the historical reality of that individual; but we cannot simply assume this to be true. There are other options.

Let us turn back to the Talmudic stories about Elisha, on which our image of the man is largely based. As I have indicated, there are two collections of these stories: one in the *Palestinian Talmud*, one in the *Babylonian*. The two collections are plainly related and share many of their materials—with, however, very significant differences. Certain regular features mark the Babylonian version over against the Palestinian. The Babylonian version, for example, consistently calls Elisha by the strange name Aher, "the other one", whose precise meaning continues to baffle scholars. (The *Babylonian Talmud* provides a fanciful tale to explain how he came by that name.) Elisha is called Aher also in most versions of the *baraita*, including the one quoted in the *Palestinian Talmud*. Yet, with the exception of one passage, the Palestinian version avoids this name, choosing instead to speak of "Elisha" or "Elisha ben Avuya".

There is a more significant distinction between the two versions, from the perspective of Elisha's relation—and, indeed, the relation of all of the Four—to *merkavah* mysticism. The Babylonian version proceeds from the assumption that Elisha has travelled to heaven, where he beholds the angel Metatron and mistakes him for a second deity. Surely, we might think, this is a key to understanding the heresy of the historical Elisha: in the course of a mystical experience, apparently, he became a (Gnostic?) dualist. But we must reckon also with the *Palestinian* materials. This version of the Elisha stories, which may well be the older, is innocent of any belief in either his dualism or his heavenly journey (Halperin, 1980)! This will perhaps suggest that dualism and heavenly ascensions are indeed important in understanding one branch of the Elisha traditions—*but not in understanding the historical Elisha.* Their historical context may not be the second-century Palestine where Elisha ben Avuya lived, but the sixth-century Babylonia where the Talmud was edited.

The effect of all this is plain enough. The more closely we examine the stories of Elisha ben Avuya, the more the figure of Elisha himself retreats into obscurity. We cannot doubt that the man existed, or that there was something unconventional about his beliefs and scandalous about his behaviour that made him an appropriate figure around which Talmudic storytellers could construct their fascinating image of a faithless "anti-rabbi".[2] But, as historians and philologists, we find ourselves without the tools we need to retrieve the man himself from the web of fictions that later generations spun about him.

The Judaica scholar we have imagined, with her orientation towards history and philology, is painfully aware of all this. She knows that similar problems stand in the way of her approach to Elisha's three companions. They are not quite the same as the problems I have described in connection with Elisha—there is no shortage of Talmudic data relating to the famous Akiva, for example, but rather a huge mass of material that does not well lend itself to being shaped into a coherent human personality—but they are not a great deal more tractable. The roads leading back to the mysterious garden, and to the four rabbis who are said to have entered it, will seem to her blocked by every kind of obstacle. She does not despair of the possibility of removing these obstacles. But she will expect to see them removed, by the

[2] Both the Palestinian and Babylonian versions of the Elisha stories, it seems to me, have as their true protagonist—not Elisha himself, nor his orthodox pupil Rabbi Meir—but, rather, the *Elisha–Meir pair.* The two men, who are inseparable through these stories, are best understood as representing two opposed aspects of the rabbinic personality: the conventionally pious (Meir) on the one side, the questioning and heretical (Elisha) on the other. This reading of the stories—which I intend to develop in greater detail in a separate study—does nothing to bring us closer to the historical Elisha. On the contrary, it increases our distance, in that it implies that our main sources of information about Elisha are the fictions of anonymous but extremely gifted and creative storytellers with an overriding agenda of their own. These fictions may give us profound insight into the ambivalent presence of faith and faithlessness in the soul of rabbinic Judaism and yet tell us little or nothing about the real Elisha ben Avuya.

familiar historical and philological tools of her craft, before she will trust anyone who claims to tell her what the garden was, how the Four responded to it, and what we can learn from their responses.

This is why she is likely to respond to Ostow's paper with some perplexity and frustration. It will not be easy for her to criticize it in any detail, for its agenda of questions and modes of response are vastly different from hers. Her overall comment, however, is likely to be that Ostow puts the cart before the horse. She may grant that it is possible to make psychological statements about people of the remote past, on the basis of analogy with modern clinical evidence. (Some Biblicists, as I observed near the beginning of this chapter, regard the contrary position as axiomatic.) But surely the historical and philological work has to be done first; surely psychological statements only have a chance of being correct if we have some prior mode of gaining information about the people of whom they are made. Let Ostow first grapple with the sources, she will say. Let him first establish solid biographical information about the Four. Only then can he proceed to the next level and add the prefix that turns biography into psychobiography.

* * *

There, however, is the rub.

If there is anything that has emerged clearly from over a century of scholarly fascination with the story of the Four (see Liebes, 1990, and Bregman's scholarly commentary in Schwartz & Bregman, 1995), it is that our standard historical and philological modes of investigation are more or less helpless before it. The overwhelming nature of the methodological difficulties, as I have sketched them, do perhaps suggest that Ostow has underestimated his task. But they also suggest that the more conventional methods of approach, which are his competitors, may be inadequate to that task; and that perhaps he has begun the work of finding a new and more effective method.

Ostow may perhaps be unconscious of the historical assumptions he is obliged to make in his analysis, and this may indeed constitute a flaw in his work. But I think that perhaps our imagined Judaica specialist suffers from a corresponding unconsciousness relating to the psychological assumptions she makes in her own analyses. For—*pace* the Biblicist I quoted near the beginning of this essay—historical and philological investigations cannot possibly "prescind from psychology".

If we are obliged, for example, to choose between several competing versions of an incident, we find ourselves asking which version is the most plausible, in terms of what we know—or, rather, what we assume—about the ways human beings may be expected to behave. In deciding whether to discard some detail as inauthentic, we ask, *Did anyone have a motive to invent it?* If we can conceive such a motive, we will feel ourselves able to explain and thus to dismiss the detail. If, on the contrary, we can imagine no such motive, we will be apt to accept the detail's veracity. How can we decide what an acceptable motive might be, unless we have some model of human psychology on which to base our decision? Even the text-critical work that is so basic to rabbinic scholarship involves questions of motive. (Is it easier to imagine a scribe replacing Reading A with Reading B, or the other way round?) It therefore rests ultimately on psychological presuppositions.

It follows that our Judaica scholar needs a psychological model of some sort to guide her at nearly every step she takes, along every path that might lead back to the historical Elisha ben Avuya. For this purpose she will probably use an everyday common-sense psychology, a psychology of ordinary consciousness. *But it is precisely Ostow's point that this model is inadequate for the purpose.* This is why he cannot satisfy her challenge that he first recover reliable biographical details about the Four who entered the garden, and only then apply to them his own psychology—the psychology of the unconscious. It is as if she were to say to him, *"You must first solve the textual and historical problems of the sources on the basis of the psychological model I am prepared to use; only then are you permitted to approach them on the basis of the model you prefer to use"*. He must, in other words, succeed in solving the riddle in accord with her rules before he can begin to solve it in accord with his own. Put this way, the demand cannot be met. Ostow's not having met it cannot be used as grounds to discredit his work.

Seen in this light, Ostow is justified in having side-stepped—for the time being—the historical, text-critical, and literary-critical problems involved in the story of the Four. These problems must be tackled eventually, but at a later stage. Ostow's contribution is more fundamental. He has applied his rich theoretical knowledge and practical experience of psychoanalysis to the construction of a fresh perspective on what is plausible, what motives are reasonable and expectable, when we are considering the lives and creations of the ancient rabbis.

This perspective necessarily has a provisional, "as if" quality about it. We have not, after all, yet established the relevant historical details on any firm basis. But, granting this, we are equipped with a new set of (provisional) criteria that we can use when we turn to the literary sources from which we must educe these details. We can use these (provisional) criteria as we reason out the sources' relationship to one another, and to the human beings who were their authors and subjects.

Our hypothetical Judaica scholar's idea of what constitutes proper method is, thereby, in a sense, turned on its head. She believes that we must first elicit reliable facts from the extant sources, on the basis of standard historical and philological criteria, before we can consider them in the light of psychoanalytic awareness. We now find ourselves contemplating a procedure that seems to be the reverse. First we apply (as Ostow has done) psychoanalytic awareness to a provisional set of "facts", the reliability of which we have not yet been able to secure. We then undertake a fresh approach to the sources, weighing their relation to one another and to historical reality on the basis of criteria that have emerged from our provisional exercise in psychohistory. Now, perhaps, the sources will more readily yield their secrets; and the paths that lead from them to the realities that shaped them will open up for us. If this happens, the quotation marks that currently enclose our "facts" will fade away. The result will be an appreciation, both historical and psychoanalytic, of the Four who entered the garden; and this appreciation will have a reasonable chance of representing the historical and psychological truth.

By taking this approach, we do not in reality discard the standard historical method. Nor do we discount the objections that must be made to Ostow's work from the standpoint of that method. We seek, instead, to incorporate and transcend them. We do not aim for a linear, step-by-step progression, in which we move first from text to history, then from history to psychology.

We are prepared, instead, to oscillate between psychological and historical–philological perspectives, continually using each of these modes of reasoning to check the other. We begin with the "facts" of our inquiry very much in quotation marks. But, as we work back and forth from "facts" to textual sources to "facts", these quotation marks gradually disappear.

* * *

I shall follow up these general remarks with a specific example of how a problem raised by the historical–philological investigation of ancient Jewish texts, and normally discussed only by the standard canons of this investigation, may be solved if we take Ostow's insights as the starting-point of our approach.

A very early Jewish apocalypse (late third or early second-century BC?), the "Book of Watchers" that constitutes chapters 1–36 of the *Ethiopic Book of Enoch*, includes the following account of a heavenly ascent. The antediluvian patriarch Enoch is the speaker.

> And behold I saw the clouds: And they were calling me in a vision; and the fogs were calling me; and the course of the stars and the lightnings were rushing me and . . . the winds were causing me to fly and rushing me high up into heaven. And I . . . approached a wall which was built of white marble and surrounded by tongues of fire; and it began to frighten me. And I came into the tongues of the fire and drew near to a great house which was built of white marble . . . the floor of crystal, the ceiling like the path of the stars and lightnings between which (stood) fiery cherubim and their heaven of water; and flaming fire surrounded the wall(s), and its gates were burning with fire. And I entered into the house, which was hot like fire and cold like ice, and there was nothing inside it [an important textual variant has here, "there was no pleasure of life in it"]; (so) fear covered me and trembling seized me. . . . And behold there was an opening before me (and) a second house which is greater than the former and everything was built with tongues of fire. . . . And I observed and saw inside it a lofty throne—its appearance was like crystal and its wheels like the shining sun . . . and from beneath the throne were issuing streams of flaming fire. It was difficult to look at it. And the Great Glory was sitting

> upon it—as for his gown, which was shining more brightly than the sun, it was whiter than any snow. None of the angels was able to come in and see the face of the Excellent and Glorious One; and no one of the flesh can see him—the flaming fire was round about him, and a great fire stood before him. No one could come near unto him from among those that surrounded the tens of millions (that stood) before him. He needed no council, but the most holy ones who are near to him neither go far away at night nor move away from him. Until then I was prostrate on my face covered and trembling. And the Lord called me with his own mouth and said to me, "Come near to me, Enoch, and to my holy Word." And he lifted me up and brought me near to the gate, but I (continued) to look down with my face. [1 Enoch, chapter 14; translated by E. Isaac, in Charlesworth, 1983, pp. 20–21]

This passage is not among the texts that Ostow discusses in chapter five. But it seems reasonable to suppose that he would see, in Enoch's entry into a house and then into a second house within, a clear allusion to a fantasy of return to the maternal claustrum. That the claustrum is so monstrously unpleasant—"hot like fire and cold like ice", "no pleasure of life in it"—may be explained by Ostow's postulate of "an affect-regulating system that automatically acts to oppose an impulse of excessive strength, in fact, to activate an opposite tendency. Too strong a desire to move towards one goal, or too presumptuous a move, either in reality or fantasy, automatically elicits an equally vigorous tendency to move towards its opposite" (pp. 175–176). Enoch is indeed able to enter the longed-for claustrum. But, when he does, he finds it almost unendurable.

Judaica scholars who discuss this passage (e.g. Rowland, 1982, pp. 219–222; Halperin, 1988, pp. 79–85; Himmelfarb, 1993, pp. 13–23) must account for the same features that confront the psychoanalytic investigator. But the paths they take to find an explanation, and the sort of explanation they find compelling, are radically different. They will not look to perennial features of the human psyche, but to the immediate social and political context of the author of the "Book of Watchers"; and to the literary sources—most obviously, the Hebrew Scriptures—that he presumably had before him.

The feature of Enoch's house-within-a-house that will most strike them, for example, will be its obvious resemblance to the Jerusalem Temple. (The latter was divided into an outer Holy Place and a Holy of Holies.) Correlating this with other priestly elements of Enoch's heaven, they will suppose that the writer has created his image of heaven by projecting the Temple into the skies. They may interpret his doing so in the light of David Suter's suggestion (1979) that the fallen angels of the "Book of Watchers" are representations of the contemporary Jerusalem priesthood, which the author perceived as debased and corrupt. To the historian, all of this will sound far more concrete, far more relevant to normal historical concerns, than any talk about a maternal claustrum.

The fantastic details of the heavenly structure—its impossible mixture of fire and ice, for example—also demand explanation. Here the Judaica scholar's instinct is to turn to the Hebrew Bible and to look there for passages describing God and His surroundings, which the Enochian writer may be assumed to have creatively synthesized. One obvious source will be the *merkavah* vision of Ezek. 1, which Ostow has discussed in his chapter. But there are others. I have argued, for example, that the theme of mixed fire and ice is based ultimately on Ps. 104:1–4, which the writer has elaborated in accord with a midrashic process attested also in rabbinic literature (Halperin, 1988, pp. 82–84). We take the author's veneration of the older Scriptures entirely for granted and suppose that this postulate can be used to provide a convincing explanation of the thought processes that resulted in his own creations.

Moreover, the vision of God in Dan. 7:9–10 is so strongly reminiscent of the Enochian account that we can hardly doubt some direct link between the two.

> As I looked, thrones were placed and one that was ancient of days took his seat; his raiment was white as snow, and the hair of his head like pure wool; his throne was fiery flames, its wheels were burning fire. A stream of fire issued and came forth from before him; a thousand thousands served him, and ten thousand times ten thousand stood before him; a court sat in judgment, and books were opened. [RSV]

Our first thought might be to suppose that this is another of the Biblical passages upon which the Enochian author has drawn. But here problems begin to arise. Historical allusions in Dan. 7 permit us to date it, with some confidence, to the years 167–164 BC. Fragments of the "Book of Watchers" found in the Dead Sea caves seem (from the style of handwriting) to date from the middle or early years of the second century BC; and the date of these manuscripts is necessarily the latest possible date for the book's authorship. (It might, of course, be decades or centuries older.) When we add to this that the "Book of Watchers" seems to have developed in stages into its present form, and that the vision quoted above does not appear to belong to the last of these stages, it is difficult to avoid the conclusion that the vision in the "Book of Watchers" was, in fact, written *before* Daniel's. The apparent links between Dan. 7 and 1 Enoch 14 require some other explanation.

Shall we simply reverse the dependent relationship and suppose that Dan. 7 drew upon 1 Enoch 14 (Rowland, 1982, pp. 255–258)? Or shall we look (as I prefer) to shared exegetical traditions based on the older Scriptures? The influence of Ezekiel's *merkavah*, on both writers' description of the divine throne, is clear. Both, I have suggested (Halperin, 1988, p. 83), draw the detail of God's snowy white garment from Ps. 104:2. But what of the most striking parallel, the stream or streams of fire that issue from beneath God's fiery throne? There is no clear Biblical source for this detail; and to say that Enoch borrowed it from Daniel or vice versa does little to clear up the problem of its origin.

The fiery streams, says Martha Himmelfarb,

> . . . have their origins in the ancient traditions of the divine council. The mountain of El at which the council meets in Ugaritic literature has two rivers at its base. The rivers of Canaanite myth are not fiery, but Israelite (and Canaanite) traditions of fiery theophanies could easily suggest fiery rivers. Like other features of the Canaanite traditions of the abode of the gods, the rivers at the base of the cosmic mountain have been transferred in biblical literature to the temple mount, as in the concluding vision of the Book of Ezekiel (47:1–12). [1993, p. 17]

This explanation, whatever its merits, does practically nothing to explain the most remarkable detail of the rivers: that they are fiery. In my own discussion of the problem, I (like

Himmelfarb) called attention to Ezek. 47:1–12; and, like her, I glided over the issue of the rivers' fiery character. "As for the river of fire", I wrote, "if it is a celestial projection of the river that flows from the restored Temple in Ezek. 47:1–12 (as seems likely), we must assume that the shared tradition [shared, that is, by Dan. 7 and 1 Enoch 14] already had some orientation toward the Temple" (Halperin, 1988, p. 82).

Christopher Rowland (1982) has grappled with the problem more directly than either Himmelfarb or myself.

> The origin of this [fiery river] imagery is not easily explained, though a verse like Ezek. 1.13 (". . . out of the fire went forth lightning") could easily have provided the basis for this development within the throne–chariot vision itself. Also the description of the theophany at Sinai in Exod. 19.16 provided material which could form the basis of the belief in the fiery elements which proceeded from God's immediate presence. Indeed, in Revelation 4.5 an allusion to Exodus 19.16 replaces the reference to the fiery stream. [p. 221]

A few pages later, Rowland takes up again the question of how the theme manifests itself in the Book of Revelation.

> . . . there is a clear indication that John [the author of Revelation] does know of the fiery stream, as we find in Revelation 22.1 a reference to "a river of living water as clear as crystal" coming out of God's throne. Despite the pastoral setting, and whatever the influence of passages like Ezek. 47.1 and Zech. 14.8, the river is to be connected with the fiery stream because of the close link that exists between it and the throne of God. What has happened here is that the threatening aspect, which the fiery stream presents to those who enter the divine presence (Rev. 15.2ff.), has been replaced with the life-giving water which flows through the new Jerusalem and renews the inheritors of the new age. The barrier which had hitherto existed between God and man has now been removed (Rev. 21.3), and so it is entirely appropriate that all that might appear to separate man from God should be removed. [Rowland, 1982, p. 224]

I have quoted these scholars (including myself) at some length, inasmuch as they set forth the best explanations that conventional historical–philological methods have so far been able to give for the fiery rivers of Daniel and Enoch. These explanations are remarkably hesitant and unpersuasive. It follows that the methods that produced them are significantly limited. We must ask again whether Ostow's insights about the maternal claustrum in apocalyptic visions, when combined with the more traditional methods, may not get us farther.

It seems clear to me (Rowland to the contrary) that Revelation's description of "the river of the water of life" flowing from the throne of God (Rev. 22:1–2) is based primarily on Ezek. 47:1–12, perhaps with some influence of midrashic traditions concerning the latter passage (e.g. Tosefta Sukkah 3:3–10). The detail of the trees on the river's banks, with their monthly yield of fruit and their healing leaves (Ezek. 47:12, Rev. 22:2), seems to me to guarantee this. Revelation's claim, that the river flows "from the throne of God and of the Lamb", will then make explicit what is implicit in Ezek. 47:1, where the river flows from the inside of the Temple.

This observation encourages me to stand by the view I earlier expressed, which I share with Himmelfarb. The life-giving river of Ezek. 47:1–12 was the inspiration for all three apocalyptic writers we have considered: the authors of 1 Enoch 14, Dan. 7, and Rev. 22. The author of Revelation left the river more or less as Ezekiel had described it. The other two writers—or a tradition followed by both—transformed it into fire. Why?

In my most recent study of Ezekiel (Halperin, 1993, pp. 211, 228), I proposed that the restored Temple functioned for Ezekiel as an unconscious representation of the good, chaste, nurturant mother for whom he longed. This is why her eastern gate is forever sealed, to be entered only by Yahweh (her proper husband) and by the "prince" (the foetus, Ezekiel's self-representation), who is to be nourished within it (Ezek. 44:1–3). This "gate", the entrance to the nurturing and protective womb, appears in Ezek. 47:1–12 as the source of the nurturing and healing river. We may take it that the river functions for Ezekiel as a parallel representation of the good mother: vast and engulfing (Ezek. 47:5), yet nevertheless benevolent and life-giving (Ezek. 47:9).

This is the latent content of Ezekiel's fantasy of the river of life. All three apocalyptic writers were certainly familiar with the vision's manifest content. We may suppose that they were unconsciously aware of its latent content as well (cf. Halperin, 1995). The author of Revelation was comfortable with this latent content and therefore left the river as Ezekiel had described it.

The Enochian writer and the author of Daniel were not comfortable with it. The underlying fantasy, of reincorporation in the mother, was too powerful and dangerous. The authors had come, perhaps, to believe that techniques existed by which they might undertake an ecstatic journey to heaven. Their yearning to return to the maternal womb—with its overtones of the incestuous and the tabooed—thus ceased to be a deliciously remote fantasy and became a tangible and frightening possibility. They consequently inhibited their own quest and repressed their own secret desires, by transforming a welcoming fantasy of infantile delight into a forbidding image of terror. Ezekiel's river thus changed from water to fire, from pleasure to agony.[3]

The reader will observe that this process is nearly the reverse of the process postulated by Rowland, in explaining how the fiery river of Daniel and Enoch was transformed into the watery river of Revelation. His explanation, resting as it did on conventional theological postulates, was able to explain transformation from fire into water, but not the reverse. Rowland was therefore obliged to disregard what seems the most reasonable reconstruction of the relationship among the several sources. If we are to preserve this relationship and still explain the river(s) of fire, we must seek a framework that will enable us to explain a transformation from water to fire. The psychoanalytic postulates set forth by Ostow will provide this framework.

* * *

Let us recapitulate. The parallel apocalyptic visions in Dan. 7 and 1 Enoch 14 provide at least one detail that resists explanation by the conventional explanatory modes (such as historical

---

[3]The *Babylonian Talmud*, Hagigah 13b, explains that Daniel's fiery river originates "from the sweat of the *hayyot* [the living creatures of Ezekiel 1, who carry the divine throne], and . . . is poured out . . . upon the heads of the sinners in Gehenna." Cf. Revelation's negative counterpart to the river of life, the "lake that burns with fire and brimstone, which is the second death", and in which sinners are tormented (Rev. 20:10, 15, 21:8).

context and literary influence) available to the historically and philologically trained scholar of Judaica. The most adequate solution to the problem—*that the transformation of a welcoming and life-giving river into a forbidding and destructive river was the outcome of an unconscious reaction against the latent content of the original fantasy*—can be stated only in psychoanalytic terms, on the basis of the premises Ostow has set forth in this volume.

In order to be true to our own craft, therefore, we Judaica scholars must be prepared to incorporate the insights of trained psychoanalysts like Ostow into our work. We have no justification for treating their offerings as a distinct "psychoanalytic" genre of explanation with which we have nothing to do, irrelevant to us because it responds to questions that we have decided not to put on our agenda. Our agenda itself requires some revision.

Psychoanalytic experts, however, need to understand that the Judaica specialist will often have legitimate reservations, of the sort I have sketched above, about their contributions. They must take care not to collude in their own alienation by seeming to disregard the historical problems that the specialist correctly perceives as essential.

It is necessary, in other words, that I take care to listen to the people in the other camp and do not allow my eyes to glaze over when I hear what is alien to my habitual concerns. But I must also take care to speak in language that will address the habitual concerns of the other camp and that will make my way of viewing the data seem as little alien to them as possible.

Ostow's chapters four and five may be seen as starting-points for a vital and productive collaboration between two groups of creative thinkers who have often had rather little to say to one another.

It is in this way that the tremendous potential of his work may come to be realized.

Comments

Mortimer Ostow

ON HALPERIN'S "METHODOLOGICAL REFLECTIONS"

Professor Halperin has presented the case for psychoanalytic input to the study of old and ancient documents most persuasively. I appreciate his confidence in my method—as well as his many listed and unlisted contributions to this volume. I appreciate, too, the importance of his cautions about the need to respect historical and philological data. The purpose of this note is to elaborate his model of the basis for collaboration between students of these texts and psychoanalysts.

"We are prepared", Halperin says, "to oscillate between psychological and historical-philological perspectives, continually using each of these modes of reasoning to check the other". In my opinion these two methods of investigation do not merely check or add to each other. They each contribute a dimension so as to form together a two-dimensional picture. The historical-philological approach gives us the sources of the ancient images and fantasies, the sources in the real world of culture, history, economics, geography, and so on, and sometimes even the sources in the psychology of conscious motivation. What the psychoanalytic approach offers is the motivational explanation for why these specific materials were selected from the many, many data and images in the surrounding landscape.

Professor Halperin mentions the terms "manifest content" and "latent content"—terms proposed by Freud for distinguishing the unconscious motivating impulse and fantasies of the dream (latent content), from the overt dream itself (manifest content). In doing so, Halperin seems to be implying that the scholarly puzzles in which we all share an interest are best approached as one would approach the interpretation of a dream. I think this is a valuable suggestion.

Let us go back to the dream of C (p. 169), the fourth dream given in the essay on *merkavah* mysticism. As I understand it, the historical method of explication would elicit the following observations. Madison Square Garden was mentioned because C had attended a number of sporting events there. Squash courts were mentioned because in the past he had played squash. The terrain that reminded him of the ruins of Machu Picchu was included because he had recently returned from a visit to that spot. The large chair reminded him that he was accepting some furniture from his mother, who was moving into smaller quarters (and I believe it referred to the analytic chair as well). He had, indeed, visited a square in Rome that the grassy area of the dream reminded him of, and he had seen there the building from which Mussolini had addressed the crowds. He believed there was also a church. Kneeling suggests to him a religious act. These are the authentic historical data.

The memories and associations tell us the source of some of the elements that appear in the manifest dream, but the collection of these facts does not constitute an "interpretation" or even an "explanation" of the dream. Why were these details selected for reproduction in the dream from among the countless impressions that he had encountered in recent weeks?

Let us now take note of some of the psychological data, motivating affects, and conflicts. First, in recent weeks, it had become known that his mother faced the prospect of surgery for a serious illness, and so he became more affectionate with his mother and protective of her. Second, he was eager to find a suitable candidate for marriage, and he was dismayed to observe that he was unable to work up enthusiasm for any of the young women whom he met, some of whom seemed to be quite eligible, objectively considered. His brothers, who were recently married, were starting families. Recent business success had created the conflicts that success often does. Moreover, since his father had died a few years ago, he had assumed the role of *pater familias*.

Let us acknowledge now that the dream resembles in form typical *hekhalot* images. The dreamer wishes to enter and take possession of his mother despite the threatening opposition of his father. But the father is dead. He does not appear in the hekhal. So is Mussolini; the powerful leader has been defeated, deposed and is gone. Those who constructed the Peruvian ruins are gone too; only the ruins of their edifices remain. The dreamer is in a position to triumph, to take possession of the woman whom he encounters as he kneels on the "throne"–chair. But he fails; he withdraws at the last moment, as he has been withdrawing from women in waking life. This dream differs from the typical *hekhalot* fantasy in that the father has been eliminated. The son now seeks to take possession of the father's throne—that is, the mother—but he fails because he is inhibited. (For evidence that the throne symbolizes mother, see Scholem's comments about the *Bahir* image in chapter five.)

We now have an "interpretation" of the dream. C would like to pursue his natural desires at this point in his life and to take advantage of the prestige and material comfort that he has achieved. But oedipal conflict prevents him from enjoying the fruits of his success. His mother's illness creates a desire to move closer to her emotionally, whereas since childhood he had always held her at arm's length. Knowledge of the meaning of the *hekhalot* fantasy and recognition of it permit us to understand why the specific images from the recent past were included in the dream. And knowledge of the patient's life situation has permitted us to understand what purpose is served by the invocation of the *hekhalot* complex.

Let us return now to the problem of the fiery rivers of the *Ethiopic Book of Enoch*. The hypothetical adversarial scholar whom Halperin has created would have collected the sources of the images of the fantasy correctly. But these are not sufficient to "interpret" the fantasy or even to explain certain variants of the original images that are introduced into the text. However, if we invoke the conflict that usually accompanies the *hekhalot* fantasy, we will understand why the components of the image include elements that are essentially ambivalent, like fiery water and houses that are simultaneously too hot and too cold. The account reminds us that the decision to approach too closely to God and to look at Him incurs mortal danger. Our psychoanalytic approach explains that the expectation of danger arises from our own guilt and anxiety elicited by the yearning to violate a prohibition that somehow appeared early in childhood. The explicit textual images constitute the manifest content, but the latent content can be ascertained only when the underlying dynamics are exposed. Proper understanding or "interpretation" requires the coordination of the two.

Halperin's selection has proved to be felicitous. But the optimal result would be obtained, not from alternating the historical–philological with the psychoanalytic approach, but from coordinating them. The one establishes the basis in the real world for the selection of the images presented in the text, and the other attempts to discern, by examining what can be ascertained of the psychodynamics, why these elements were selected and how they relate to each other and to the writer's personal agenda. The recognition of universal archetypical complexes can contribute strongly to the solution of these problems.

If only a scholar intimately familiar with the historical and philological materials is qualified to attempt to solve the problems inherent in the ancient texts, and if only an analyst with clinical experience obtained from long and intense practice is qualified to offer psychodynamic hypotheses, then satisfactory studies can be achieved only by cooperation rather than by individual study. If this volume helps to encourage such cooperative endeavours, it will have achieved one of its major purposes.

* * *

Let me add a parenthetical comment addressed, not to the argument, but to the illustrative text that Halperin drew to our attention. I refer to the image of a stream issuing from beneath a throne. That certainly corresponds to no real historical throne or stream.

Halperin quotes Himmelfarb, who relates the fiery stream to the Mountain of El, mentioned in Ugaritic literature, at the base of which two streams run. There is nothing remarkable about streams that flow at the bottom of a mountain. Halperin himself then observes that the stream issuing from the Temple mount, as described in Ezekiel 47:1–12, can be seen as derived from the streams found at the base of the Ugaritic cosmic mountain. Here, too, since the Temple stands on an elevated platform, it would not be that unusual to find a stream issuing from its base. Its miraculously increasing its vigour with distance, and its miraculous fructifying properties can be attributed to prophetic hyperbole. But in Daniel 7 and Revelation 22, we encounter streams issuing from beneath a throne. That is an unnatural image.

Let me call attention to a few clues to what seems to me a reasonable guess about the significance of this strange fantasy. (1) I have noted that the mystical fantasies reproduce fantasies of childhood. The mystic tends to reproduce, in his imagery, impressions of physical closeness to parents. These often or usually deal with anatomical details—for example, God's phallus. The *Shiur Qomah*, which I mentioned in chapter five, does this with absurd precision. (2) Dr. Galenson informs us that in their earliest years, children exhibit intense interest in their parents' toilet functions. (3) Halperin quotes Hagigah 13b to the effect that Daniel's river originates from the sweat of the chimerical creatures of Ezekiel 1, and that the sweat is poured out upon the sinners in Gehenna. Halperin compares this fantasy to Revelation's negative counterpart of the river of life, namely the "lake that teems with fire and brimstone, which is the second death", and in which sinners are tormented (20: 10, 15; 21:8). (4) Both Ezekiel 47 and Revelation 22 emphasize the purity of the water.

Given these clues, it is difficult to avoid the conclusion that the unconscious fantasy that gives rise to the image of the stream issuing from under the throne may be the image of God's urinary stream—an image approximated fairly closely by the explanation given in Hagigah 13b. Depending upon its context, the stream may come to be seen as pure and fructifying (human excreta—"night soil"—are used to fertilize food crops), or foul and poisonous. This idea may seem less outrageous if we consider that (1) human excreta—"night soil"—are commonly used in less developed countries to fertilize food crops; (2) that brimstone shares with human faeces the penetrating sulphurous odour; and that, as noted above, Ezekiel reports that God instructed him to cook his food over human faeces used as fuel. If that is correct, then in addition to the other determinants of the fiery quality attributed to the stream, the experience of suffering an acute urinary infection or even a chronic prostatitis, which I assume was fairly common in ancient times, certainly combines the impression of fire and water.

In short, the image of the fiery stream issuing from under the throne leads us right to the matter of our central concern—ultimate intimacy.

SEX AND GENDER IN THE KABBALAH

Introduction

Kabbalah proper, or mediaeval Jewish mysticism, is a set of systems of theosophy and cosmology. Two terse mystical books appeared in Western Europe, the first, *Sefer Yezirah*, perhaps between the third and sixth centuries, and the second, *Sefer ha-Bahir*, during the twelfth century. The former constructed a cosmology based upon combinations of numbers and letters that purported to reveal a harmony in the universe, all a product of God's calculations and construction. The latter uses the approach of numerology and of letter mysticism, together with verses from the Bible, to construct a more personal cosmos completely occupied by an omnipresent God. With these as a foundation, the kabbalists elaborated more and more complex systems. The definitive formulation appeared in a book called *Sefer ha-Zohar*, referred to briefly as the *Zohar*. It appeared in Spain towards the end of the thirteenth century and is attributed by Gershom Scholem to Moses b. Shem Tov de Leon. This is a very large work comprising several sections, not all of the same quality and therefore probably including sections from other authors. The major part is constructed as a systematic sequential commentary on the Pentateuch. It, too, establishes a cosmology, a theory of the nature of the Godhead, and a reassurance that divine love and justice continue to govern mankind's destiny. The propositions of the *Zohar* constitute a kind of mythic system that was subsequently elaborated by various kabbalistic authors and in kabbalistic circles. In the sixteenth century, Safed became the centre of kabbalistic study and Isaac Luria became the dominating figure. He proposed a more developed and original mythic system that seemingly took account of exile, of evil, and of the possibility of restitution.

In Kabbalah, the Godhead is conceived as far more abstract than it is in normative Judaism, unapproachable and, in fact, inconceivable. In His most recondite form, He is called *En Sof*, or "Infinite". It is only in a series of progressively "lower" and more concrete grades that He can be known to mankind. Ten *Sefirot* are attributed to *En Sof*. There is no one English word that properly translates the word *Sefirah*. The word probably derives from the Hebrew word for number. In essence, the ten *Sefirot* are probably unknowable by mankind, but their manifestations in the universe can be recognized. They are conceived as arranged in a structured pattern suggesting the frame of the human being, with four mid-line structures and three lateral pairs. Of the mid-line structures of the diagram, the lowest is called *Malkhuth* or kingship, sometimes known as *Shekhinah*, or the feminine component of God. In some kabbalistic accounts it is considered a female component of the total structure and one that is necessary for its completeness. The mid-line structure immediately above it, *Yesod* or foundation, is generally acknowledged as the phallus, the reproductive organ, and the direct source for processes of rebirth. We have already mentioned, in chapter one, Luria's concept of the cosmic catastrophe, the bursting of the vessels containing the holy sparks, and his emphasis on the possibility of *tikkun* or restoration. This is accomplished by the combined efforts of all Jews in the performance of good deeds [*mitzvot*], prayer, and study—that is, study of classical texts, presumably as illuminated by Kabbalah.

There is thus a congruence between the divine anthropos and the human. As a result, God becomes, at least in His operative functions, knowable and familiar to humans. Secondly, the congruence seems to imply the possibility of connectedness, so that human behaviour can influence the divine anthropos. As we shall see, this principle is the basis for speculations about the divine sexuality.

What is mystical about these ideas? The mystic is trying to escape from the feeling of living in an inhospitable universe. He overcomes that feeling by entering into a reconstructed cosmos in which the Godhead is assumed to possess characteristics similar to those of humans and is therefore familiar, comprehensible, and subject to influence. The Kabbalah established the possibility of intimate knowledge of, if not actual intimacy with, the Divine. It is this pursuit of intimacy that distinguishes Kabbalah from the antecedent non-mystical mythology of Talmud and Midrash. Presumably, intimacy can be obtained by the three modalities we just mentioned—good deeds, prayer, and study, and especially the study of kabbalistic cosmology. Wolfson (1993a) observes that theosophic study can induce mystical ecstasy. Intimacy is also achieved by viewing one's own behaviour as participation in the cosmic system. Everything one thinks and does can be a link to a warm, vital, and hospitable cosmos.

The idea that the human and the divine anthropos exert a mutual influence upon each other provides the opportunity for the sense of power and the possibility of exerting a magical influence on the universe. It is this idea that has led to the notion that the Kabbalah confers magical powers.

No aspect of human life, mental or physical, is excluded from Kabbalah. Idel and Wolfson have provided us with two splendid and comprehensive essays on sexuality in kabbalistic theory, with the expectation that that subject would offer the most immediate correlation with psychoanalytic theory.

Kabbalah is concerned with sexuality for two reasons. In the first place, sexuality is the path that leads directly to procreation—that is, the possibility of birth and rebirth. Secondly, sexuality, like mysticism, is powerfully directed towards union and reunion. The mystic hopes to reunite with a non-material surrogate for mother, while the sexually motivated individual strives towards physical union with a partner. But I see also a third motivation—namely, to foreclose the possibility that the sexual drive, which is always individual, might divert one from religious behaviour and complete commitment to the religious group. Kabbalah does not simply attempt to prevent competition between sexuality and commitment to worthy behaviour; it actually exploits sexuality to conduce to commitment.

To illustrate the use of sexuality in Kabbalah, let me quote a particularly transparent passage taken from the section of the *Zohar* called *Idra Zuta* (Margalioth, 1960, 3:296a):

> Then His physical thighs expand, enclosing between them the two kidneys and two testicles within which are accumulated all of the oil (secretions?) and greatness and bodily strength, and from which the strength which is to be released is released, and ejaculated from the orifice of the penis. These thighs are called Hosts, Victory and Majesty. Beauty is the Lord. Victory and Majesty are the Hosts and therefore He is called Lord of Hosts. The male phallus, the completion of the entire body is called Foundation, and this is the grade that gratifies the female. All of the desire of the male is for the female. With this foundation he enters the female, into the place called Zion, which is the concealed genital of the female, and which is homologous to the womb of the mortal woman. And therefore the Lord of Hosts is called Foundation.

I would infer from the explicitness of this account that sexuality is not used here as a metaphor for union between the human and the divine, so much as a vehicle; the sexual quest carries with it the quest for union with the Godhead.

A comparable passage from *The Autobiographical Life of St. Teresa of Jesus* (quoted in Underhill, 1961, pp. 292f):

> Though I have visions of angels frequently, yet I see them only by an intellectual vision. It was Our Lord's will that in this vision I should see an angel in this wise. He was not large, but small in stature, and most beautiful—his face burning, as if he were one of the highest angels, who seem to be all on fire. . . . I saw in his hand a long spear of gold, and at the iron's point there seemed to be a little fire. He appeared to me to be thrusting it at times into my heart and to pierce my very entrails; when he drew it out, he seemed to draw them out also and to leave me all on fire with a great love of God. The pain was so great that it made me moan; and yet so surpassing was the sweetness of this excessive pain that I could not wish to be rid of it. The soul is satisfied now with nothing less than God.

Note that the former account purports to be an account of divine experience, the latter a personal experience. In the first account, the female is almost incidental; in the latter, the female is the principal. Most important, however, is the fact that the former account is quite explicitly genital and sexual, while in the latter account the genitality and sexuality are symbolic. St. Teresa does not permit herself to acknowledge that she is enjoying a sexual experience. To the extent that St. Teresa's report is characteristic of Christian mysticism, and to the extent that this account from the Idra Zuta is characteristic of kabbalistic mysticism, we can understand that the former can be autobiographical and exoteric, whereas the latter is didactic and esoteric.

Both Idel's and Wolfson's chapters are fairly technical, but they will give the reader an idea of the nature of kabbalistic thinking. Idel summarizes kabbalistic thought about the relation between divine and human sexuality. Wolfson describes the asymmetrical attitude of Kabbalah towards the two sexes. He makes a clear distinction between biological sexuality and culturally assigned gender.

In an interesting paper on circumcision, Nunberg (1949) reported the case of a patient who was circumcised at the age of 5. He thought of the loss of the foreskin as a loss of femininity and a strengthening of his masculinity. He imagined that his 1-year-old sister had acquired his foreskin and that he could retrieve it by marrying her. He strove in other ways to undo separations and divisions, namely, to reunite what was separated. Nunberg does not report any mystical affect, but the mythic fantasy reminds us of kabbalistic material reported by Wolfson—namely, that biological sexuality does not limit fantasy of gender identity, and that sexual union promotes feelings of identity and wholeness. The child's fear of loss and his need to reunite what had been separated led him to androgynous fantasies and yearnings for sexual contact. He had been circumcised because the glans and the foreskin had been chronically irritated. His penis required his mother's frequent attention for cleaning. After the circumcision, he requested his mother to renew her attentions, but since there was no objective need, she refused. It was then that he developed the fantasy that his sister was actually a twin, and as a result of his circumcision, she had acquired his foreskin. Therefore by sexual contact with her he would not only reacquire the foreskin but also restore his original androgynous state. The myth of androgyny is calculated to ameliorate the pain of separation and loss (Nunberg, 1949).

That brings us to a seeming contradiction between Idel and Wolfson. Idel informs us that the Kabbalah does not accept the myths of androgyny of Gnosticism, nor of some early Christian views of transformation of one sex into the other. Wolfson contends that in Kabbalah the female and male may exchange qualities, so that in some circumstances the concept of the female and the concept of the male are combined, or contained within each other. The Kabbalah leaves no ambiguity about the physical differences between the sexes, both among humans and within the divine anthropos. Wolfson shows us that the Kabbalah assigns a gender value to each individual in relation to certain functions.

What these essays demonstrate is that, given the need to establish a feeling of intimacy or union, one can enrich the prosaic experiences of daily life by an act of deliberate reorientation, especially in the company of others determined to accomplish the same task. Sexuality lends itself especially to this endeavour because its striving is towards actual physical union. The quest for intimacy, physical and emotional, is easily reconciled with and recruited into the service of the mystical quest for union with the Godhead.

Each of these essays presents a series of propositions and extensive documentation for each proposition. Most readers will find the terms and concepts unfamiliar. For both reasons, the reading may be slow and difficult if one attempts to follow the arguments closely. It may help if the reader keeps in mind the principle that the intent of the mystical enterprise is always to augment the availability of the Divine to the human mystic. In addition, it is well to remember that in most instances the author is talking, not about literal human beings and literal sexuality, but about the concepts of people and their sexual activities. Idel correctly emphasizes the metaphoric quality of the ideas described. It will be of interest to take note of the many quoted comments that emphasize that everything is united and combined, everything is one. The reader who comes to this material from the domain of psychoanalysis will find a number of instances in which the kabbalists correctly apprehend the unconscious symbolic equivalence of archetypes—for example, that sacred space usually signifies mother.

Finally, let me emphasize that Kabbalah is not a fixed structure, either in content or in history. To ask what Kabbalah says about a given subject is like asking what psychoanalysis says about a subject. In each case one must specify who the authority is, when he wrote and where, and at what point in his own development the specific views were formulated.

Jacob Arlow comments on Idel's chapter. He tries to show that the introduction of the feminine into the image of the Godhead alleviates some of the sexual tension that is involved in the male worshiper's submitting completely to a male God. Neubauer, commenting on Wolfson's chapter, examines how the propositions of gender transcendence apply to psychoanalytic propositions of development and observes that not all myth fantasies are consistent with each other with respect to phase of development. I think that such consistency is not pursued by mystics. The most archaic fantasies of reunion by incorporation and identification appear side by side with phallic sexual union and group cohesiveness.

CHAPTER SEVEN

Sexual metaphors and praxis in the Kabbalah

Moshe Idel

Two major usages of sexual imagery, metaphors and praxis, occur in the kabbalistic literature. For describing these usages, it is reasonable to divide various types of sexual discussions into two main parts, according to their referents on the theological or theosophical plan. (1) When the relationship symbolized by the sexual imagery or praxis is between humans and God, I refer to it as "vertical symbolism". (2) When the relation the sexual imagery or praxis is pointing to is a process taking place between entities found on the same level, it is referred to as "horizontal symbolism". "Vertical symbolism" can be found in two main kabbalistic schools: the theosophical kabbalah, whose main chef d'oeuvre is the thirteenth-century *Zohar*, and in the ecstatic kabbalah, represented by the thirteenth-century writings of R. Abraham Abulafia and his followers; the "horizontal symbolism" recurs almost exclusively in the theosophical kabbalah.

Roughly speaking, the two main types of symbols occur already in the classical rabbinic texts—the Talmud and the midrash. However, the mediaeval kabbalists, who adopted the already existing sexual motifs, elaborated on details of rabbinic thoughts concerning sexual issues and sometimes integrated philosophical ideas, which contributed mainly to the formations occurring in the ecstatic kabbalah.

Let us begin with the vertical symbolism. This type of symbolism includes two differing kinds of symbols.[1] The theosophical kabbalah refers to the divine manifestations as female partner, whereas the kabbalists or the ideal figures of the remote antiquity (biblical or rabbinic heroes) are conceived of as playing the role of the male in their relation to the Divine. The ecstatic kabbalah, on the other hand, presents the mystic or his spiritual faculties as the female, whereas the supernal powers (viz. the active intellect or God Himself) are viewed as the male partner. I would refer to the theosophical usage of vertical as well as horizontal symbolism as "descending symbolism".

This term, which was proposed and defined by Erich Kahler (1960, p. 65), indicates a case when

> symbolic representation detaches itself, descends to us, from a prior and higher reality, a reality determining, and therefore superior to, its symbolic meaning. That is to say, genuinely mythical and cultic works are not intended as symbolic representation, they are meant to describe real happenings.

In our case, the "higher reality" is the processes taking place in the infradivine world, namely, the domain of the *sephirot* ("the potencies and modes of action of the living God"—see Scholem, 1965, p. 100) which serve as archetypes for both the vertical and horizontal processes.

On the other hand, the vertical symbolism of the ecstatic kabbalah will be referred to as "ascending symbolism",[2] this

[1] I shall limit myself to self-evident *sexual* discussions in kabbalah, leaving aside a whole series of *erotic* imagery. Some of them were studied by Vajda (1957) or Wirszubski (1975, pp. 13–23); see also Langer, 1923, and nn. 5 and 50 below.

[2] This term occurs also in Kahler's essay—however, in speculative contexts other than those discussed here; and I prefer, therefore, to propose my own definition for this phrase; cf. Kahler, 1960, pp. 67–68.

phrase expressing the elevation of a corporeal, human sexual act to the status of a metaphor for the relationship between the human soul and supernal entities.

I shall start with an analysis of the history of the vertical ascending symbolism.

Vertical ascending symbolism

It is a commonplace that mystical literature is inclined to express the relationship between the mystic soul and the divine by means of erotic imagery (see, e.g., Waite, 1915, esp. pp. 126ff.). All the classical bodies of mystical writings can easily provide numerous examples, sometimes striking ones, wherein sexual images are openly and often employed. Kabbalah has nothing unique on this issue; it also extensively uses sexual images and metaphors. However, there is something novel in this body of literature that transcends the more common usage of erotic and sexual motifs. The difference lies not so much in the texts, but in their sociological contexts.

Unlike their Christian correspondents, the Jewish mystics who adopted sexual imagery in order to describe their experience of the divine shared with other Jews the conviction that actual marriage and fulfilment of the command to multiply are religious imperatives and, accordingly, the kabbalists could hardly be regarded as persons who employed sexual metaphors as a compensation for the frustration of "real" erotic experiences (see Leuba, 1925, pp. 116ff.). Abraham Abulafia, Isaac of Acre, or any other kabbalists who will be mentioned later were seemingly married or, at least, persons who viewed sexual relations as religiously licit. Therefore, the very recurrence of this type of imagery in Jewish sources is evidence that the relatively common explanations offered by some scholars to the genesis of sexual imagery in the repressed libido can be no more than a partial solution.

A short survey of the vertical ascending symbolism evinces that it occurs in two major types of texts: the ancient classical Jewish literature and mediaeval kabbalistic literature. In the Bible and the talmudic–midrashic texts, the relationship between God and the Jewish people, sometimes designated as *Knesset Israel*, is described as the relation between husband and wife. This was also the main avenue adopted in the exegetical literature of the Song of Songs in mediaeval texts, which regarded the plain meaning of the biblical text to be concerned with the people of Israel and God. This is obviously a part of the national myth, which changes the entire nation into one entity standing in sexual relation to the other entity—the Divinity. This mythical relationship has little to do with mysticism; it is interested primarily in the whole nation as a unit, whereas the particular Jew is rather neglected as a meaningful factor. The individual, according to classical Jewish texts, can take part in this bond with God by his participation in the significant great unity, *Knesset Israel* [the community of Israel]. His activity, therefore, must be focused on becoming a part of this larger body. The erotic and sexual imagery occurs, in my opinion, solely on this plane: the relation of the mythical *Knesset Israel* with God. This bond mediates between the individual Jew and the Divinity whenever this relation is expressed in sexual terms. It is only later, in the mediaeval period, that in addition to this mythical bond, expressed in marital terminology, a mystical relation between the individual and God made its appearance. The human soul—or, sometimes, the human intellect—was conceived of as female in its relation to a supernal "male" entity, be it the active intellect—viewed as a cosmic force—or God Himself.[3] This is the pattern adopted since the late twelfth century by Jewish philosophers, and from them it infiltrated into the ecstatic kabbalah.

To illustrate this, I have chosen examples that permit us to perceive the neutralization of the mythical aspect of *Knesset Israel* as it appears in classical rabbinic texts or in the theo-

[3] I consciously delete any discussion of Philo's parallel views because his literary *corpus* did not apparently influence kabbalah. Phenomenologically, the structure of Philo's thought is close to that of Abulafia's, both employing vertical ascending symbolism together with Greek philosophical terminology; again, in their writings, a neutralization of mythical elements is obvious. On Greek sexual puritanism, see Dodds, 1951, pp. 154–155; see also, on Plotinus's usage of erotic imagery and its influence on the Renaissance, Wind, 1967, pp. 61–68.

sophical kabbalah,[4] and its transformation into an allegory of a human spiritual capacity.

In his *Gan Naul*, Abraham Abulafia writes:

> The Song of Songs is only an allegory to *Knesset Israel* and God, the latter being a perfect bridegroom to her, and she is for Him a perfect bride, He—on the divine plane—she—on the human plane . . . and the human love does not unite with the divine one except after long studies and after comprehension of wisdom and reception of prophecy. [Ms. MBS 58 fol. 323][5]

Therefore, the attainment of "prophecy"—namely, of ecstatic experience—is tantamount to the union of a bride and her bridegroom. The nature of the bridegroom is obvious: God; the bride, however, named *Knesset Israel*, is human. On the basis of this passage alone it seems evident that *Knesset Israel* is conceived as an individual entity; after all, the reception of prophecy is, commonly, an individual experience. Furthermore, Abulafia let us know, in another work, that

> the secret of *Knesset Israel* is . . . *Knesset I-Sar-El* (that which is gathered by the Prince removed ten [sephirotic] stages from God), since the perfect man brings everything together, he is called the community of Jacob. [*Imre Shefer*, Ms. BPNH 777, p. 57]

The transition from the perfect nation as the partner of God to the individual soul is evident in this comment. The wise man stands for the whole "community of Jacob", for he includes

---

[4] See our treatment of R. Jehudah ben Yakar's passage later in this chapter in our discussion of "Horizontal Descending Symbolism".

[5] Scholem's statement that "older Kabbalists never interpreted the 'Song of Songs' as a dialogue between God and the Soul, i.e. an allegorical description of the path to *unio mystica*" (Scholem, 1967, p. 226) must therefore be corrected. Abulafia indeed proposed such an allegorical interpretation, the ultimate aim of which is the *unio mystica*; his perception is closer to the philosophical interpretations than to the early kabbalistic one. However, he differs also from the philosophers, for he strove for an actual realization of the *unio mystica*, and thus allegorical interpretation turns into what I propose to call a spiritual interpretation or hermeneutic. On the philosophical perceptions of the Song of Songs, see Halkin, 1950, pp. 389–424; Vajda, 1957.

Knesset in his mind, the Active Intellect, which is represented by the word *Israel*. This ecstatic experience is described by Abulafia, again using strong erotic themes, as *unio mystica*:

> This is the power of man: he can link the lower part with the higher one and the lower (part) will ascend to and unite with the supernal (part) and the higher (part) will descend and will kiss the entity ascending towards it, like a bridegroom actually kisses his bride, out of his great and real desire, characteristic of the delight of both, coming from the power of God (or His Name). [*Or ha-Sekhel*. Ms. VBAE, 233 fol. 115]

According to Abulafia, the final aim of ecstasy is the "pleasure of the bridegroom and bride"—an expression recurring several times in his writings (see, e.g., Abulafia's *Hayye ha Nefesh*, Ms. MBS 408 fol. 65). This union of the human and Divine represents a clear shift not only from the mythical to mystical, from national to individual, but also from the traditional terminology to the philosophical one. According to an anonymous treatise from the Abulafian school, "the rational faculty, named the rational soul, which received the divine influx, is called *Knesset Israel*, whose secret is the Active Intellect" (*Or ha-Menorah*, Ms. JNL 8 1303 fol. 28b).[6]

Therefore "Israel", or "*Knesset Israel*", represents the human intellect, which is related, in a secret way, to the supernal Intellect. The nature of the secret seems to be the gematria,[7] *Israel* being tantamount to *Sekhel ha-Po'el* [the active intellect].[8]

Let us summarize the shift from the classical to the speculative view of *Knesset Israel* as the spouse of God: only when it was interpreted as referring to the individual was this term related to the mystical union between two monads. Only then could the kabbalist see himself as the "female" into whom the divine spark is sown and the spiritual son born. That is, a transmutation of

---

[6] Compare to the collectanea stemming from the Abulafia circle found in Ms. NYJTSA Mic. 1771 fol. 34, where, again, *Knesset Israel* is connected to the rational soul.

[7] An equation of the numerical value of the Hebrew letters in each word or phrase.

[8] Both having the value of 541; on other philosophical allegorizations of *Israel*, see Saperstein, 1980, pp. 100, 248.

the human spirit takes place as a result of contact with the Divine (see Idel, 1985, pp. 190–203; cf. Baer, 1970, pp. 55–64). It is important also to remark that the epithalamic symbolism[9] used by Abulafia is sometimes transcended by the occurrence of unitive symbolism.[10] For example, the passage previously quoted from *Or ha-Sekhel* appears immediately after the following passage:

> The Name [of God] is composed from two parts[11] since there are two parts of love [divided between] two lovers, and the [parts of] love turn one (entity) when love became actuated. The divine intellectual love and the human intellectual love are conjuncted, being one. [Ms. VBAE 233 fol. 115]

Before leaving this type of metaphor, it must be emphasized that an actual experience of a sexual contact is not essential for the ecstatic kabbalist. He may have experienced it or not in the past or still enjoy it (or not) in the present; the very act of sexual union plays no ritualistic role in the mystical experience.[12] By its nature, ecstatic kabbalah is mostly interested in spiritual processes for which the corporeal actions would be only a hindrance.

---

[9] Cf. Scholem's view of mystical "communion", which is characteristic of Jewish mysticism (Scholem, 1972, pp. 203–205).

[10] On *unio mystica* in Abulafia's doctrine, see Idel, 1988c, pp. 5–12, where additional material is quoted to substantiate the thesis that Abulafia asserted that total fusion with a higher entity—sometimes being God—is possible.

[11] The value of the letters of the Tetragrammaton is 26, which is formed from 13 +13; now "13" is the value of *Ehad*, that is, "one", and *Ahavah*, that is, "love". By the way of gematria, Abulafia evinces that it is possible to attain mystical union (One, One) with God (Tetragrammaton) by means of love [*Ahavah*].

[12] Nevertheless, marriage or sexual relationship is never presented by Abulafia or his disciples as an obstacle for attaining a mystical experience. We know for sure that Abulafia himself was married, and in his list of requirements for an ideal student (see *Hayye ha-Olam ha-Ba*, Ms. OBL 1582, fol. 33v–35r) no reference to sexual impurity can be found. See also Idel, 1988c, pp. 143–144, on the non-ascetic characteristic of Abulafia's mysticism.

Vertical descending symbolism

"If a man and woman are worthwhile, the divine presence dwells between them, if not—they shall be consumed by fire" (b. Sotah 17a).[13] What is the significance of this talmudic dictum? Is it merely a warning intended to strengthen the laws of purity? Perhaps. This possibility notwithstanding, I should like to propose a more elaborate interpretation, which regards the act of union between husband and wife, when performed according to the Jewish ritual, as fraught with theurgical[14] meaning. Or, to put it a different way, the perfect sexual union[15] actually influences the Divine Presence, causing it to dwell with the worthy pair. When the union is performed by impure persons, on the other hand, the result is fatal: fire will devour them.

The pairs of opposites, the favourable presence of divinity versus the devouring fire, reminds us of the possibility inherent in another situation: the entrance into the innermost Jewish sanctuary. Moses was able to hear the divine voice from between the cherubim in the Tabernacle, whereas Nadav and Abihu were consumed by fire as they entered the sanctuary (Lev. 10:1).[16] Is this parallelism a sheer coincidence? Is there any significant

---

[13] Cf. Pirke de-R. Eliezer, ch. 12, and R. Tuviah ben Eliezer's Lekah Tov on Gen., 2:23. M. Kasher, *Torah Shelemah, XXII*, Appendix, p. 18, has already pointed out the possible connection between this dictum and the cherubim. See also Louis Ginzberg's apologetical view that this dictum reflects "another pagan conception which, in refined form, passed into the Cabala through the Talmud" (1970, p. 190).

[14] *Theurgy*, in this essay, stands for the conception that human actions, mostly the commandments, are intended to change processes taking place in the supernal divine system. For more on my view of this concept, see Idel, 1988b, ch. 7–8.

[15] The formulation of R. Akiva's dictum does not explicitly refer to sexual union; however, this is the way the dictum was understood by the classical commentators, for example, by Rashi. See also the rabbinic view that God participates in the process of producing the infant together with his father and mother (b. Niddah 31a and parallels). The affinity between these two rabbinic views was perceived and exploited by the anonymous kabbalist who composed the famous *Epistle on the Sexual Conjunction* attributed to Nachmanides; see the edition of C. Chavel in *Kitve ha-Ramban* (Jerusalem, 1964, II, pp. 324–325).

[16] Here, as in the Sotah quotation, the verb *'achal* is used in order to express the idea of consummation by fire.

affinity between the pure sexual union and the sanctuary? It seems to me that the answer is yes. The divine presence was conceived as dwelling between the two cherubim (Num. 7:89). This biblical view was elaborated in the Talmud: the cherubim turn towards each other when Israel performs the *mitzvot*, but when they sin the cherubim turn their faces away from each other (see b. Baba Batra 99a).[17] Therefore, by the fulfilment of the divine will the cherubim change their position, as apparently described in another talmudic passage:

> When Israel used to make the pilgrimage, they (i.e. the priests) would roll up for them the *Parokhet* [curtain] and show them the Cherubim which were intertwined with one another, and say to them: "Behold! Your love before God is like the love of male and female." [b. Yoma 54a][18]

It seems, therefore, that the fulfilment of the divine will and the love of God for Israel find their expression in the sexually oriented position of the cherubim. But God's love for Israel is not tantamount to the love of one cherub for another; the cherubim do not stand for God and Israel. Only the nature of the love of male and female is a metaphor of the divine love.

The dwelling of the divine presence between the cherubim and between the pure husband and wife are but particular cases of a more general intention, expressed by the midrashic statement: "The natural place of the Shekhinah was below" (*Genesis Rabba 19*, 7, p. 176; *Midrash Rabba* on Song of Songs, 5, 1).[19]

---

[17] Interestingly enough, the two positions of the cherubim—separate or united—stand, according to some mediaeval interpreters of the Talmud, respectively, for the curse and blessing occurring in the talmudic discussion of the cherubim in b. Yoma 54b; see R. Shemuel Edeles, *Novellae*, where he quotes R. Yom Tov Ashvili's view. Has this presumably later conception something to do with the perception of the cherubim as the two divine attributes, as found already in Philo?

[18] See the interesting proposal of Menahem Kasher that this text may be connected to the perception that regards the Song of Songs as the holy of holies, and the secrets of the forbidden sexual unions in Mishnah Hagigah 2:1, as an esoteric topic; see "*Zohar*" (Maimon, 1958, pp. 55–56). This argument merits a more elaborate analysis.

[19] See also *Bereshit Rabba*, p. 177, where it is implied that the righteous are persons who can cause the descent of the *Shekhinah*, who has left our world because of the sins of the sinners; cf. also *Hebrew Enoch*, Ch. 5.

The building of the Temple or the performance of the commandments—and in our case those connected to the sexual act—are intended to restore the pristine state of the divine presence.

Interestingly enough, a most important talmudic discussion on the imperative to prepare a residence for the *Shekhinah* is again explicitly connected to procreation (Yevamot 63b–64a). There Ben Azai's refusal to marry in order to devote himself to the study of Torah is sharply condemned by some early sages; R. Eliezer even proclaims that whoever abstains from procreation will be punished by death, on the basis of the example of Nadav and Avihu, who died, according to this interpretation, because "they had no children" (Num. 3:4).[20] An alternative explanation for the transgression of abstention is the fact that such an abstention causes the retraction of the *Shekhinah* from Israel, this view being sustained by the verse, "to be a God unto thee and to thy seed after thee" (Gen. 17:7). The anonymous sage continues: "[w]henever thy seed is after thee, the Shekhinah dwells [below], [whenever] there is no seed after thee, upon whom will the Shekhinah dwell? Upon trees and upon stones." Therefore, procreation is indispensable for attainment of the ideal state of the *Shekhinah*. Not only is She present during the very act of union between husband and wife (cf. *Bereshit Rabba*, 8; 9, p. 63; 22, 2, p. 206), but, owing to the productive nature of this act, She continues to dwell below.

The affinity between the presence of the *Shekhinah* on the cherubim in the Temple and Her dwelling on the pure human pair is, in my opinion, highly significant. It seems as if the religious role of the cherubim was transferred to human pairs; when the Temple was destroyed, its function was partially preserved by the human activity. This transfer was seemingly facilitated by the existence of a very ancient conception of the Holy of Holies as a bedroom. According to a Gnostic treatise preserved in Nag Hammadi:

> The mysteries of truth are revealed, though in type and image; the bridal chamber however, remains hidden. It is the holy in the holy. The veil at first concealed how God controlled the creation, but when the veil is rent and the things

---

[20] On this issue see Shinan, 1983, pp. 182–183.

> inside are revealed, this house will be left desolate. [*Gospel of Philip*, 1984, p. 150][21]

Or

> There were three buildings specially for sacrifice in Jerusalem. The one facing west was called the "Holy." Another facing the south was called the "Holy of the Holy." The third facing east was called the "Holy of the Holiest" . . . the Holy of the Holies is the bridal chamber. [*Gospel of Philip*, p. 142][22]

It seems that these Gnostic texts reflect an already existing Jewish perception of the Temple. According to *Midrash Tanhuma*, commenting on the reference to the royal bed in Song of Songs 3:7, the anonymous commentator asserts that "'his [Solomon's] bed'—this is the Temple. And why is the Temple compared to the bed? Just as this bed serves fruitfulness and multiplication, so too the Temple, everything that was in it was fruitful and multiplied" (Buber's version, Num. fol. 17).[23]

Let us focus on the assertion that the veil "concealed how God controlled the creation". It seems plausible to assume that the Gnostic author intended to hint at a sexual act taking place in the holy of the holiest, for the latter is viewed as "a bridal chamber". At the same time, in this "bridal chamber" the way the world is governed can be visualized. The entities that were seen in the holy of holiest were related on the one hand to the cherubim—because of the sexual overtones—and on the other hand to the two attributes of God, *Middat ha-Rahamim* [mercy]

---

[21] Some affinities between this treatise and Jewish concepts were pointed out by Liebes (1982, pp. 230–232) and Idel (forthcoming). It is important to stress the fact that the relatively positive attitude towards sexuality and marriage occurring in Gnostic texts, as in this Gospel and parts of *Corpus Hermeticum*, seem to be the result of Jewish influence.

[22] See also p. 150: "The holies of holies were revealed and the bridal chamber invited us in" (see also Grant, 1961, pp. 129–140; Sevrin, 1974, pp. 143–193; Sevrin, 1982, pp. 448–450).

[23] Cf. Patai, 1947, pp. 89–92, and on the perception of the holy of holies as *cletoris* in the *Zohar*, see Liebes, 1982, p. 194. It seems plausible that the midrashic connection between *Apirion* [litter for a wedding procession] mentioned in the Song of Songs III and the Temple and Tabernacle may have something to do also to with sexuality and fertility; see *Song of Songs Rabbah* III, 15–19 (Dunski, 1980, pp. 93–96).

and *Middat ha-Din* [stern judgement], which represent the manner in which God "controls the creation". This thesis is based on the fact that Philo of Alexandria already identified the cherubim with the divine attributes (see Goodenough, 1935, pp. 25–26, 359–369; 1954, IV, p. 132). In addition, identifications of the cherubim with masculine and feminine powers were known in ancient times even beyond the boundaries of Judaism (see Stroumsa, 1981, pp. 46–47). Though the influence of Philo on the *Gospel of Philip* is possible, this thesis is by no means the only probable solution for the explanation as to how Jewish views of the holy of holies reached the Gnostic author. It is equally possible that Jewish traditions, contemporary to Philo but possibly independent of his writings, were known by the anonymous author.[24] We may conclude that a sexual perception of the holy of holies was in existence in ancient Judaism.

Shortly after the destruction of the Temple, we learn about a substitute for the Temple as the place where the *Shekhinah* may dwell. According to a view found in the talmudic context discussed earlier (b. Yevamot, 64a.), the presence of the *Shekhinah* requires the existence of at least twenty-two thousand children of Israel,[25] and each and every one has to contribute to the maintenance of this figure. The people of Israel are viewed, either as individuals or as a nation, as *Imago Templi*—a theme that extended its influence into both Christianity and Islam.

According to this conception, the pure union of male and female functions as a restorative act, enabling the *Shekhinah* to keep Her natural place amid the Jewish nation. At least partially, procreation is done for the sake of the divinity, it being an effort to reestablish the harmony that existed during the period the Temple was functioning. It seems, therefore, reasonable to suppose that the mediaeval kabbalistic dictum, "The dwelling of the Shekhinah below (or among Israel) is for Her (own) sake"[26]

---

[24] Liebes (1982, p. 231), even asserts that the anonymous Gnostic author was of Jewish extraction.

[25] This figure recurs in midrashic texts: see Goldberg, 1969, pp. 357–359, 508–509.

[26] See Nachmanides, *Commentary on Exodus*, 29:46, and a long series of other kabbalists afterwards; compare also to R. Joseph Gikatilla's expression "the need of Shekhinah" in *Sha're Orah*, ed. J. ben Shlomo (Jerusalem, 1970), I, 67.

faithfully reflects a more ancient perception, which was only more clearly articulated by the kabbalists.

Let us elaborate upon another kabbalistic view of this theme. According to the classical rabbinic sources discussed earlier, the presence of the *Shekhinah* during the sexual act is conditioned by the ritual purity of the participants. No requisite of *kavvanah* [proper intention] is mentioned in these contexts. But the requirement of pure intention, described by the kabbalists as aiming to raise human thought to its supernal source while causing the descent of the *Shekhinah* afterward, was added in one of the early and most influential kabbalistic texts, *Iggeret ha-Kodesh*:

> It is well known to the masters of Kabbalah that human thought stems from the intellectual soul, which has descended from above. And human thought has the ability to strip itself [from alien issues] and to ascend to and arrive at the place of its source.[27] Then, it will unite with the supernal entity,[28] whence it comes, and it [i.e. the thought] and it [i.e. its source] become one entity.[29] And when the thought returns downward from above, something similar to a line appears, and with it the supernal light descends, under the influence of the thought that draws it downward, and consequently it draws the Shekhinah downward. Then the brilliant[30] light comes and increases upon the place where the owner of the thought stands . . . and since this is the case, our ancient sages had to state that when the husband copulates with his wife, and his thought unites with the supernal entities, that very thought draws the supernal light downward, and it (the light) dwells upon the drop [of semen] upon which he directs his intention and thought . . . that very drop

[27] This view was taken over by the anonymous author of the *Iggeret* from Geronese Kabbalah (see Scholem, 1962, pp. 320–321). Our author is, seemingly, original in applying the already existing view of *elevatio mentis* to the procreative sexual process.

[28] Literally, "secret"—"*sod*".

[29] On this expression, see Scholem, 1962, p. 322, n. 192.

[30] The expression "the light of the Shekhinah" [*or ha-Shekhinah*], which might influence this text, was in existence several centuries before the author of the *Iggeret*; see Vajda, 1975, pp. 133–135, to which we may add *Midrash Tadshe*, ch. 11 (Epstein, 1887, p. 156), and Goldberg, 1969, pp. 318–319.

> is permanently linked with the brilliant light . . . since he thought on it [the drop] is linked to the supernal entities it draws the brilliant light downward. [Chavel, *Kitve ha-Ramban*, II, 373.]

Therefore, the human mystical intention that has to accompany the sexual union can cause the supernal light—and the *Shekhinah* as well[31]—to descend on man during sexual intercourse. The husband has to elevate his thought to its source, to achieve a *unio mystica*, which will be followed by the descent of supernal spiritual forces on the *semen virile*.[32] Here *ascensio mentis, unio mystica*, and *reversio* are prerequisite stages of the ideal conception.[33]

It is worthwhile to compare this mystical conception of the sexual act to the tantric view. In both cases, the sexual act must be performed in a very mindful manner; a certain mystical consciousness is attained alongside the corporeal act. However, the usage of intercourse as a vehicle for spiritual experiences is evidently different. The mystical union of thought with its source is, in kabbalah, instrumental to the main goal—conception; the spiritual attainment is solely a preparatory phase in the process of procreation, which has to be performed with the cooperation of the *Shekhinah*. In the tantric systems, the mystical consciousness, the *bodhicitta*, is an aim in itself, whereas the perfect state is obtained by the immobilization of the flow of *semen virile* (see Eliade, 1969, pp. 118–119; 1971, pp. 248–249, 266–68). The sexual act is regarded by the kabbalists as a life-

---

[31] The presence of the *Shekhinah* is induced by the pure thought of the husband according to some additional statements (Goldberg, 1969, p. 332), one of them asserting that whoever thinks of the exterior beauty of his wife does not think according to the "supernal pure thought", and thereby causes the *Shekhinah* to leave the pair.

[32] I assume that to the ancient rabbinic view, concerning the presence of the *Shekhinah* during intercourse, the kabbalists supplied a certain magical perception. According to several mediaeval sources, man is able to prepare below an appropriate substratum, upon which he can draw a supernal influx named *Ruhaniat* in Arabic or *Ruhaniut* in Hebrew. In our text, the *semen virile* stands for the substratum that is prepared to collect the supernal influx, named here "brilliant light" or *Shekhinah*.

[33] Compare this view, which considers *unio mystica* as a means, to R. Isaac of Acre's view, discussed later, where only after the corporeal relations is severed, the "higher" spiritual status of union is achieved.

giving act; with the tantric masters, the ejaculation is viewed as "death" (see Eliade, 1971, p. 249). The kabbalists put mystical union in the service of procreation; tantra put fruitless intercourse into the service of mystical consciousness.

For the theosophical kabbalists, intercourse is not an aim in itself. The final goal or goals are procreation and preparation of appropriate *substrata*—human beings—to serve as residences for the *Shekhinah*. Either the human couple or its descendants come into direct contact with the *Shekhinah*, which descends on the man who performs the sexual act in purity. Therefore, a contact is evidently established between the human and the divine, during which the former retains his masculine nature.

In the texts analysed earlier, the *Shekhinah* descends during proper intercourse. However, She does not play the role of the female, and no mention of sexual relations between the male and the *Shekhinah* can be discerned in these discussions. It seems that the *Zohar* contributed an important concept in the domain of sexual motifs;[34] for the first time in a Jewish source,[35] the righteous person is portrayed as standing between two females (see Tishby, 1963, I, 149): the human one—that is, the spouse—and the supernal one—the *Shekhinah*. The man is able to attain this status only when marrying a human woman, but afterwards he is compensated by the presence of the *Shekhinah* whenever he separates from his earthly wife. This sexual description of human contact with the *Shekhinah* is primarily attributed to Moses, "*Ish ha-Elohim*" [lit. "the man of God"], a phrase interpreted by the kabbalists as "the husband of the Shekhinah" (see Idel, 1985a, p. 56, notes 117, 119, 120). However, even other religious men are sometimes described in similar terms. According to the *Zohar*, marriage bestows the righteous not only with the opportunity to fulfil the requirement of procreation, but it also enables him to attain the mythical status of the human husband of "the world of the Womanhood" [*Alma de-nukba*]. It is worthwhile to focus on this view—the ritualistic marriage is a prerequisite for the acquirement of the role of the mythical husband. The actual consummation of marriage is a *sine qua*

---

[34] On the importance of sexual symbolism in the *Zohar*, see Scholem, 1967, pp. 225–229; Tishby, 1963, II, 607–626; Waite, 1990, pp. 377–405.

[35] A parallel concept occurs also in Sufic material; see Idel, 1985a, p. 56, n. 117.

non for it. However, afterwards it may sometimes become an obstacle for the attainment of the spiritual experience. Note, for example, the opinion of R. Isaac of Acre:

> Jacob, our ancestor, as long as he was [living] with the corporeal Rachel, outside the land of Israel, his soul could not unite with the supernal Rachel, the latter's residence being in the Holy Land; but as soon as he has reached the Holy Land, the lower Rachel died, and his soul united with the higher Rachel's. [*Ozar Hayyim*, Ms. M–G 774 fol. 73; in Idel, 1985a, p. 56. n. 117]

This combination of corporeal marriage as a first step, with the spiritual one as the second step, seemingly points to a synthesis of the theosophical importance of the marriage with the emphasis that the ecstatic kabbalah puts on the spiritual nature of the relation between man and God.[36]

Horizontal descending symbolism

The sexual symbolism that describes the relationship between the righteous and the *Shekhinah* assumes the female nature of the *Shekhinah*. The evolution of this concept is a complex issue, which cannot be discussed in this chapter.[37] However, it is

---

[36] Compare the explanations offered by R. Moshe de Leon and the *Zohar* on the death of Rachel before Jacob's entrance to the Land of Israel. According to these texts, the interdiction to marry two sisters who are alive is stressed. Therefore, the ritualistic conception is chosen rather than the spiritual one. (See Tishby, 1982, p. 45.) The transition from a corporeal concept of relation to women to a spiritual one is also evident in an important parable adduced by R. Isaac, on the "daughter of the King"; see Idel, 1985a, pp. 53–54; see also n. 33 above.

[37] The generally accepted view of the *Shekhinah*, in ancient sources, as identical with the divinity and therefore without any feminine characteristic, was formulated by G. Scholem and E. E. Urbach and endorsed by Goldberg in his monograph. On the other hand, Patai (1978) proposed a radically different conception of the *Shekhinah* as a separate feminine entity, without, however, providing solid evidence. It seems that though the first view represents the common view of classical rabbinical sources, the second view is not totally absent.

important to stress that, for the kabbalists, the feminine characteristic of the divine manifestation is only secondarily associated with her relation with righteous humans. Primarily, she is viewed as the feminine partner of the system of nine *sephirot*, which are regarded as the "world of the male" or of their representatives, the sephirot *Tiferet* or *Yesod*. Righteous humans, therefore, are imitating the parallel relationship between the supernal righteous entities, *Yesod* and *Shekhinah*. The real, archetypical processes take place in the divine world; here below we only reflect the mysterious dynamics of the infradivine world. Like righteous humans, who stand between two females—the human and the divine—so, too, the divine female stands between two males—the human and the divine (cf. *Zohar* I, 153b; Liebes, 1982, pp. 122, 179 n. 314; 205 n. 407).

Because the relationship between righteous humans and the *Shekhinah* is, with the kabbalists, basically a mimesis of a supernal process, we may conceive it as being expressed by a "descending symbolism": The most important process takes place above,[38] and we use this symbolism in order to reflect a parallel phenomenon below. Thus, the vertical descending symbolism is rooted, according to the kabbalists, in the horizontal descending symbolism. The harmonious relation between *Tifereth* and *Malkhut*—or, as this relation was more commonly called, "*Yihud Kudsha Berikh Hu u-Shekhintei*" [the unification of the Holy One, blessed be He, and His Divine Presence]—is crucial for the welfare of the world. Only when the union between the two divine powers is achieved can the influx stemming from the *Eyn Sof* [the infinite one] be transmitted to the lower world. This harmony, which was disturbed by the primordial sin, as well as by sins in general, can be restored by the kabbalistic performance of the *mitzvot*, one of the most important of these

[38] Compare Bertil Gärtner (1961, p. 253): "[I]n the Gnostic systems the man–woman relationship is motivated basically by the structure of the heavenly world, the male and female powers which are striving after unity." The kabbalists also accepted, at least *de jure*, this rationale for their sexual behaviour; de facto, they visualized the higher worlds as ruled by the human sexual relationship as it was moulded by the halakic regulations. Or, to put it differently, kabbalists viewed symbolism as a "descending symbolism", whereas, at least from a modern perspective, this symbolism is an ascending one. See also n. 50.

being pure sexual relations. The human pair performing the sexual union is able to induce a state of harmony above. The sexual act is conceived as fraught with theurgical powers. With most of the kabbalists, this human act both reflects the higher structure and influences it. Therefore, marriage and sexual union have a tremendous impact on the upper worlds. This perception is one of the most important contributions kabbalah has made to the Jewish *modus vivendi*: Marriage and sex were transformed into a mystery that reflects a mysterious marriage above, whose success is crucial for both the divine cosmos and the lower universe. Reproduction, as the ultimate goal of the marital relations, became, in the kabbalistic *Weltanschauung*, a secondary goal; although still most important for the human pair—mostly for the husband—the theurgical significance became more and more central as kabbalistic thought developed.

One of the earliest kabbalists, R. Jehudah ben Yakar (late twelfth to early thirteenth centuries), expressed the "descending" perception of the sexual union in a very concise manner:

> and the commandment of union which concerns us is connected also to what G–d said to Shabbat:[39] Knesset Israel will be your spouse and it [Shabbat] is the Righteous, the foundation of the world (cf. Prov. 10:26), and therefrom all the spirits and souls come[40] . . . this is the reason people are accustomed to celebrate the marriage on Shabbat. [Jerushalmi, 1979, pt. II, p. 42][41]

---

[39] See *Genesis Rabba* XI, 8, pp. 95–96, adduced by R. Jehudah immediately afterward.

[40] Compare to a parallel view occurring in *Sefer ha-Bahir* (Margaliot, 1978a, par. 157): "The Righteous is alone in his world . . . and he is the foundation of all souls . . . and Scripture [supports this in saying (Ex. 31:17)]: On the seventh he rested and was refreshed [= *vayinafash*; the same Hebrew root forms the word soul = *nefesh*]."

[41] On Shabbat as a propitious time for sexual relations, see T. Ketubot 62b, the *Zohar* (several times), and the text of R. Moshe Cordovero, n. 72. It seems that the kabbalist has a quasi-astrological perception of Shabbat; because it was regarded as the divine potency, namely, the *sephirah* [*yesod*], which presides over the process of fertility, it was thought that Shabbat is particularly proper for sexual activity (and see Fromm, 1951, pp. 241–249).

Here, *Knesset Israel* is conceived of as the bride of the Shabbat, which seemingly symbolized the ninth *sefirah*, *Yesod* [= bridegroom]. Therefore, the human union, which generates the body, reflects the higher union, in the realm of the sephirot, wherefrom the souls emerge. We witness here, then, an interesting example of the transformation of an early midrash dealing with two mythic entities—*Knesset Israel* and Shabbat—into a full-fledged theosophical myth. One important factor in this shift is the overemphasis of the sexual polarity, which is apparently secondary in the midrash. Interestingly enough, one hundred years ago M. Joel pointed out the possibility that this midrash might have been composed based on the background of the Gnostic theory of syzygies [couples or pairs of entities, hierarchically arranged] (Joel, 1880, I, 107, 160–161); the mediaeval kabbalists exploited the mythical potentialities of this midrashic passage in order to elaborate their own mythical theosophy. The commandment of union is, according to R. Jehudah, an imitation of the supernal union, not only on the sexual level, but also as a custom that views Shabbat as propitious for such a union.

I would like to dwell on the way such a sexual reshaping took place. According to the wording of the midrash, Shabbat is implicitly viewed as a feminine entity whereas *Knesset Israel* is explicitly referred to as masculine: *Ben Zug* ["the (male) partner"]. However the roles change in the kabbalistic casting of this issue. Is this an arbitrary departure from the midrash, motivated by theosophic speculations? Indeed, as we have noted, Shabbat is viewed as masculine even in another early kabbalistic text, the *Book of Bahir*. However, it seems that we must also look for a more ancient conception, found, again, in the midrash. According to another passage in *Genesis Rabba* (XVII, 4, p. 156),[42] Adam could not find an appropriate mate among animals, and he exclaimed (like Shabbat), "each being has its partner, while I have no one". Here, the male is described as

[42] See Tishby, 1945, p. 17, and n. 15. It is highly probable that the identification of the cherubim with the two divine attributes is a continuation of an ancient tradition, found already in Philo and in *Midrash Tadshe* (see Goodenough, 1935, pp. 25–26; 1954, IV, p. 132; and Patai, 1978, p. 82). This issue will be elaborated in a separate study.

searching for a female mate. Therefore, I assume that this paradigm moulded the kabbalistic apperception of the relationship between Shabbat and *Knesset Israel*.

The description of the union of the sephirot *Tiferet* or *Yesod* and *Malkhut* were labelled earlier as sexual horizontal descending symbolism. According to the definition offered by Kahler of "descending symbolism", adduced at the beginning of this chapter, this term denotes a process that is symbolized by a system that is rooted in a higher level. As far as the lower sephirot are concerned, their relationship, expressed in sexual imagery, reflects an even higher sexual dichotomy described in the earliest kabbalistic treatises, where the sephirot *Hesed* and *Gevurah* were conceived of, respectively, as a pair of masculine and feminine powers. Such is the case in R. Abraham ben David of Posquieres, who regarded the two divine attributes, seemingly *Hesed* and *Gevurah*, as *du-parzufim* [possessing dual characteristics]—that is, apparently as masculine and feminine (see Scholem, 1962, pp. 232–233). Therefore, the lower sephirot reflect a higher syzygy. Indeed, a close scrutiny of the evolution of early kabbalistic symbolism evinces that the probably earlier sexual relationship of the two divine attributes, *Hesed* and *Gevurah*, influenced the same type of perception of the lower sephirot (see Idel, forthcoming). Again, this sexual understanding of the relation between *Hesed* and *Gevurah* may reflect a still higher syzygy of sephirot: *Hokhmah* and *Binah*, which were regarded, respectively, as "father" and "mother". As the lower sephirot have to be in the status of *Yehud* ["union"], so, too, do the higher sephirot, in order to attain the condition of "higher union".[43] According to important kabbalist sources, the two higher sephirot are mediated by a peculiar sephirah, *Da'at*, whose sexual overtones are almost explicit (*da'at* [knowledge] being the biblical term for sexual familiarity), mostly in the Lurianic kabbalah (see *Iggeret ha-Kodesh*, *Kitve ha-Ramban*, II, p 324). Therefore, sexual imagery played a most important role in the description of the nature of most of the divine attributes and the relations between them. Furthermore, according to the kabbalists, the existence of the syzygies in the divine world is a

[43] On the two levels of *Yehud*, or unification, see Tishby, 1963, II, pp. 261 ff.

sine qua non for the achievement of the balance that ensures the existence of the divine structure. Thus, the masculine–feminine relationship is presented by them as an all-comprehensive dynamic, which pervades the entire divine world. The human sexual relationship is, therefore, viewed as a "participation mystique" in the divine hierogamy, both by reflecting it and by influencing the divine processes.

Moreover, some of the emanational phases in the autogenesis of the divine system are described in striking sexual symbolism. The seven lower sephirot were generated out of the union between *Hokhmah* and *Binah*, the seven sephirot being commonly considered the "sons" of the higher sephirot. According to a sixteenth-century kabbalist, the whole process of emanation can be described as the successive impregnations and births of the sephirot from one another, beginning with *Causa Causarum* and ending with the last sephirah (see Abraham ben Eliezer ha-Levi's *Masoret ha-Hokhmah*, in Scholem, 1925–1926, pp. 129–130).[44] According to R. Moshe Cordovero, a leading kabbalist of Safed:

> The issue of sexual union between the divine attributes is truly symbolized by our sexual union, after the corporeal part of it has been completely deleted; the conjunction of two attributes and their desire of union can be compared to, and explained by, their comprehension of the [supernal] spiritual season which consists in the influx of the light of *Eyn Sof* onto the attributes, and they [i.e. the attributes] love each other and desire each other exactly like the desire of man for his bride, after the corporeal part of it is deleted. [See *Shiur Komah*, p. 26]

Here the relationship between the divine attributes is not only compared to the structure of the human sexual act, but also described as depending on a higher process taking place between the *Eyn Sof* and the sephirot. The usage of the term *onah* [season] has overt sexual overtones (see Ex. 21:10), and the "light" symbolizes the semen[45] that the sephirot *qua* feminine entity receive from above. I assume that the supernal season is

---

[44] On the conception of the sexual life in the work of a contemporary of Cordovero, see the important discussion of Werblowsky (1977, pp. 133–139).

[45] Compare the tantric view referred to by Eliade (1969, pp. 40–41).

the eve of Shabbat, which was considered by the kabbalists as particularly proper for sexual relations.[46]

The anonymous author of *Iggeret ha-Kodesh* summarized the kabbalistic descending symbolism when he wrote:

> All the issues we discussed[47] are the secret of the system of the order of the world and its structure, and the prototype of male and female [which are] the secret of the donor [of the influx] and [its] receiver,[48] and behold, the worthy union of man and his wife, is in the likeness of heaven and earth. [*Kitve ha-Ramban* II, 325][49]

The mainstream of kabbalah, the theosophical kabbalah, articulated earlier Jewish perceptions of human and divine existence, employing a multiplicity of sexual factors. Elements associated with the creation of humans in the Bible and midrash, with the cherubim in midrashic texts and perhaps with the divine attributes in Philo and talmudic–midrashic texts, were all structured into a comprehensive system that was apparently already evident in the very first kabbalistic sources.[50]

---

[46] See discussion of R. Jehudah ben Yakar's text above, as well as my discussion of Cordovero (Idel, 1982, pp. 54–55).

[47] Seemingly the divine powers that form the supernal *Merkavah*, namely the sephirotic realm; see *Kitve ha-Ramban* II, p. 324.

[48] *Mashpia u-mekabbel*; these terms for masculine and feminine functioning entities are widespread in R. Joseph Gikatilla's later works.

[49] These words may symbolically refer to the sephirot *Tipheret*, and *Malkhut*. Compare to the Upanishadic parallel referred to by Eliade (1971, p. 254). It is worth remarking that already in the midrash, *Numbers Rabbah* par. 2, the cherubim stand for heaven and earth.

[50] See, e.g., the conception expressed in the *Alphabet of R. Akiba* (in Wertheimer, 1955, II, p. 357): "All of the creatures that we will in the future create are [to be created] one male and one female", and see the sources adduced in idem, n. 38. This view was adopted by R. Eleazar of Worms and R. Jacob ben Sheshet (see Ben Sheshet's *Meshiv Devarim Nekhohim*, Vajda, 1969, p. 114). The issue of sexual polarity in supernal worlds in the views of the Ashkenazi Hasidism of the twelfth and thirteenth centuries is an important topic that must be meticulously inspected, because it may constitute one of the main bridges between ancient Jewish views of sexuality and early kabbalah (see also n. 51 and Harris, 1959, pp. 13–44).

It seems indeed that kabbalistic material influenced Leone Ebreo's thought, which was described as "the radical polarization of the entire universe in terms of male and female symbols" (see Perry, 1980, p. 15; see also Idel, 1985b, pp. 89–93).

This correlation between the various levels of reality permitted the kabbalists to regard the sexual union as an *imitatio Dei* from one perspective and as a theurgical act intended to induce a harmonious state in the supernal entities from another.

Moreover, kabbalists used these principles, as well as already existing motifs, in order to construct a bisexual system of the powers of evil. So, Sammael and Lilith are the "apes of God" who try to imitate the divine union in the demonic counterpart structure (see Werblowsky, 1972, II, 318–325; Dan, 1980, pp. 17–25).[51]

A comparison between the various Jewish views on the sexual relationship and some ancient Christian and Gnostic views is pertinent at this final stage of our discussion.[52] The Philonic, the talmudic-midrashic, and the kabbalistic perceptions of sexuality are all unambiguously positive. The existence of two sexes is accepted as a fact that enables humankind to perpetuate itself without any pejorative insinuation of the nature of the sexual act. The return to the primal androgyne state of humans, which was commonly described by Gnostics,[53] or the endeavour to transcend the feminine plight by mystic transformations of the female into a "male" recurring in ancient Christian thought[54] and Gnosticism (Baer, 1970, pp. 69–71),

[51] The story of the development of the demonic bisexual structure has to be reconsidered, in my opinion, in the direction of an earlier appearance of the sexual relations between the heads of demons.

[52] I consciously ignore the possibly more interesting comparison between the kabbalistic approach to sexuality and Hindu views, for I am interested in comparing conceptions that flourished in the same geographical region and could influence each other. Moreover, Gnosticism and kabbalah share the vision of the pleroma as being composed from syzygies and having hierogamic relations between them. Against this background, the discrepancies between them are even more startling.

[53] See, e.g., the *Gospel of Thomas* and the *Gospel of Philip*. The pertinent texts were adduced in Eliade, 1969, pp. 105–107; Baer, 1970, pp. 72–74; Robinson, 1970, pp. 111–117; Meeks, 1974, pp. 188–197.

[54] See *Gal.* 3:28; Meeks, 1974; Jung, 1977, pp. 373–374. This motif is well known already in Philo but, in my opinion, is unknown in Hebrew texts; see Baer, 1970, pp. 45–55. See, however, his standard Jewish attitude towards marriage (idem, pp. 75, 94–95). Philo's views on "masculinity" and "virginity" as a mystical ideal were highly influential on the patristic literature and thereby on Christian thought in general (see Cline Horowitz, 1979, pp. 190–204).

is alien to talmudic and theosophical kabbalistic *Weltanschauung.*[55]

The cherubim can be viewed when intertwined, but they can also separate from each other. Human beings can unite in the sexual act without losing their specific sexual nature. The supernal divine manifestations are supposed to attain their ideal state when the opposite divine powers are united, a union that is explicitly described in sexual imagery. Nevertheless, nowhere is this union regarded as an annihilation of two sephirot and the emergence of one, androgynous, alternative divine power. What is characteristic of the kabbalistic view is the emphasis on the attainment of a harmonious relationship between opposing principles, whose separate existence is indispensable for the welfare of the entire cosmos. Or, to put it in other words, theosophical kabbalah was not interested in a drastic restructuring of existence by either the transformation of the feminine into masculine or by their final fusion into a bisexual or asexual entity. Rather, the kabbalists were striving for an improvement of the processes going on between polar elements composing the terrestrial and the divine universes.

The kabbalists transported the human sexual relationship—not only the sexual polarity—into the supernal world; the pro-

---

[55] As Meeks (1974, p. 186) properly remarks: "In Judaism the myth (of androgyne) serves only to solve an exegetical dilemma and to support monogamy." However, the ecstatic kabbalah sometimes employs androgynous imagery, under the influence of Greek philosophy, mediated by Maimonides' works. Nevertheless, no ascetic movement emerged from this trend of thought; see n. 3 above. Another crucial difference between the Jewish and Greek view of androgyny is the positive Jewish perception of the separation between the male and female, whereas with Plato this separation is viewed as a punishment. Cf., however, Boman (1960, pp. 96–97): "the form of the myth is quite different from that in Gen. 2, but the meaning is exactly the same"! [my emphasis]. See also the Gnostic *Apocalypse of Adam* (tr. G. Macrae, in Charlesworth, 1983, I, p. 712): "God, the ruler of the aeons, and the powers, separated us wrathfully. Then we became two aeons, and the glory in our hearts deserted us, me and your mother Eve." Compare also the accusation of a *matrona* that God created woman "by thievery" (Gen., Rabba, XVII, 7, p. 158) versus the answer of R. Jose, who stresses God's benevolence. On the possible Gnostic background of this passage, see Gershenzon-Eliezer Slomovic, 1985, pp. 20–22.

cesses there had to conform to human sexual behaviour. The Gnostic view attempted to copy the higher rule of androgyneity or asexuality in the lower world.[56] Gnostic—and to a certain extent also Christian—attitudes towards sexuality represent an important aspect of their more comprehensive rejection of this world (see Meeks, 1974, p. 207). The Gnostic and Christian eschatologies present a spiritual escapism that aims at the restoring of the paradisiac androgyny or asexual status of the believer. At least in the Gnostic case, the uneasiness extends beyond this world to its evil creator, sexuality being regarded as an instrument implanted by him into humans in order to perpetuate his evil world. Christian asceticism is but a milder attitude towards the temporary plight of the world until the second arrival of the Saviour. The sexual instinct was either suppressed or partially sublimated in the form of love of Christ.

Under the impact of the halakhic views, kabbalah dealt with the regulation of the libido rather than with its suppression or sublimation. This attitude towards sex and sexuality is generally this-world-oriented; the main effort was invested in their attempt to find the golden mean between the sexual asceticism cultivated by the Christian mystics and an uncommon emphasis on the centrality of the sexual processes, which could explode the regular texture of the family life.[57] The danger that haunted Jewish mediaeval kabbalah was not an exaggerated spirituality that disregarded "carnal" love, but an outburst of positively perceived sexual relationships beyond the boundaries of halakhah.

---

[56] Or, as Jung put it very adequately, "Gnosticism . . . endeavoured in all seriousness to subordinate the physiological to the metaphysical" (1959, p. 177). Meeks (1974, p. 207) uses the phrase "metaphysical rebellion" in his description of androgynous tendencies in Christian and Gnostic circles. It seems that with kabbalah the situation was completely different.

[57] See the various midrashic discussions of God's ongoing pairing couples since the end of the creation of the world, collected, translated, and analysed by Agus (1980, pp. 18–30). Though Agus may indeed be right in his emphasis of the anti-Gnostic character of the rabbinic perception of God as an *arche-Shadkhen*, some anti-Christian tendencies may also have contributed to the emergence of this view. I hope to deal elsewhere with this problem. (See also Gershenzon-Slomovic, 1985, pp. 28–29.)

The balance between a positive and natural attitude towards sexuality and its perception as a reflection of the supernal hierogamy also had its problems. When the halakhic regulations weakened, one of the main and immediate results was a removal of the sexual inhibitions. Shabbateanism and Frankism, two sects connected with mystical Judaism, deviated from kabbalah mainly by their transgression of incest interdictions—transgressions that were interpreted as the imitation of unrestrained relations in the divine world (see Scholem, 1972, pp. 136–137). Both extreme Shabbateans and Frankists based their licentious behaviour on classical kabbalistic texts.[58] Like the Gnostics,[59] the Shabbateans viewed the perfect man—in their case Shabbatai Zevi—as being free from all moral restrictions and as belonging to Gan Eden, a paradisiac state, as opposed to the lower world, described as "the heart" of the demonic world.[60] Moreover the very core of Shabbatai Zevi's activity was once described as the restoration of the glory of sexuality, seemingly of the unrestrained sort:

> The patriarchs came into the world to restore the senses and this they did to four of them. Then came Shabbatai Zevi and restored the fifth, the sense of touch, which, according to Aristotle (*Nicomachean Ethics*, III, 10, 1118b) and Maimonides (see *Guide of the Perplexed* II, 36, 40; III, 8, 49), is a source of shame for us, but which now has been raised by him to a place of honour and glory. [Quoted in Jacob Emden, *Sefer hit'abekut* (Lvov, 1877) 6a, in Scholem, 1972, p. 117][61]

We witness here a clear case where metaphysics—in this case, kabbalistic theosophy—turned into an independent factor that shaped the behaviour of persons. When put into the service

---

[58] They were designated as *Zoharisten* because of their frequent leaning on this work.

[59] On the phenomenological affinity between radical forms of Shabbateanism and Gnosticism, see, e.g., Scholem, 1972, pp. 132–133.

[60] See Natan ha-Azati's *Treatise on the Menorah* (printed in Scholem, 1934, p. 102); see also Scholem, 1973, pp. 810, 311–312.

[61] The presentation of Shabbatai Zevi as the redeemer of the sense of touch is rather curious. Almost all the kabbalists refuted Maimonides's view and agreed on a positive perception of the sexual act; see the stand of *Iggeret ha-Kodesh*, ch. 2 (Chavel, 1967, pp. 323–324).

of the metaphysical "idea", with ordinary sexual modes obliterated, orgiastic practices turned into a *via mystica* of the new aeon. No wonder the next important development of Jewish mysticism—Hasidism—was much more reticent in using sexual symbolism.

Finally, a remark on the metamorphosis of the above-mentioned attitudes towards sexuality in our own period may be pertinent. The ancient Jewish attitude towards sexuality as a mystery, as represented by midrashim describing the holy of holies, had a profound impact on Judaism in general and on kabbalah in particular. The supernal hierogamy and its lower reflection in the marital relations became one of the basic tenets of kabbalistic lore; at least on this point, kabbalah elaborated on an already existing Jewish topic.[62] This unequivocal view of sexuality had an important repercussion in modern psychoanalysis through Freud's appreciation of the libido.[63]

On the other hand, the reticent and sometimes ambiguous attitude towards sexuality and marriage in Christianity and Gnosticism found its expression in the works of Carl Jung and Mircea Eliade.[64] These scholars were not only deeply interested in the Gnostic mythology, but they even seem to have adopted several Gnostic *mythologoumena*, as atemporal truths[65] or even

[62] This most important insight, shared by several authors, was ignored by the founders of the scholarly study of kabbalah such as Scholem and Tishby; cf. Patai, 1978, pp. 119ff; M. Kasher (in n. 18); Baer,1975, pp. 101–104.

[63] David Bakan's assertion that Jewish mystical tradition had indeed influenced Freud's views seems to be a sound approach, notwithstanding the author's difficulties when he attempted to prove it by using historical arguments. It is enough to recognize that, at least regarding sexuality, the Jewish "non-mystical" attitude was not so far from the kabbalistic one and that the general positive approach to this issue was a common denominator for most of the Jews.

[64] I refer primarily to their acceptance of the hermaphrodite or androgynic idea as a symbol for human perfection; see their works referred to in nn. 53, 54, and 56; Eliade, 1971; see especially Eliade's discussion of androgynization (1969, pp. 111–114).

[65] Jung's perception of the androgyne as archetype is a fine example; according to him, androgyny as a "primordial idea has become a symbol of the creative union of opposites, a 'uniting symbol' in the literal sense" (see Jung, 1959, p. 174).

as spiritual guidance for our age.[66] Individual perfection is the ultimate goal of their idealization of androgyneity, as opposed to the creative interest, be it procreation or restoration of divine harmony, in the theosophical kabbalah. Any further comment would be superfluous.

---

[66] See Eliade, 1969, p. 100, where he refers to androgyny as a symbol for the "wholeness resulting from the fusion of the sexes", "a new type of humanity in which the fusion of the sexes produces a new unpolarized consciousness"; and also p. 114. Compare his sympathetic description of orgiastic rituals (Eliade, 1963, pp. 356ff., especially p. 361). For Eliade as a creative hermeneut who attempted to further a spiritual discipline, see Branneman, Yarian, & Olson, 1982, pp. 57–71.

Comments

Jacob A. Arlow

BISEXUALITY IN JEWISH MYSTICISM

It takes more than a degree of daring to apply the techniques of psychoanalytic interpretation to Jewish mysticism and the Kabbalah. Yet we are encouraged, even urged on, by the sentence with which Gershom Scholem concludes his book, *On the Kaballah and Its Symbolism.* He says, ". . . the historian's task ends where the psychologist's begins" (Scholem, 1965, p. 204).

In this chapter Idel essentially confronts the issue of androgyny or bisexuality in Jewish mysticism, although he does not state the issue in these terms until the last page. He begins, instead, by stating, "It is a commonplace that mystical literature is inclined to express the relationship between the mystic soul and the divine by means of erotic imagery. All the classical bodies of mystical writings can easily provide numerous examples, sometimes striking ones, wherein sexual images are openly and often employed. Kabbalah has nothing unique on this issue; it also extensively uses sexual images and metaphors. However, there is something novel in this body of literature that transcends the more common usage of erotic and sexual motifs. The difference lies not so much in the texts, but in their sociological context" (p. 219). According to the author, in the ecstatic kabbalah the mystic or his spiritual faculties are presented as female, whereas the divine powers (viz., the active intellect of God Himself) are viewed as the male partner.

From the psychological point of view, certain problems become apparent immediately. While it is true that Kabbalistic writings, in common with other mystical literatures, express the relationship between the individual mystic and the Divine by means of erotic imagery, what is striking is that such imagery and metaphor should be used in *Jewish* mystical writings. In Jewish tradition, explicit imagery of male and female erotic interaction depicting the relationship between the mystic and the Divine is from many points of view a startling phenomenon. Such concepts were foreign indeed to the moulders of Jewish religious thought, certainly in the rabbinic tradition. As Idel clearly indicates,

> In the Bible and the talmudic–midrashic texts, the relationship between God and the Jewish people, sometimes designated as *Knesset Israel*, is described as the relation between husband and wife. This was also the main avenue adopted in the exegetical literature of the Song of Songs in mediaeval texts, which regarded the plain meaning of the Biblical text to be concerned with the people of Israel and God. This is obviously a part of the national myth, which changes the entire nation into one entity standing in sexual relation to the other entity—the Divinity. This mythical relationship has little to do with mysticism; it is interested primarily in the whole nation as a unit, whereas the particular Jew is rather neglected as a meaningful factor. The individual, according to classical Jewish texts, can take part in this bond with God by his participation in the significant great unity, *Knesset Israel* [the community of Israel]. . . . This bond mediates between the individual Jew and the Divinity whenever this relation is expressed in sexual terms. [pp. 219–220]

While the love of God, the wish to be at one with Him, to be united in loving kindness, acceptance, and forgiveness, is richly expressed in the Biblical and rabbinic literature, an explicit demarcation of the role of the individual's relationship to the

Godhead in sexual terms, using precise erotic imagery, is unknown.

In Jewish tradition, God is always described and referred to as masculine. A female goddess equal in power and importance to the male god, sharing dominion over the fate of man, does not appear. How significant a role the female goddess Ishtar, referred to in several places in the preachings of the prophets, played at any time in the history of the Hebrew people is difficult to determine. Neither she nor any similar figure ever loomed as a competitor or a participant in the authority of the divine Yahweh. A female image connected with the Godhead seems to have disappeared quite early in the course of Jewish theological development.

It has been suggested that the oft-repeated yearning for the land of Israel, for the city of Jerusalem, and for the Holy Temple served as substitute expressions of love for the mother. Be that as it may, Judaism differed from most of the other religions alongside which it developed. No place was accorded the Great Mother as a consort of the divine power. It can hardly be doubted that the absence of a mother goddess in Jewish moral and religious tradition must have played some role in shaping the character and personality of the Jews.

Personal identity is an amalgam of both male and female elements—a natural consequence of the nature of the family and the fact that most individuals are raised by both a mother and a father. The consolidation of the mature sexual identity is by no means a simple process, and it does not reach its culmination until sometime during the period of adolescence. A mature sexual identity is usually organized in keeping with the social mores, consistent with the obvious anatomical nature of the individual. Nevertheless, certain psychological features and wishes appropriate to the opposite sex remain, and, although subordinated to the manifest sexual identity, they are nonetheless incorporated into the final personality structure. Clinical experience teaches us that the process of achieving a mature, relatively conflict-free sexual identity is beset by many difficulties. Conflicts over identification with the opposite sex may arise in different individuals to a greater or lesser degree, depending upon the nature of their endowment, their early life experience, and, of course, the social milieu in which they were raised. The social mores control and limit the employment and gratification of opposite-sex tendencies in the individual identity. Conflicts of this sort are by no means unusual. The practices of different religions frequently afford an outlet for conflicts of this kind, such as the celibate Catholic priest attired in feminine garb. Judaism, on the other hand, offers fewer organized outlets for opposite-gender wishes and aspirations.

Because Judaism developed largely as a masculine enterprise, righteousness, the path to God's love, was concretely experienced as obedience to God's commandments, unquestioning submission to His will, and finding grace in His eyes. Of the 613 commandments or rules that the Jew was called upon to honour, only three applied only to women—the lighting of the Sabbath candles, the challah and its sacrificial portion, and, specifically, the rules of sexual purity. The latter two could clearly be conceived of as in the husbands' interests. In effect, women were physically and spiritually dependent upon their husbands' relationship to a male God. In the case of the individual man, his fortune in life articulated God's love or disapproval. In the case of the nation, the vicissitudes of history represented the divine judgement on the merits or sins of the nation. As in the case of the individual, the suffering and the disasters of Jewish history constituted proof manifest that the people had sinned. Suffering, instead of expiating guilt, only intensified it (Arlow, 1987). The relationship of God to both the individual and to His chosen people was one of moral judgement, not one of erotic sensibility. By fulfilling His commandments, one attained His grace. There was little room, if any, for the sensuous and the erotic in this relationship. Sensuality and physical pleasure were to be avoided.

For example, according to rabbinic literature, if you cease your studies in order to admire the beauties of nature, it is almost as if you had forfeited your soul. The relationship to the Divine perforce had to become a masochistic one, structuralized within a code of commandments to be obeyed. This type of masochism, however, was not perverse, nor manifestly sensuous. Physical flagellation and submitting to actual pain was not part of the tradition. On the other hand, for the individual, the alternative of a sensuous, erotic relationship to the Godhead was equally unacceptable, since it would be connected with the fear and danger of homosexual submission. Such a combination of factors clearly would foster the development of moral masochistic character formation.

In one of his pithy, all-encompassing observations, Freud noted that moral masochism represents a regression from true morality to negative Oedipus complex (1924c). This statement deserves more elaboration than is possible at this point. Briefly put, moral masochism as a rule develops in the following way. At a certain stage in his development, the male child, under special conditions, adopts a loving, feminine, passive, submissive attitude towards the father. Since sexual submission, however, is unacceptable, this trend is opposed and may be replaced by a painful but nevertheless more acceptable compromise formation; instead of wishing to submit sexually in the manner of a woman, the individual substitutes the wish to be beaten physically. At this level one outcome could be the development of a masochistic perversion. However, in a further defensive manoeuvre, the wish to be beaten physically is replaced by a tendency to be oppressed by moral strictures. At first these strictures may be experienced as emanating from the father figure. In turn, however, they may be replaced by the laws and commandments imposed by God and experienced as a constant inner moral imperative.

To be sure, moral masochism is an important dynamic in almost every religion—more in some than in others, more perhaps in Protestantism than in Catholicism. In Judaism, however, the absence of some representation of the female principle in the Godhead, I would suggest, facilitates the development of moral masochism.

Religions that have a divine presence female in nature afford an opportunity to invoke the protection of a loving mother figure, an intercessor with a more punitive male Godhead. In such religions, the presence of a female principle also makes it possible for the individual to overcome guilt in a spirit of loving reunion with the female goddess or her substitute. Religious experience thus can become more manifestly erotic in nature and at the same time less threatening to the individual male. In Catholicism, for example, this only serves as a stopgap, because the final judge and arbiter is the unquestioned male image of God. But through His son, who embodies many qualities characteristically or historically associated with the female nature—that is, tenderness, compassion, forgiveness—through this ambiguous sexual identity, the fear of passive sexual submission to a male God is mitigated.

Accordingly, from the psychoanalytic point of view, the manifest sexualized relationship between the individual mystic and God would represent an undoing of the defensive compromise of moral masochism, leading it back to its antecedent stage of sexual love and submission. (While we have many accounts of the sexual sensations experienced by Christian mystics, particularly women, vis-à-vis the Godhead, there are no comparable detailed expositions of sexual elements in the ecstasy of Jewish mysticism that have come to my attention.) Accordingly, I would suggest that the introduction of the concept of the *Shekhinah* as a representative of the female aspect of the divinity and the more manifest role of sexuality in ordering the universe must have proved to be an appealing escape from the rigours of moral masochism. Undoubtedly, this must have played some role in the fact that Hasidism readily responded to and incorporated mysticism and Kabbalah as part of life and thought. To quote Scholem (1965),

> This discovery of a feminine element in God, which the Kabbalists tried to justify by gnostic exegesis, is of course one of the most significant steps they took, often regarded with the utmost misgiving by strictly Rabbinical non-Kabbalistic Jews. Often distorted into inoffensiveness by embarrassed Kabbalistic apologists, this mystical conception of the feminine principle of the *Shekhinah* as a providential guide of creation achieved enormous popularity among the masses of the Jewish people, so showing that here the Kabbalists had uncovered one of the primordial religious impulses still latent in Judaism. [p. 105]

The concept of the *Shekhinah* accordingly introduced or re-introduced sensuality and sexuality into Jewish theosophy. Whenever or wherever the *Shekhinah* abided, there was the awareness of some feminine erotic principle. How to view the significance of the role of the *Shekhinah* from the point of view of psychoanalytic psychology would be quite difficult. We are faced with the question as to what extent the feminine sexual components in mystical and Kabbalistic thinking constituted an awareness, by way of the mechanism of projection of the repressed, feminine, sexual components in the mystic's psychology. Idel comes close to this issue but then backs away. For example, he states, "The ecstatic kabbalah, on the other hand, presents the mystic or his spiritual faculties as the female, whereas the supernal powers (viz. the active intellect of God Himself) are viewed as the male partner" (p. 218). But, as if to counter any suggestion of feminine *sexual* tendencies in the mystic, Idel emphasizes that "Jewish mystics . . . shared with other Jews the conviction that actual marriage and fulfilment of the command to multiply are religious imperatives and, accordingly, the kabbalists could hardly be regarded as persons who employed sexual metaphors as a compensation for the frustration of 'real' erotic experiences" (p. 219). He goes on to cite several leading Kabbalists who were married or who at least viewed sexual relations as permissible and desirable as evidence that the "relatively common explanations offered by some scholars to the genesis of sexual imagery in the repressed libido can be no more than a partial solution" (p. 219).

This point would be well taken if only typical *heterosexual* impulses were concerned, but we know from experience that there are other non-heterosexual desires that each individual may possess to a greater or lesser degree and which he may try to master in a variety of ways. Sexual imagery permitting identification with the female in religious mystical experience could represent one way out of such dilemmas. In some way, Idel is aware of this when he goes on to say that in the mediaeval period a mystical relationship between the individual and God made its appearance, and the human *soul* was conceived as female in relation to the divine male entity. A further example of this awareness on the part of the author occurs when he states, ". . . the shift from the classical to the speculative view of *Knesset Israel* as the spouse of God: only when it was interpreted as referring to the individual was this term related to the mystical union between two monads. Only then could the kabbalist see himself as the 'female' into whom the divine spark is sown and the spiritual son born. That is, a transmutation of the human spirit takes place as a result of contact with the Divine" (pp. 222–223).

In his efforts to buttress his arguments opposing the concepts of androgyny—or, as we psychoanalysts would prefer to say, psychic bisexuality—Idel maintains that the actual experience of sexual contact is not essential for the ecstasy and that the act of sexual union plays no ritualistic role in the mystical experience. "By its nature, ecstatic kabbalah is mostly interested in spiritual processes for which the corporeal actions would be only a hindrance" (p. 223).

In much of the material, one can discern references to an equation of the Ark and the Holy of Holies, on one hand, and the female genital on the other. The Ark of the Covenant, the Holy of Holies, and the Land of Israel "was a place where the female principle, the Shekhinah, dwells". Following the logic of this concept, a pure union of male and female serves as a restorative act, enabling the *Shekhinah* to keep her natural place amid the Jewish union. Intercourse and procreation are done for the sake of the divinity, an effort to reestablish the harmony that existed when the Temple was functioning. Alongside this sexual imagery concerning God and the people of Israel is the parallel representation of the mystical qualities of sexual intercourse between a man and his wife. According to the Kaballah, the pure intentions required during sexual intercourse may eventuate in raising human thought to a superior source, and thus causing the descent of *Shekhinah*. According to the Kabbalists, the *Shekhinah* descends upon the couple during proper intercourse. However, Idel states that the *Shekhinah* does not play the role of the female, and no mention of sexual relations between the male and the *Shekhinah* can be discerned in reference to this issue. In spite of these disavowals, the imagery created is that of three presences—the male, the female, and the *Shekhinah*—the latter definitely a female representation. It should strike us as at least challenging that a third party becomes a member of this very intimate relationship. In the course of psychoanalytic therapy, third-party situations of this sort make their appearance in many forms. Not infrequently during the act of intercourse an individual may think or fantasize about someone other than the partner in the sexual act at the time. Furthermore, the situation suggests a type of dream that is quite common during the course of psychoanalytic experience. These are dreams in which the patient sees himself or herself in the treatment situation with the analyst present when a third party walks in. As a rule, the intruding third party is an unwelcome presence, because it represents a repudiated aspect of the patient's wishful thinking, one that threatens the emergence of anxiety and/or guilt. Accordingly, the presence of the *Shekhinah* during sexual intercourse may be viewed as representing the intrusion of the mystic's feminine wishes. In the same spirit, actual sexual experiences in which a couple and a third party participate most often reveal, upon analysis, an underlying homosexual wish. Viewed in this manner, the presence of the *Shekhinah* could represent a means of mastering the anxiety associated with homosexual impulses through the process of idealization of the feminine urges. Or, to put it another way, through its connection with divine purpose, feminine wishes represented by the *Shekhinah* as projections of the individual mystic's homosexual urges are made acceptable and welcome. Accordingly, one could generalize from this point to state that the impetus for ecstatic mystical experience could represent for many individuals a "sublimation" of sexual wishes for a divine God-father image. By immersing themselves in Kabbalah and mysticism, certain individuals may have found an adaptive resolution of their bisexual conflicts. Often enough, as we know from history, such efforts failed in their purpose, with the result that many leading figures in the Jewish community felt that the study of Kabbalah and mysticism should be the province of the emotionally mature and the mentally strong. On the other hand, the recognition of the value of mystical experience, of the role of ecstasy and sensuousness in the life of the individual, may have eased to some extent the moral burden of observing the commandments and, in fact, might have prepared the way, as has been suggested, for Hasidism, a movement that is both spiritual and joyous.

CHAPTER EIGHT

Crossing gender boundaries in kabbalistic ritual and myth

Elliot Wolfson

Despite the acknowledged fact that the trend of mediaeval Jewish mysticism known as "theosophic kabbalah" is distinguished in the religious history of Judaism by the explicit and repeated use of gender symbolism to characterize the nature of the divine, the state of research in this area is still somewhat rudimentary. Indeed, the majority of previous studies on gender in the relevant kabbalistic literature have been marred by a conspicuous lack of sophistication. Most scholars who have written on issues relevant to this subject-matter have taken for granted that the occurrence of gender images should be interpreted within a framework of what may be called a naive biologism—that is, the presumption that the differences between male and female are linked essentially and exclusively to biological functions. Needless to say, such an orientation fails to recognize that the latter in and of themselves are indicators of sexual but not gender differentiation. While there obviously is a correlation between biological sex and gender identity, the two are not equivalent, as recent scholars in the fields of cultural anthropology and feminist psychology have emphasized. Gender identity is engendered by cultural assumptions concerning maleness and femaleness that interpret the body. In that respect we should speak of gender as a sociocultural construction that is a matter of semiology (reading cultural signs) rather than physiology (marking bodily organs). The body is a sign whose signification is determined by the ideological assumptions of a given society. There is no body without culture, as there is no culture without body.[1]

In this study I will attempt to illuminate the role of gender in kabbalistic symbolism by exploring the phenomenon of crossing gender boundaries—that is, the transformation of the feminine into the masculine and the masculine into the feminine. An examination of these phenomena will disclose that the theosophic myth that informed kabbalistic symbolism and ritual reflects the androcentric and patriarchical norms of mediaeval society in general and that of rabbinic culture more particularly. Even though the kabbalists consistently speak of the unity and perfection of God in terms of the union of masculine and feminine, the idea of ultimate wholeness or oneness is predicated on a reconstituted male androgyne.[2] The kabbalistic representation of androgyny, therefore, is that of the one male force who represents the ideal anthropos that comprises both masculine and feminine traits. Applying the mythic account of the creation of man and woman in the second chapter of Genesis to the Divine, the kabbalists posit that the female is part of the male. Just as the Yahwist version of creation depicts woman, who comes

---

[1] See Bynum, 1986, p. 7; Epstein & Straub, 1991, p. 3.

[2] See Wolfson, 1994f, pp. 166–204; see also Wolfson, 1995a, pp. 79–121, and notes to this chapter. In those studies, as well as here, I do not deny that some kabbalists describe the Infinite [*Ein–Sof*] in terms that would suggest a transcendence of gender. I contend, however, that the neuter Infinite reflects an attempt to portray the kabbalistic myth in philosophically acceptable terms. I do not consider the philosophical transformation of the myth in political terms as a kind of intellectual dishonesty of acquiescence. On the contrary, theosophic kabbalists of the Middle Ages were living in environments that incorporated, to one degree or another, philosophical modes of religious discourse. The main point, however, is that alongside these more speculative formulations is a deep structured myth predicated on a gendered Infinite, as I have argued at length in the aforementioned studies. The personal character of the *Ein-Sof* in kabbalistic writings has been emphasized recently by a number of scholars; see references in Wolfson, 1995a, p. 194 n. 201.

from man, as secondary and derivative, so in the kabbalistic theosophic appropriation of that myth the feminine aspect of the Godhead is supplementary and ontically inferior to the masculine.[3] The privileging of the male will become evident in both forms of gender transformation discussed in this chapter.

On being male

Ontic containment of the feminine in the masculine

The theoretical presumption underlying the possibility of the female becoming male is the notion that femaleness is, in fact, only an aspect of masculinity. The ontic inclusion of the feminine in the masculine is a recurring and fundamental motif in theosophic kabbalah from the incipient stage of its literary manifestation.[4] Consider, for example, the following description of the sefirotic pleroma:

> Therefore [the sixth emanation] is called the median line, and corresponding to it below is the Foundation (*Yesod*) which is the phallus (*berit*) and the end of the body (*sof ha-guf*). Endurance (*Neṣaḥ*) and Majesty (*Hod*) correspond to the thighs, Endurance is the right leg and Majesty the left

[3] To be more precise, it must be noted that the kabbalists read the Priestly version of the creation of man and woman (especially as mediated through the rabbinic conception of the androgyne) in light of the Yahwistic version. That is, there is no appreciable difference in orientation between the two creation accounts. On the contrary, the secondary status accorded the woman in the Yahwistic version is used to interpret the ostensibly more egalitarian approach of the Priestly version. For discussion of the two creation narratives from the vantage point of human sexuality and gender, see Bird, 1991, pp. 11–34. On the appropriation of the Yawhistic account in Christian literature in the patristic and mediaeval period, see Bloch, 1991, pp. 22–29.

[4] See Tishby, 1989, p. 289. Tishby notes that the feminine *Shekhinah*, the last of the ten *sefirot*, is not to be regarded as a "second man" but rather as the "completion of the male image". Tishby nevertheless speaks of the "harmonious partnership of male and female" and thus does not appreciate the extent of the androcentric representation of the female in kabbalistic symbolism.

> leg. Thus you have the form of an anthropos fixed in the ten *sefirot*. . . . The Foundation is called the Righteous (*Ṣaddiq*) . . . and it corresponds to the phallus (*berit*) and it is the one that unites the secret of circumcision for it is joined to the Kingdom (*Malkhut*) which is the tenth that is the Crown (*'Atarah*). Therefore, the rabbis, blessed be their memory, said that the Community of Israel is the mate of Beauty (*Tif'eret*). The Crown is symbolized by the tongue, and she is this world, for she is [assigned] the governance of this world by means of the overflow that reaches her from the Foundation. [Ms. NYJTSA, Mic. 2194, fols. 25a–b]

The divine potencies [*sefirot*] are circumscribed within the shape of an anthropos. That the sex of that anthropos is male is obvious from the explicit reference to the penis. By contrast, no mention is made of a corresponding feminine form or even of the female genitals. The aspect of the divine that corresponds to the feminine, the tenth gradation, is linked anatomically to the tongue of the singular masculine form.[5]

---

[5]It is of interest to note that in the diagram accompanying this text (Ms. NYJTSA Mic. 2194, fol. 25a), the sefirotic potencies are configured in a shape that resembles that of a penis extended upward. The significance of this graphic depiction is that the *sefirot* collectively constitute one phallic entity. No independent place is accorded the feminine. Compare the depiction of the *sefirot* in the shape of a phallus in the version of the anonymous thirteenth-century *Sefer ha-Yiḥud* in Ms. VBAE 236, fol. 174a. Interestingly, the Infinite is represented by a black circle that crowns a line extending upward from the first *sefirah* designated as *'Ayin*. It is hardly coincidental that the black circle resembles the corona of a penis. Cf. Ms. VBAE 274, fol. 167a. According to the drawing of the sefirotic hypostases in this manuscript, there is similarly one form that constitutes a phallic representation of the divine. The feminine, or the last of the emanations, is depicted as the foot of this one form rather than a separate entity. It is also noteworthy that the first of the emanations is portrayed as the head of the penis, thus lending credence to my conjecture concerning an upper phallus. What is here graphically represented is expressed in other kabbalistic documents. See, e.g., the phallic description of *Keter* in the anonymous commentary on the *sefirot* in Ms. NYJTSA Mic. 1805, fol. 15b. See below, n. 65. The phallic character of *Keter* is highlighted in the Idrot sections of the *Zohar*. See, e.g., the description of the skull [*gulgalta'*] in *Zohar* 2:128b–130a, 135b–136a (*'Idra' Rabba'*) and the description of the thirteen adornments of the beard of *'Arikh 'Anpin* in ibid., 130b–134b. For parallel discussions see *Zohar* 3:288a–289b, 292b–293b (*'Idra' Zuta'*). In particular, the image of the oil overflowing

The ontological dependence of the female on the male is expressed in a striking way in a kabbalistic commentary on the secret of illicit sexual relations [*sod 'arayot*], which reflects the unique terminology and thought of the kabbalist, Joseph of

---

from the curls of the beard has a strikingly phallic connotation. See *Zohar* 3, 139a where the homoerotic implication of this symbolism is evident: "When the holy flowing oil goes down from the supernal glorious beard of the Holy Ancient One, who is concealed and hidden from everything, to the beard of *Ze'eir 'Anpin*, his beard is arrayed in nine adornments." The homoerotic element seems also to be implied in the depiction of the ocular gaze in *Zohar* 3, 128b: "When *Ze'eir 'Anpin* looks at ['*Arikh 'Anpin*] everything below is arrayed, and his countenances extend and spread out at that time, but not all the time as [is the case with] *'Atiqa'*." The extension of the face is a euphemism for the elongated phallus. See *Zohar* 3, 133b: "When the two apples are revealed *Ze'eir 'Anpin* appears to be happy and all the lights below are joyous." It appears that in that context the apples symbolically represent the testicles (see nn. 114 and 115 below). The phallic signification may also underlie the designation of the beard of *'Arikh 'Anpin* as *mazzal*, which is connected etymologically in the kabbalistic imagination with the root *nzl* [to overflow]. Cf. *Zohar* 3, 134a and 289a–b. The phallic implications of many of these images are developed along similar, but not always identical, lines in the writings of other kabbalists who may have been involved in the zoharic circle, e.g. Joseph of Hamadan, especially his *Sefer Tashaq* (see Zwelling, 1975) and a fragment of an Aramaic text extant in Ms. JM 134, fols. 124a–131b, David ben Yehudah he-Ḥasid, especially in *Sefer ha-Gevul*, his translation of and commentary on a section of the *'Idra' Rabba'* (on the phallic nature of *Keter*, cf. *The Book of Mirrors: Sefer Mar'ot ha-Ẓove'ot by R. David ben Yehudah he-Ḥasid* (Matt, 1982, pp. 94, 220), and Joseph Gikatilla, especially in his *Sod Yod-Gimmel Middot ha-Nove'ot min ha-Keter 'Elyon* (Scholem, 1930, pp. 219–225; see esp. 221–222). See Liebes, 1993, pp. 103–134. The phallic character of the uppermost aspect of God according to the symbolism of the Idrot is depicted iconically in *Sefer ha-Gevul*. To mention a few salient examples from two manuscript versions that I examined: In Ms. NYJTSA Mic. 2193, fol. 2b, there is a depiction of the skull [*gulgolet*] that extends downward from the supernal crown [*keter 'elyon*] through the path [*netiv*] to the world of the righteous [*'olam ha-ṣaddiqim*]. The shape of this diagram is that of a phallus pointing downward, for the flow of semen goes from top to bottom. In the same manuscript, fol. 4a, *'Arikh 'Anpin* and *Ze'eir 'Anpin* are configured in the shape of a phallus pointing upward. The head of the phallus, or the corona, is labelled *'Arikh 'Anpin* and the base of the phallus consists of the thirty-two paths of *Ze'eir 'Anpin*. Cf. *Sefer ha-Gevul*, Ms. NYJTSA Mic. 2197, fols. 6b, 8b, 9a, 13a, 16b, 20b, 30a.

Hamadan, active in the late-thirteenth and early-fourteenth centuries:

> In the middle of a person are two orifices that separate him into two things . . . sometimes male and sometimes female. Similarly, his face and his back are two faces, the great face and the small face. Thus is God and His equanimous unity, His name and His essence are one thing, for there are two faces, the great face and the small face, *ze'eir 'anpin* and *rav 'anpin*, the face that is illuminated and the face that is not illuminated, the speculum that shines and the speculum that does not shine. . . . This was the form of the cherubim, the form of male and female. [Ms. OBL[6] 1565, fol. 15b]

It is evident from this text that the male and female aspects of the divine, represented, respectively, by the technical terms "great face" and "small face", *rav 'anpin* and *ze'eir 'anpin*,[7] are comprised within one anthropomorphic figure. The two faces are respectively the front and back of that one form. Moreover, genital dimorphism is attributed not to a pair of independent organs, but, rather, to the two orifices found in one body.

In spite of the fact that Joseph of Hamadan's writings are replete with graphic and dramatic descriptions of the feminine persona who complements and receives the overflow from the masculine,[8] it can be shown that he, too, posited one divine form that is an androgynous male. Thus, for example, in one passage he writes:

> The secret of the letter *dalet* and [the letter] *gimmel* is one image of the body of the holy King, for the *gimmel* reveals the head, neck, right arm, and part of the body, [symbolized by

[6] See also Ms. NYJTSA Mic. 1777, fol. 15a

[7] On the shift in meaning of these terms in Joseph of Hamadan as compared to the zoharic literature, see Idel, 1988b, pp. 134–135; Liebes, 1993, pp. 105–107; Mopsik, 1992, p. 214 n. 34.

[8] See Idel, 1988a, pp. 47–55. Joseph of Hamadan was especially fond of the image of the cherubim which he uses constantly to relate the erotic dynamic between the ninth and tenth gradations. Moreover, one finds in his writings graphic descriptions of the female anatomy that go beyond what one finds even in the more recondite strata of zoharic literature. See, e.g., "Joseph of Hamadan's *Sefer Tashak*" (Zwelling, 1975), pp. 123–124, 296ff.

> the letter] *yod*, and the letter *dalet* the image of the whole body and the left arm. Thus the whole body is completed by these two letters. . . . The head, arms, and body are complete, but the holy legs are not revealed except in the letter *he'* for it has two holy legs. And the *he'* is called the Matrona. ["Joseph of Hamadan's *Sefer Tashak*", Zwelling, 1975, p. 152][9]

The complete body of the divine anthropos is represented by the vertical alignment of the contiguous letters *gimmel*, *dalet*, and *he'*. Significantly, the feminine character, designated by the technical term *Matrona*, is located in the legs of this corporeal form. Although no mention is made of the male genitals, it is fairly obvious that the upper part of the anthropomorphic figure is masculine, referred to specifically as the "body of the holy King". The divine anthropos consists of the unity of the masculine and the feminine, but the latter is portrayed as an aspect of the former—that is, the two together comprise the singular image of the body of the King.[10] The goal of the *hieros gamos* is to

---

[9] On the masculine and feminine symbolism connected respectively with *gimmel* and *dalet*, see ibid., pp. 147–148.

[10] The androgynous quality of the phallus is also alluded to in the remarks of Joseph of Hamadan that the *gimmel* symbolizes both the masculine King (pp. 148–149) and the *Matrona* sitting upon a throne (p. 150). It is of interest to note the following observation of Joseph of Hamadan in his commentary on the *sefirot*, Ms. OBL 1678, fol. 66b:

> This attribute [*Ḥokhmah*] forever overflows, for from the side of *Binah* and onwards there is masculinity and femininity, emanating from one side and receiving from another side. But [in] the attribute of *Ḥokhmah* everything is conjoined to one another, and masculinity and femininity are not yet discernible, i.e. it is not known in what side it emanates and in what side it receives. Therefore this attribute does not emanate and receive but rather only emanates.

(See ibid., fols. 67a–b, where *Binah* is likewise described as comprising masculinity and femininity, bestowing and receiving, and is called by the name androgynous.) Even though gender is said not to apply to *Ḥokhmah*, the latter is described as overflowing or emanating, traits that are valorized as decidedly masculine. One may conclude, therefore, that the aspect of the Godhead beyond sexual differentiation is still characterized in essentially male terms (Ms. VBAE 236, fol. 168a). Concerning this work of Joseph of Hamadan, see Idel, 1979, pp. 74–84. The unisexual character of the divine anthropos is affirmed in slightly different imagery overcome the apparent sexual duality so that the female is reintegrated into the male.[11] Joseph of Hamadan conveys this notion in his artful interpretation of the verse, "Draw me after you, let us run! The king has brought me to his chambers. Let

---

in "Joseph of Hamadan's *Sefer Tashak*" (Zwelling, 1975), p. 136: "When the holy name YHWH appears, the head of the Holy One, blessed be He, and all of the holy body are manifest, and the Matrona is His crown." The feminine aspect of the Godhead is identified as the crown of the masculine form (symbolized by the Tetragrammaton). The eschatological application of this model is evident in ibid., p. 145: "In the days of King Messiah when the Holy One, blessed be He, will build his Temple, He will be crowned in His crowns and He will sit on the throne of His royalty. He will be perfected from all the holy sides like the letter *gimmel*, which has a crown and a throne." The portrait painted by Joseph of Hamadan of the crowned king sitting on his throne is meant to convey the reintegration of the feminine—manifest in the double aspect of crown and throne—to the masculine. Hence, God is symbolically represented by the *gimmel*, which comprises the three elements of the crown, the body, and the throne. It is likely, moreover, that this letter stands for the *gid*, or the phallus. The eschatological future, therefore, is marked by the reconstitution of the androgynous phallus. Cf. ibid., pp. 151–152. See also the description of the ontological status of the Jews given on p. 270: "they are all bound to the holy crown of the Master of the world". The conception of the male androgyne is also affirmed in the following passage of Joseph of Hamadan, ibid., pp. 161–162: "Therefore these four letters [YHWH] join together. The *yod* is the image of the head of the Holy One, blessed be He; the *he'* is the right arm and the [right] side of the body; the *waw* is the body in its entirety, the thighs, the feet, the knees, and the holy phallus; and the *he'* is the left arm and the *Shekhinah*."

[11]Conversely, the mystical significance of the commandment forbidding illicit sexual relationships turns on the presumption that these relations result in the separation of the masculine and feminine potencies of the divine. See Joseph of Hamadan, *Sefer Ta'ame ha-Miṣwot*, negative commandments (no. 30), Ms. BPNH 817, fol. 155a:

> They are called *'arayot* because the attribute of *Ṣaddiq* is contained in the attribute of *Malkhut* and the attribute of *Malkhut* in the *Ṣaddiq* like a flame bound to the coal, and so too the rest of the attributes. Thus "the Lord shall be one and His name one" (Zech. 14:9). The one who transgresses any of the illicit sexual acts discloses [the nakedness of] *Ḥokhmah* in relation to *Binah* and thereby separates these two attributes, and similarly between *Ṣaddiq* and *Malkhut*.

The image from *Sefer Yeṣirah* of the flame bound to the coal is used repeatedly by Joseph of Hamadan to depict the union of the masculine and feminine, specifically *Yesod* and *Shekhinah*. Cf. "Joseph of Hamadan's *Sefer Tashak*", Zwelling, 1975, pp. 37, 55, 66, 72, 93.

us delight and rejoice in your love, Savoring it more than wine—Like new wine they love you!" (Song of Songs 1:4):

> By way of kabbalah this alludes to the second cherub that corresponds to the Bride, the Community of Israel, who is perfect in all the perfections and comprises all beauty. She began to praise the bridegroom who is the King, Lord of the hosts, for everything is one, blessed be He. Concerning the one who separates these two attributes the verse says, "You shall not make for yourself a sculptured image, or any likeness" [Exod. 20:4]. How is this so? Since God, blessed be He, is one, he creates a division within Him by making the attribute of Kingdom separate. It is like one who takes a stick and with his knife cuts it and makes from it two things. Therefore, the verse says, "You shall not make for yourself a sculptured image, or any likeness", [the word *pesel*, sculptured image] indicates that one should not cut (*yifsol*) in a place where it is not appropriate. Therefore, it is written, "You should not have other gods" [Exod. 20:3], for everything is one matter, blessed be He. . . . Thus, the Bride, the Community of Israel, says before the Bridegroom, "Draw me after you, let us run!"—i.e. [the meaning of] "draw me" (*mashkheni*) is spread your wings over me and cover me with skin, from the [Aramaic] word [for skin] *mashkha'*, as I have alluded—"and pour forth your good anointing oil over me." "Let us delight" [the plural signifies] the Bridegroom and the Bride together. "The king has brought me to his chambers", the chambers of the nuptial canopy. "Let us delight in you", in the attribute of the *Ṣaddiq*. "Savoring it more than wine", for he pours forth the good oil. ["Joseph of Hamadan's *Sefer Tashak*", Zwelling, 1975, pp. 22–23]

The myth of sexual coupling as it took shape within the monistic framework of kabbalistic speculation, combined with an androcentricism rooted both in classical Jewish sources and mediaeval European society more generally, produced the idea well formulated by Joseph of Hamadan: the yearning of the feminine potency to receive the *semen virile* from the masculine translates theologically to the desire to avoid positing two divine powers. Idolatry, or the making of a sculpted image, is essentially the psychological tendency to reify the feminine as a distinct deity.[12] Ironically, the eroticized language of the verse from Song of Songs underscores the reintegration of the female in the male rather than affirming the ontic autonomy of the bride over and against the bridegroom.

The point is also epitomized in the following comment in an anonymous kabbalistic text:

> These two cherubim are *Tif'eret Yisra'el* and his *Malkhut*, and they are two-faced (*du-parṣufim*). Concerning them it is said according to the hidden meaning (*nistar*), "Male and female He created them" [Gen. 1:27]. This is the perfect

---

[12] Cf. ibid., pp. 257–258:

> Therefore the Torah said, "You shall not wear cloth combining wool and linen" (Deut. 22:11), for these are the garments of the Matrona, and one is forbidden to wear them, as it is written, "for you must not worship any other god" (Exod. 34:14), this corresponds to the Matrona. He who wears the garments of Matrona seems as if he worships her, and thus it is written, "You shall not wear cloth combining wool and linen." And this is the secret of "a man shall not wear woman's clothing" (Deut. 22:5), this refers to the Matrona, and a person should not wear her garments which are a mixture of wool and linen.

A similar explanation of this prohibition is given by Joseph of Hamadan in his *Sefer Ta'ame ha-Miṣwot*, negative commandments, Ms. PBNH 817, fol. 145a. For his more general explanation of idolatry as the spiritual and psychological reification of the feminine, cf. "Joseph of Hamadan's *Sefer Tashak*", Zwelling, 1975, p. 274, and *Sefer Ta'ame ha-Miṣwot*, negative commandments, Ms. PBNH. 817, fol. 141b:

> Know that this matter "You shall not have other gods besides Me" (Exod. 20:3) corresponds to *Ze'eir 'Anpin*, the attribute of *Malkhut*, which is the secret of the Bride. One should not separate her from the Bridegroom who is the King, Lord of the Hosts, and one should not make of her an independent form or an independent god. One should not cut the shoots.

In the continuation of this text (fols. 141b–142a) Joseph of Hamadan discusses the prohibition of making idols, which he explains kabbalistically in terms of the same phenomenon of separating the masculine and the feminine potencies in the Godhead. This is precisely how kabbalists explained the major transgressions recorded in the Bible. Examples of this are, Adam and Eve eating the fruit of the Tree of Knowledge, the drunkenness of Noah, the construction of the Tower of Babel, and the worshipping of the Golden Calf. All of these sins, and indeed the very nature of sin in general, involve the separation of the male and female that results from reifying the female as an autonomous potency.

> human (*ha-'adam ha-shalem*), and the cherubim depicted in the Sanctuary were in their pattern. They were made of one hammered work[13] to indicate the perfect unity (*ha-yiḥud ha-shalem*). In their pattern Adam and Eve were created, and this is the secret of "Let us make Adam in our image and in our likeness" [Gen. 1:26]. . . . You already know that these two countenances are the Written Torah and the Oral Torah, and they are one Torah for them. [Ms. VBAE[14] 504, fol. 312b]

Just as the two cherubim of gold were made from one material substance, so, too, the corresponding *sefirot* above, as well as the man and woman below in the earthly sphere, derive from one ontic source, and that source is the masculine anthropos. Analogously, we can speak of a Written and an Oral Torah, but in essence they are one. The union of the Written Torah and the Oral Torah is, in effect, the reintegration of the feminine in the masculine. As the anonymous author of *Sefer ha-Yiḥud* put it:

> I have already informed you that the Written Torah is the form of *Tif'eret*. . . . [W]hen a person reads the Written Torah alone and he does not merit to read the Oral Torah, concerning him it says "a querulous one alienates his friend", *we-nirggan mafrid 'alluf* [Prov. 16:28]. This is like the situation of the bridegroom being in the nuptial chamber while the bride is still standing in her father's house. . . . He is like a person who has no God for he divides the one power into two powers. But the true unity is in *Tif'eret* to establish the Written Torah with the Oral Torah as one. When a person is involved with the two Torot and harmonizes them as one, then the two countenances that were turned back-to-back face one another face-to-face. . . . [T]hen all attributes of judgment disappear . . . and the white face, the face of mercy, is merciful, and the blessing is found in all the lower realities. . . . This is the true and perfect unity, and this unity depends on *Tif'eret*. [Ms. VBAE 236, fol. 168a]

The union of male and female is predicated ultimately on the absorption or containment of the left side (passive, judgemental, constraining female) in the right side (active, merciful, overflow-

---

[13] Cf. Exod. 25:18.
[14] See also fol. 308b.

ing male).[15] Indeed, the negative valorization of the feminine in certain kabbalistic texts, especially the zoharic literature, is underscored by the fact that when the female potency is separated from the masculine, the potential exists that she will evolve into a punitive or even demonic force.[16] Sexual coupling of male and female is indicative of an androgynous unity that has been fractured. In the ideal state gender differentiation is neutralized and the female is absorbed back into the male. As Reuven Sarfati expressed the matter:

> The statement "they felt no shame" [Gen. 3:1] was before the sin because they were in the pattern of above for "in the image of God He created them,[17] male and female He created them" [Gen. 1:27]. That is, as we have said, they were created in the pattern that is above. Before the fruit was

---

[15] See Wolfson, 1986, pp. 27–52. It should be noted that, in accordance with another ontological principle articulated by the kabbalists, each attribute is contained in and interacts with its opposite. It is thus possible to speak of the containment of the right in the left just as one can speak of the containment of the left in the right. See, e.g., Jacob ben Sheshet's reflection in *Sefer ha-'Emunah we-ha-Biṭṭahon* on why the divine names sometimes have feminine verbs and sometimes masculine:

> The reason for this is that even though there is a distinction in names between the attribute of judgement and the attribute of mercy, everything that is in the one is in the other. Therefore, the attribute of judgement changes into the attribute of mercy and the attribute of mercy into the attribute of judgement . . . for if the attributes were not all contained one in the other one could not be changed into the other. . . . These names sometimes are in the masculine form and sometimes in the feminine. The Holy One, blessed be He, is unified in all of them [*meyuḥad be-khullan*] and all of them are unified in Him [*we-khullan meyuḥadim bo*]

Cf. *Kitve Ramban*, ed. C. D. Chavel, Jerusalem, 1964, 2, pp. 359. There is, however, a qualitative difference between the containment of the left in the right and the right in the left, for in both cases the distinctive character of the left is altered by its containment in the right.

[16] See, e.g., *Zohar* 3:59b. Cf. the description of the *Shekhinah* in the commentary on the *sefirot* in Ms. NYJTSA Mic. 1805, fol. 16b: "If, God forbid, she is separated from the [phallic] All, then 'The Lord has a sword; it is sated with blood' (Isa. 34:6). She is aroused to judge the world by harsh punishments and severe judgements."

[17] The biblical text here reads "him", but I have translated the passage as it appears in the manuscript citation.

> separated from the tree they had no [sexual] desire at all . . . they experienced no arousal through the genitals. "Male and female He created them" in the pattern that is above. The allusion is to the androgyne (*du-parṣufim*). The moon was not yet diminished and there was none to give or receive for the chain was doubled in itself (*ha-shalshelet haytah kefulah be-'aṣmo*), that is, they were created as twins in the pattern that is above. [Ms. OBL, 1923, fol. 93a]

Prior to the sin of Adam and Eve, there was no sexual lust, because male and female were not separate entities. On the contrary, Adam and Eve were in the pattern of the androgyne above. In the ideal state there was no gender bifurcation, no distinction between that which gives and that which receives. The locus of masculinity and femininity was in the phallus, a point alluded to by the statement that the "chain was doubled in itself"—that is, the divine grade that corresponds to the male organ comprised both masculine and feminine. The task of *homo religiosus* is to restore the feminine to the masculine, to unite the two in a bond that overcomes gender differentiation by establishing the complete male who embodies masculine and feminine. Ontologically, there is only one gender in kabbalistic theosophy, for the female is part of the male. The reintegration of the feminine in the masculine facilitated by traditional religious observance mimics the ontological situation of the Godhead prior to the primordial cleft or fission of the male androgyne into a division of sexes.[18]

---

[18] In some kabbalistic sources, including the *Zohar*, one finds a retrieval of the ancient myth of parthenogenesis involving the primal splitting of the cosmic egg that gives birth by fission rather than through union (see Liebes, 1993, pp. 65–92, esp. 82–88). In the relevant kabbalistic sources, however, the primordial cleft is not a splitting of the mother as one finds in the ancient myths (see Loraux, 1992, pp. 38–39), but, rather, the rupture of the male androgyne into a father and mother, who then procreate through union. The privileging of the male gender in the first of the emanations that is above sexual differentiation is evident, e.g. in "Joseph of Hamadan's *Sefer Tashak*" (Zwelling, 1975, p. 73), where it is stated that from *Keter* "judgment and mercy separate but He, blessed be He, is entirely merciful". In light of the correlation of mercy and masculinity, one must assume that the kabbalistic symbolism implies the masculine character of the Godhead even in an ontological state that precedes the duality of male and female. See n. 9, above.

Androgynous phallus and the eclipse of the feminine

The theological imagination of kabbalists has been completely dominated by phallocentricity. The point is epitomized in the following comment included in *collectanea* of kabbalistic exegesis, *Shibbolet shel Leqeṭ*, arranged by Moses Zacuto: "The essence of the Creator is *Yesod* for the *Nuqba'* is only a receptacle that receives the semen that *Yesod* gives her, and she is the speculum that does not shine" (Ms. OBL 1782, fol. 14a).[19] The author of this passage has stated in no uncertain terms that the divine nature is principally and essentially linked to *Yesod*; the feminine is but a vessel that receives the seminal drop from the phallus, and thus what is significant about her is judged exclusively from the vantage point of the phallus. The force of the phallocentric mentality on the part of the kabbalists goes even farther, for according to the engendering myth of kabbalistic theosophy the locus of the feminine is the phallus—that is, the aspect of the divine that is the ontic source of both masculinity and femininity corresponds to the male organ. The point is made quite simply in one of the first kabbalistic works to surface in twelfth-century Provence, *Sefer ha-Bahir*: in one passage we read that the letter *ṣaddi* (which stands for the *Ṣaddiq*, the Righteous one who is in the position of the phallus in the divine anthropos) can be broken orthographically into a *yod* on top of a *nun*, the former symbolizing the male potency (the sign of the covenant of circumcision) and the latter the female (perhaps related to the word *neqevah*) (*Sefer ha-Bahir*, § 61).[20] Contained within the one letter is the duality of male and female. One should speak, therefore, of an androgynous phallus. The symbolism of the bi-sexual phallus is operative in other bahiric passages as well—for example, in the description of both the final *nun* and the open *mem* comprising male and female (*Sefer ha-Bahir*, §§ 83–84). One of the most interesting expressions of this motif is found in the following passage:

---

[19] See OBL 1782, fol. 2b: "All of the power of the female and the essence of her lights and potencies are all hidden within *Ze'eir 'Anpin* in the manner that the female is the fulfilment of *Ze'eir 'Anpin*."

[20] Margaliot, 1978a. For a more extended discussion of this passage, see Wolfson, 1993b, pp. 70–71.

> Another explanation: "[I am awed, O Lord,] by Your deeds. Renew them in these years" [Hab. 3:2]. To what may this be compared? To a king who has a precious stone, and it is the delight of his kingdom. In the time of his joy he embraces it and kisses it, places it upon his head and loves it. Habakuk said, even though the kings[21] are with you, that precious stone is a treasure in your world. Therefore [it says] "Renew them in these years." What is the meaning of the expression "years"? As it says, "God said, 'Let there be light'" [Gen. 1:3]. There is no light but day, as it is written, "the greater light to dominate the day and the lesser light to dominate the night" [ibid., 16]. The "years" are from the "days", as it is written, "Renew them in these years", in the midst of that very jewel that gives birth to the years. And it is written, "From the east I will bring forth your seed" [Isa. 43:5]. The sun shines in the east. You said that the jewel is the day!? I only said, "And there was evening and there was morning, a first day" [Gen. 1:5], as it is written, "When the Lord God made earth and heaven" [ibid., 2:4]. [*Sefer ha-Bahir*, §§ 72–73]

Scholem noted that in this passage, as well as other bahiric texts, the image of the precious stone is a symbol for the *Shekhinah*, the feminine aspect of the divine. Historically, wrote Scholem, this symbolism could be explained

> either as reflecting aggadic symbolism, where the Torah appears as a jewel in God's treasure and where the soul is compared to a pearl, or—equally well—as a reversion to the language of Gnosticism, where the Sophia or soul is likewise described as a gem or pearl. [Scholem, 1962, p. 174][22]

While it is undoubtedly correct that the image of the jewel here and elsewhere serves as a symbol for the feminine potency, in this particular redactional context it is the androgynous nature of the jewel that is emphasized.[23] This is underscored by the

---

[21] I have followed the reading in Ms. MBS 209, fol. 19a, *melakhim*, as opposed to the printed text, *mal'akhim*, angels.

[22] Cf. Scholem, 1991, p. 176.

[23] The interpretation I have proposed is further confirmation of my thesis (1993b) that the idea of the androgynous phallus belongs to the final redactional stage of the *Bahir* in Provence. It is of interest to note that

end of the passage that connects the image of the precious stone that gives birth to the motif of the seed coming forth from the east. From other contexts in the *Bahir* it is evident that the latter is a phallic image.[24] Hence, the introduction of this motif in this setting indicates that the masculine potency, the sun shining in the east, is paired with the feminine. Indeed, from the verses cited in the concluding part of the paragraph it is clear that all duality is removed, since the male and female together constitute one entity that is the phallus, the precious stone that is the day comprising morning and night, a union symbolized as well by the two divine names, YHWH and Elohim. Time itself—in its double aspect of darkness and light—ensues from the androgynous phallus.[25]

---

in *Sefer ha-Bahir*, §§ 91–93, the reference to the crown that is made of the precious stone is immediately followed by a discussion of the blue in the fringe garment that culminates with the description of the two signs [*simanim*], one belonging to the king and the other to his daughter. The blue of the fringe garment is the seal [*ḥotam*] of God that comprises two elements, the masculine and the feminine. It seems fairly obvious that in this context as well the symbolic allusion is to the bi-sexual phallus.

[24] Cf. *Sefer ha-Bahir*, §§ 155, 159; Scholem, 1962, p. 154.

[25] See, by contrast, Scholem (1991, p, 196), who refers to the relevant bahiric passage and suggests that it indicates that time flows from the primal time gathered in the feminine *Shekhinah*. Scholem thus compares this to an Indian symbol that the idea of femininity produces the motion of time. In my opinion, it is the masculine potency—and, more specifically, the phallic impulse—that is the ground of time in kabbalistic symbolism, the feminine element being linked to space. For a preliminary discussion, see Wolfson, 1995b. The linkage of time and the masculine gender is underscored in the following comment on Ḥayyim Vital, *Sha'ar Ma'amere Rashbi*, 2d:

> Another reason [for the rabbinic ruling that women are exempt from positive commandments that are time-bound] can be explained from what I have informed you [regarding the fact] that *Nuqba' di-Ze'eir 'Anpin* emanated from the back of *Ze'eir 'Anpin*, from the chest and below, and there they are joined together. This place is called "time" (*zeman*) because "time" is a word that applies to the reality of day and night, and you know that *Ze'eir 'Anpin* is called day and his *Nuqba'* is called night. The positive commandments correspond to the 248 limbs. Therefore, all the commandments that are attached to the place that was mentioned, which is called "time" and which is from the chest and below, are called positive commandments that are time-bound, for there is participation of the male and female who are called "day" and "night". Since the man has already performed the commandment whose source is there,

The contextualization of the feminine in the phallus is considered by Joseph of Hamadan to be one of the mysteries of Torah. More specifically, this secret is linked by Hamadan to the aggadic tradition that in the age of R. Joshua ben Levi the rainbow was not seen.[26] That is to say, in the generation of righteousness the masculine and feminine aspects of the divine are so perfectly united that neither is seen in isolation from the other. In the final analysis, the feminine is itself part of the divine grade that corresponds to the male organ:[27]

> there is no need for the woman to perform it as well, for she is contained in him at the moment that he performs this commandment. Her 248 limbs are contained in his limbs and from him she is made and all of her anatomy is established.

Cf. parallel in Ḥayyim Vital, *Sefer Ta'ame ha-Miṣwot*, p. 35. Even though the aspect of time comprises both masculine and feminine, day and night, it is obvious that the latter is contained in the former. The concept of time expressed here is another example of the myth of the androgynous phallus. It is my intention to write a full study on the phenomenology of time in kabbalistic sources.

[26] Cf. *Genesis Rabbah* 35:2, pp. 328–329.

[27] Thus see, e.g., Joseph of Hamadan's commentary on the *sefirot*, Ms. OBL 1628, fol. 69b, where, in line with earlier sources, the *Shekhinah* is referred to explicitly as the "corona of the phallus of the pure and holy supernal form". On the other hand, there are many passages wherein Hamadan describes the *Shekhinah* as the independent force, usually depicted as the bride, that receives the seminal overflow from the phallic *Yesod*, frequently characterized as the golden bowl that pours forth fine oil. Cf. Ms. OBL 1628, fol. 72a: "The tenth *sefirah* is the attribute of *Malkhut*, the secret of the woman, for the nine upper *sefirot* are the form of a male." Cf. Meier, 1974, p. 243: "Therefore, the phallus above [*berit shel ma'alah*] pours forth the good oil upon the bride, the Community of Israel, and from there the blessing comes to the world." See ibid., pp. 140, 265–266, 274, 344; "Joseph of Hamadan's *Sefer Tashak*" (Zwelling, 1975, pp. 93, 101). Needless to say, many other textual illustrations could have been adduced. From one vantage point these symbolic portrayals are contradictory, for how could the feminine be both the corona of the penis and the independent entity (symbolized as the bride or second cherub) that receives the semen from the male (the bridegroom or the first cherub), but from another perspective the opposing views are dialectically resolved, i.e. the reception of the semen transforms the female into a male, and thus there is a symbolic equivalence between the two: the female cherub that receives the semen from the male cherub is transformed into the corona of the penis. Joseph of Hamadan thus concludes the aforementioned commentary on the *sefirah* of *Malkhut* by stating that the aggadic statement

> When the supernal, holy and pure phallus [*ha-gid ha-'elyon ha-qadosh we-ha-ṭahor*] is seen in the attribute of mercy it is called the covenant [*berit*] and when it is seen in the attribute of judgement it is called the rainbow [*qeshet*]. ["Joseph of Hamadan's *Sefer Tashak*", Zwelling, 1975, p. 68][28]

---

regarding God's wearing phylacteries applies to this attribute; see Ms. OBL 1628, fol. 72b. In what sense can this image be applied to the *Shekhinah*? Obviously, from a normative halakhic perspective one would not expect the female aspect of God to be so envisioned. I submit, therefore, that the reference to the phylacteries must be decoded as an allusion to the crown, and the latter signifies the corona of the phallus, an appropriate symbol of the *Shekhinah*.

[28] It must be noted that on occasion Hamadan emphasizes the androgynous nature of the *Shekhinah*:

> Certainly the *Shekhinah*, the bride and Community of Israel, sits beneath the shade of the bridegroom, for everything is one, blessed be He. And in relation to us it is male, as the verse says, "The Lord is mindful of us, He will bless us", *yhwh zekharanu yevarekh* (Ps. 115:12). This corresponds to the *Shekhinah* who is male [*zakhar*] in relation to us . . . and in relation to the attribute above female. [p. 97]

> This alludes to the Matrona who is [sometimes] called male and sometimes female, in relation to the Holy One, blessed be He, she receives and in relation to us she overflows. [p. 356]

> This alludes to the Matrona who is the secret of the androgyne, male and female, sometimes she is called male and sometimes she is called female. [p. 436]

In similar, although not exactly identical, terms the zoharic authorship emphasizes the androgynous nature of the *Shekhinah*. (See. e.g., *Zohar* 1:232a, noted by Scholem, 1991, p. 186; see also Tishby, 1963, p. 379.) Finally, I note that on occasion Joseph of Hamadan, in line with other kabbalists, interprets the rainbow as a phallic symbol; cf. his commentary on the *sefirot* in Ms. OBL 1628, fol. 72a. In the context of explaining the ninth of the *sefirot*, *Yesod*, he writes:

> Its color is like that of the rainbow that is seen in the cloud. Therefore the [rabbis], blessed be their memory, said [B. Ḥagigah 16a], 'he who looks at the rainbow does not show respect to his Creator and it would have been better for him not to have come into this world,' for he is looking at the phallus of the Holy One, blessed be He [*she-mistakkel bi-verito shel ha-qadosh barukh hu'*].

Cf. Joseph of Hamadan's formulation in Ms. JM 134:

> It has been taught that from that holy penis ['*ammata' qaddisha'*] a myriad of worlds are suspended in the opening of the penis [*pumeih de-'amma'*], and this is the holy covenant [*berita' qaddisha'*] that is revealed

The one gradation appears either as a manifestation of the masculine mercy [the *berit*] or the feminine judgement [the *qeshet*], but both are expressions of the divine phallus.

Many sources could be cited to illustrate the notion of the androgynous phallus in kabbalistic literature, but I would like to focus on two texts in particular, for, in my view, they express succinctly the complex gender symbol that I contend is characteristic of a fundamental structure of theosophic kabbalah as it takes shape in its mediaeval European context. The first passage reads as follows: "The sword is the Foundation, and this is the saying of the rabbis, may their memory be for a blessing (*Genesis Rabbah* 21:9, p. 203), 'the fiery ever-turning sword' (Gen. 3:24), sometimes female and sometimes male" (Ms. PBNH 680, fol. 164b).[29] The fiery sword placed at the east of Eden symbolizes the attribute of God that corresponds to the phallus, the ninth gradation, called *Yesod*, that comprises both male and female. Utilizing the rabbinic description of the fiery sword in the

---

> in a cloud on a rainy day, and all of those colors that are in it are seen in the holy covenant. [fol. 124b]

The point is reiterated in the continuation of this text:

> All the colors of those holy ones that are seen in the cloud on a rainy day are engraved in the holy covenant, and from there the Sabbath has been given to Israel. . . . Therefore the rabbis, blessed be their memory, said [B. Ketubot 62b] that the [appropriate] time for scholars to perform marital intercourse is on Friday evening because the Holy One, blessed be He, reveals that holy covenant. Therefore we are circumcised because the Holy One, blessed be He, sanctifies that holy covenant, which is circumcised. [fol. 124b]

See ibid., fol. 128b. The androgynous character of the symbol of the rainbow allows Joseph of Hamadan to apply this symbol to the masculine *Yesod* and to the feminine *Malkhut*. In the final analysis, however, the *membrum virile* is the locus of both male and female aspects. On the symbol of the rainbow in kabbalistic sources, see Wolfson, 1994f, pp. 334 n. 30, 337–338 n. 40.

[29] This passage appears in the concluding section of a commentary on the account of creation in the book of Genesis attributed to the Catalonian kabbalist, Joseph bar Samuel. This commentary is printed in Jacob ben Sheshet, *Sefer Meshiv Devarim Nekhohim*, Vajda, 1968, pp. 193–196 (see p. 11 n. 3, where the Paris manuscript is mentioned) and in Isaac of Acre, *Sefer Me'irat 'Einayim* (Goldreich, 1981, pp. 16–17). The passage that I have translated, however, is not found in either of the aforementioned versions.

Garden of Eden as androgynous, the kabbalist expresses the fact that sexual duality is contextualized in the divine phallus.[30] The second citation is taken from Joseph of Hamadan reflecting on the verse, "Tell the Israelite people to bring Me gifts; you shall accept gifts for Me from every person whose heart so moves him" (Exod. 25:2):

> "To bring Me gifts", *wa-yiqḥu li terumah*, this alludes to the *Shekhinah* who is called offering (*terumah*). "From every", *me'et kol*, i.e. the upper phallus (*berit ha-'elyon*) which is the attribute of the *Ṣaddiq*. This is the attribute of the All (*middat ha-kol*) and it is called "Man" (*'ish*). From him "you shall accept gifts for Me", *mimenu tiqḥu 'et terumati*, they took two attributes, *Ṣaddiq* and the attribute of *Malkhut*, the secret of the two cherubim. From him "you shall accept gifts for Me." Until here is the explanation of the verse in the way of kabbalah. [Joseph of Hamadan's *Sefer Tashak*, Zwelling, 1975, pp. 13–14]

Significantly, this passage follows a discourse on the verse, "Let him kiss me with the kisses of his mouth" (Song of Songs 1:2), which is interpreted as a depiction of the erotic yearning of the second cherub, the female *Malkhut*, to unite with the first cherub, the male *Yesod*. Immediately after giving expression to the rich drama of the bi-sexual myth, the kabbalist articulates the ontological principle that circumscribes this myth: the female is taken from the supernal phallus.

To put the matter in slightly different terms, the kabbalistic texts offer another example of a one-sex theory that is well documented in classical, mediaeval, and renaissance sources: the feminine is but an extension of the masculine.[31] The practical religious implications of this ontology are perhaps felt nowhere more sharply than in kabbalistic accounts of the rite of circumcision, a theme that I have discussed before but to which

[30] In other kabbalistic sources the image of the fiery sword, or the "sword that wreaks vengeance for the covenant" (Lev. 26:25), is applied to the feminine Presence on account of the fact that she is a manifestation of divine judgement. See, e.g., *Zohar* 1:66b, 240b; 2:26a; Tishby, 1963, p. 1365; Joseph Gikatilla, *Sha'are 'Orah* (ed. J. Ben-Shlomo, Jerusalem, 1981), 1, p. 71; *Ma'arekhet ha-'Elohut* (Ferrara, 1558), ch. 4, 86b–87a.

[31] For discussion of this phenomenon in Western culture, see Laqueur, 1990. For a different approach to that of Laqueur, see Cadden, 1993.

my path keeps returning.[32] For example, according to an anonymous thirteenth-century kabbalistic text, circumcision "alludes to the perfect unity, and the matter of the androgyne [*du-parṣufim*] is explained in it; examine and discover with respect to the exposure of the corona" (Ms. PBNH 843, fol. 39b). The corona of the penis symbolically corresponds to the feminine *Shekhinah*—a correlation facilitated by the fact that the word *'aṭarah* [crown], is the technical name of the corona as well as one of the designations of the *Shekhinah*.[33] Insofar as the male organ is the ontic source of both masculine and feminine, the religious significance of circumcision lies in the fact that by means of this ritual the androgynous unity of God is established (see *Zohar* 1:96b; 2:60b; Tishby, 1963, pp. 1364–1365). Judged from the human vantage point, this rite affords one the opportunity to gain access to the two aspects of the divine. The matter is spelled out more clearly in his discussion of the secret of circumcision by Joseph Gikatilla:

> The secret of the covenant is the corona (*'aṭarah*), in the mystery of the glorious crown (*'aṭeret tif'eret*). When a person is circumcised and enters into the secret of the holy covenant (*berit ha-qodesh*), he enters the two gradations that are one unity (*ḥibbur 'eḥad*), the Crown (*'aṭeret*) and the Eternally Living One (*ḥei ha-'olamim*), the secret of the All. Everything is one unity. Therefore the [foreskin] is cut and [the membrane] pulled back, for these two matters are one. [Ms. VBAE 283, fol. 51a, and Ms. MBS 56, fol. 193b][34]

---

[32] See Wolfson, 1987a, pp. 77–112; 1987b, pp. 189–215

[33] See, e.g., *Zohar* 1:162a. For other references to this motif, see Wolfson, 1987b, p. 205 n. 53, to which many more sources could be added. On the phallic character of the *Shekhinah* as the *aṭeret berit*, the corona of the phallus, cf. *Sefer ha-Peli'ah* (Korets, 1784, pt. 2, 54c–d): "*Yesod* is between the thighs . . . and corresponding to *Yesod* in the physical man is the penis that stands between the thighs. Therefore it is called *Yesod*. . . . *'Aṭarah* is the end of the supernal edifice [*sof ha-binyan le-ma'alah*]. Thus, corresponding to it is the corona of the penis [*ha-'aṭarah shel ha-ma'or*], which is the end of the person." In the continuation of this passage (55a), the anonymous kabbalist notes that the prohibition of looking at either the priest's hands or the rainbow is related to the sin of focusing on the *Shekhinah* in isolation from the other (masculine) *sefirot*. The spiritual valorization of the feminine is dependent on contextualizing the female in the male organ.

[34] Cf. *Sha'are 'Orah*, 1:114–117.

Within the symbolic representation of theosophic kabbalah, the feminine is localized in the male's reproductive organ. To avoid misunderstanding on this point, let me be perfectly clear and state unequivocally that I am not saying that kabbalists are not cognizant of the obvious fact that men and women are biologically distinguished by their genitals. It is the case, moreover, that the divine feminine is described, albeit rarely, in terms of her own genitals in contradistinction to the penis. The physiological differentiation between the sexes below is thus applied to the divine hypostases above. The point I am making, however, concerns the gender valorization of the feminine over and against the masculine, and not the issue of sexual differences linked to the body. The overwhelming evidence, in my opinion, indicates that from the perspective of gender the feminine is localized in the masculine. To illustrate my claim, let me mention one zoharic passage where it says explicitly that the sign of the covenant—that is, the penis—is that which distinguishes the male from the female (*Zohar* 1:246a).[35] Precisely in that context, however, the zoharic authorship makes the point that the female is taken from the male and hence must be restored to the masculine. The symbol of reconstituted masculinity is the *'olah*, the burnt offering that is said "to rise from the feminine [*Shekhinah*] to the masculine [*Yesod*], and from that place and above everything is masculine, and from the feminine and below everything is feminine" (*Zohar* 1:246a–b). In this context the zoharic authorship clearly recognizes the distinction between the upper "world of the masculine" [*'alma' di-dekhura'*, *'olam ha-zakhar*] from *Binah* to *Yesod* and the lower "world of the feminine" [*'alma' de-nuqba'*, *'olam ha-neqevah*] that comprises the *Shekhinah* and her angelic forces.[36] Both worlds are configured in the shape of an anthropos, but in the case of the former the head is feminine and the end of the body [*siyyuma' de-gufa'*—i.e. the genitals] masculine, whereas with respect to the latter, the head and end are feminine. It is noteworthy that even in this passage, where the sexual differentiation between *Shekhinah* and the upper sefirotic potencies is clearly enunciated, the *Zohar* still describes the process by means of which

[35] Cf. *Zohar*, 2:137a.

[36] For discussion of this terminology, see Scholem, 1931, pp. 39–41.

the feminine is restored or elevated to the masculine. That the female is only a relative male is affirmed in the continuation of this passage, where an explanation is offered for why Ephraim takes the place of Joseph in the enumeration of the twelve tribes. Since the latter represent the adornments of the *Shekhinah*, which are feminine, it was necessary for Joseph, the male potency *par excellence*, to be removed. But in what sense is his substitute, Ephraim, more feminine than Joseph? Clearly not in a biological sense. It must be the case, rather, that Ephraim assumes a feminine character insofar as he symbolically represents the *Shekhinah*. This symbolic representation, I submit, implies the (relative) masculine status of the *Shekhinah* rather than the feminine status of the biblical figure.

Even in those passages that treat the female as something distinct from the male, the phallocentric orientation is evident, for the feminine is portrayed as a receptacle that conceals the penis[37] or receives the seed from the male.[38] From this vantage point the male is contained in the female. The nature of the containment, however, is fundamentally different in this case from that of the containment of the feminine in the masculine. In the latter instance, the containment signifies the absorption of that which is contained (female) in that which contains (male), whereas in the former that which is contained (male) transforms the nature of that which contains (female). The female receptacle provides the space in which the male organ extends. Theosophically, the female containing the male is the secret of the spatial dwelling of the divine, the garment in which the glory is clothed. Space in general, and sacred space in particular, partakes of the symbolic nexus of building, dwelling, and presencing, a mystery boldly described by Joseph of Hamadan:

> The matter of the Tabernacle concerning which the Torah said, "On the first of the month, the Tabernacle was set up" [Exod. 40:17]. This signifies that another Tabernacle was set up together with it.[39] This alludes to the image of the chariot,

---

[37] Cf. the description of the *Shekhinah* in *Zohar* 3:142a (*'Idra' Rabba'*) with the description of *Binah* in Moses de León, *Sheqel ha-Qodesh* (Greenup, 1911), p. 29.

[38] See, e.g., *Zohar* 1:162a–b.

[39] Cf. *Pesiqta' Rabbati* (Friedmann, 1880), 5, 22b; *Tanḥuma'*, Nasso, 18; *Numbers Rabbah* 12:12.

> for it is precisely the image of the holy, pure, supernal chariot. Therefore, the Holy One, blessed be He, said to Moses, our master: "Tell the Israelite people to bring Me gifts" [Exod. 25:2], i.e. to your God. Let them make a body and a soul and I will assume bodily form in it (*'etgashem bo*). "To bring Me", they took My Torah. They took the image of My chariot and I too "shall take", i.e. I will be garbed in the Tabernacle. [Joseph of Hamadan's *Sefer Tashak*, Zwelling, 1975, p. 13]

The Tabernacle below is in the pattern of the Tabernacle or chariot above—that is, the feminine Presence. The religious purpose of the Tabernacle is to provide a dwelling in which the divine takes shape. In this kabbalistic version of incarnation, the phenomenon of sacred space is valorized as the female axis of divinity. The role assigned to the female is to house or clothe the masculine. The gender of femininity is valued as the clearing wherein the male organ is manifest.

It may be concluded, therefore, that the experience of genderedness imparted by the mythic symbols of kabbalistic theosophy is such that the feminine is judged exclusively from the vantage point of the phallus.[40] This is a far-reaching claim that has major implications for a proper understanding of the use of masculine and feminine images to characterize the divine in theosophical kabbalah. On the surface, kabbalistic texts abound with male and female representations of God, and one might be tempted to find in them the roots for religious and/or social egalitarianism. The task, however, is to penetrate beneath the surface, so that one may appreciate the gender images in their proper historical and cultural light. When that is done, it becomes fairly obvious that the gender imagery operative in kabbalistic thought is thoroughly androcentric.

Scholem's attempt to contrast the kabbalistic viewpoint with that of the encratist tendency of ancient Gnosticism on the grounds that the former involves the conjunction of male and female as opposed to the latter which advocates the overcoming

---

[40] Even the mythic portrayal of the feminine Presence as the attribute of judgement is coloured by a phallocentric orientation. That is, the descriptions of the Presence as a warrior or as one who wields a sword suggest a phallic understanding of judgement as an active force.

of sexual differentiation by reestablishing an original androgynous state is ultimately flawed.[41] A more nuanced understanding of gender in the kabbalistic sources does not warrant such a distinction. On the contrary, the goal of gnosis expressed in the Gnostic source mentioned by Scholem, the *Gospel of Thomas*, to "make the female male",[42] is indeed an entirely appropriate slogan for the kabbalists. The union of God is predicated on the unity of male and female, but that unity is determined further by reintegrating the female in the male such that the primary male androgyne is reconstituted. Gender imagery in the kabbalistic sources reflects the binary ideology of the general mediaeval culture, as well as the specific rabbinic society, which reinforced the division of the sexes along hierarchical lines, delegating to the female a subservient role. The male is valorized as the active, dominant, primary sex and the female as the passive, dom-

[41] See Scholem, 1962, p. 142. A similar position is taken by Mopsik (1986, pp. 324–325 n. 218) and Idel (1989b, p. 211). Mopsik has recently reiterated his position (1994, pp. 16–25). In that context Mopsik explicates the nature of the androgyne in kabbalistic symbolism in light of the Pseudo-Clementine *Homily XIV* (see pp. 24–25). According to Mopsik, the ancient Judaeo-Christian text posits an idea of dual unity, i.e. a bisexual unity in which both genders are affirmed. Mopsik contrasts this text with the conception of the androgyne in other Greco–Roman sources that entail the "neutralization of sexual difference". In my view the kabbalistic understanding of the androgyne implies precisely such a neutralization of sexual differentiation. See also the formulation of Liebes (1993b, p. 106): "the dual sexuality of the divinity is the very foundation of all the doctrine of the Kabbala." To evaluate this statement more precisely, one must take into consideration the cultural construction of gender in the relevant sources. When that is done, it becomes evident that the feminine is part of the masculine, and hence the dual sexuality of the divinity is reduced to one sex that comprises two elements: the merciful male and the judgmental female. The kabbalistic orientation, as I understand, is close to the view expressed in various alchemical tracts, reflected in the psychological theory of Jung (see Zolla, 1981).

[42] See Klijn, 1962, pp. 271–278; Meyer, 1985, pp. 554–570; Brown, 1988, pp. 103–121; Vogt, 1991, pp. 172–187. On the myth of the androgyne in ancient Greco–Roman literature, see Delcourt, 1958; Brisson, 1986, pp. 27–61.

[43] See the summary account given by C. W. Bynum (1986a, p. 257): "Male and female were contrasted and asymmetrically valued as intellect/body, active/passive, rational/irrational, reason/emotion, self-control/lust, judgement/mercy, and order/disorder."

inated, and secondary one.[43] Gendered differences are transcended when the female divests herself of her essential femininity—that is, when she becomes part of the male—since the latter embodies the generic anthropos and hence represents the most basic elemental force of the divine. The female is described as being contained in rather than containing the male. While it is certainly the case that the kabbalists emphasize time and again that the complete anthropos comprises masculine and feminine, and indeed the messianic era is understood precisely in terms of the erotic union of the male and female aspects of the divine—the "secret of faith" (see *Zohar* 1:49b) or the "perfection of everything" (see *Zohar* 3:163b)—the nature of the feminine is such that this union entails the overcoming of the femaleness of the female. Redemption is a state wherein male and female are conjoined, but in that union the female is enfolded back into the male whence she derived.[44] The point is underscored in the following comment of Isaac Luria's disciple, Moses Yonah, in his *Kanfe Yonah*:

> You already know the pearl in the mouth of the kabbalists concerning [the verse] "From my flesh I shall see God" [Job 19:26]. And the rabbis, blessed be their memory, already said,[45] It is the way of him who has lost something to search and look for that which he has lost, and it is the way of the man to go after the woman. For this reason the essence of the union, that is, the essence of the arousal to have sexual union and to illustrate love is from the side of the male. [Ms. JS 993, p. 48]

The significant aspect of this kabbalistic appropriation of the talmudic dictum is the opening citation from Job. This suggests that the feminine is part of the phallus and thus sexual copulation is a means of restoring the unity of the male organ. Scholem's distinction between the conjunction of male and female and the reestablishment of a primordial androgyne cannot be upheld.

---

[44] See, e.g., *Zohar* 3:145b. For a different approach, see Mopsik, 1986, pp. 214–215. Mopsik emphasizes that according to the kabbalists the eschaton signifies the restoration of the equality between the two sexes and the end of the domination of one over the other.

[45] B. Qiddushin 2b.

Coitus as the masculinization of the female

When the complex theosophic discourse is applied to the anthropological sphere, it is evident that here, too, it is the task of the female to become male, especially through sexual union.[46] It is no doubt true that the kabbalistic interpretation of human sexu-

---

[46] Von Kellenbach (1990, p. 207), remarks that Augustine "grants woman humanity as long as she is joined by a man, 'so the whole substance may be one image.' Marriage becomes a prerequisite for women's humanity. A single woman remains essentially incomplete. The male, on the other hand, represents the divine by himself." The passage is cited in Boyarin, 1993, p. 43 n. 25. Conceptually, this description of Augustine is applicable to the kabbalistic sources and, I believe, the earlier rabbinic sources as well. While it is true that in the rabbinic materials we find evidence for the idea that sexual union restores the image of the original androgyne, and perhaps also the divine image in which this androgyne was created, it is nevertheless the case that the female is essentially incomplete without her being joined to the male, whereas the male has a sense of independent completeness or, to put the matter somewhat differently, the perfection of both the male and the female is judged from the vantage point of the male. The fact of the matter is, moreover, that the theological pronouncements of the rabbis generally and predominantly involve an imaging of God as exclusively male. This fact not only privileges the masculine but also suggests that the male alone can represent the *imago dei*. Lest I be misunderstood on this point, let me emphasize that I am not denying the presence in rabbinic texts of the view that the complete anthropos involves the union of male and female (cf. B. Yevamot 63a), nor the notion that without a wife a man is in a state of deficiency (cf. *Genesis Rabbah* 17:1, pp. 151–152). The issue is, rather, that through the union of male and female the female completes the male by affording him the opportunity to engender new life. The completeness of the female, therefore, is obviously related to procreation, which must be seen as an androcentric value in rabbinic culture. Consider the following interpretation of "Then Adam said, This one at last is bone of my bones, and flesh of my flesh. This one shall be called woman, for from man was she taken" (Gen. 2:23) in *'Avot de-Rabbi Natan*, ed. S. Schechter (Wilna, 1887), version B, ch. 8, 12a: "[This time] the woman was created from man; from now on a man will take the daughter of his fellow and he is commanded to be fruitful and multiply." The author of this comment is dealing with the obvious empirical fact that every man is born of woman rather than the other way around, as suggested by the myth of the primal Adam (cf. Anderson, 1989, pp. 125–126). From the midrashic reflection on the verse it follows that woman's role as the one who bears the child parallels her assumed original ontic status as being taken from man. That is to say, procreation is a reconstitution of the original androgynous state wherein the female was contained in the male. Consider the statement attributed

ality is based on the assumption that the male/female relationship below mirrors the relationship of the masculine and feminine potencies above.[47] As in the case of the kabbalistic understanding of rituals more generally, in the particular case of sexuality this mirroring is not merely passive, but is predicated, rather, on the notion that the acts below affect and impact on the corresponding realities in the divine realm. By means of carnal intercourse, therefore, the union of a man and his wife assists in the unification of the male and female aspects of God, especially the sixth and tenth emanations. A typical expression of this idea is found in the following zoharic text:

---

to R. Simlai in *Genesis Rabbah* 8:9, p. 63: "Originally [literally, in the past] Adam was created from the earth and Eve was created from Adam, but from that point on [it is said that man and woman were created] 'in our image and in our likeness,' for man is not [created] without woman nor woman without man, and neither of them without the *Shekhinah*." In this particular setting, the teaching of R. Simlai is presented as the internal interpretation of the key phrase in Gen. 1:26 that stands in marked contrast to the master's response to the query of the heretics [*minim*]. It is significant that the divine likeness is connected with human procreation. (I owe this insight to David Aaron, who has made this very same point in "Imagery of the Divine and the Human: On the Mythology of Genesis Rabba 8 § 1" [forthcoming].) As Theodor and Albeck note in their edition of *Genesis Rabbah*, the thematic import of R. Simlai's statement is analogous to the rabbinic teaching that there are three partners in the creation of every person: the biological parents and God (cf. B. Qiddushin 30b). That the underlying intent of the statement attributed to Simlai is as I have explained is supported by a second context in *Genesis Rabbah* 22:2, p. 206, where the relevant comment is placed in the mouth of R. Ishmael, who thus interprets the significance of the particle *'et* in the expression *wa-to'mer qaniti 'ish 'et yhwh*, "she said, 'I have gained a male child with the help of the Lord'" (Gen. 4:1): "[The significance of] *'et yhwh* is that originally Adam was created from the earth and Eve from Adam, but from that point on [it is written] 'in our image and in our likeness,' man is not [created] without woman nor woman without man, and neither of them without the *Shekhinah*." The divine likeness and image is connected to procreation, which, in turn, is a reconstitution of the originary state wherein the feminine was contained in the masculine. For a different reading of the rabbinic sources on the nature of the androgyne, see Boyarin, *Carnal Israel*, pp. 42–46.

[47] The point is well documented in scholarly literature: see Waite, 1990, pp. 377–405; Scholem, 1967, pp. 225–229; 1991, p. 183; Tishby, 1963, pp. 1355–1379; Mopsik, 1986, pp. 45–163; Idel, 1989b, pp. 207–213; see also Langer, 1989, pp. 41–57.

> The Holy One, blessed be He, praises the Community of Israel and the love of the Holy One, blessed be He, is [directed] towards her to join her. Therefore, the one who is married must praise the Holy One, blessed be He. It has been taught . . . when a man cleaves to his mate and his desire is to receive her, he worships before the holy King and arouses another union, for the desire of the Holy One, blessed be He, is to cleave to the Community of Israel. The Holy One, blessed be He, blesses the one who arouses this matter and the Community of Israel blesses him. [*Zohar* 3:37b][48]

Despite the overt affirmation of heterosexual intercourse between a man and his wife as a sacral *imitatio dei*, it can be shown from at least two vantage points that in the kabbalistic world-view the carnal coupling must be judged from a purely androcentric perspective.[49] In the first instance, it is evident that the union of male and female is intended to augment the divine

---

[48] Many of the zoharic passages that I cite in my analysis of the kabbalistic understanding of sexual intercourse have been noted by Tishby (1963, pp. 1357–1360), and the accompanying notes. Needless to say, however, my way of interpreting the texts is radically different from that of Tishby. Thus, for example, after reviewing some of the relevant sources, Tishby commented: "These passages assign a very important role to the woman in marriage. She is depicted as occupying an exalted position, since she is a reflection of the Shekhinah and also enjoys her protection" (p. 1358). Although Tishby goes on to note the negative characterization of the feminine in terms of the demonic power, he does not fully appreciate the androcentric understanding of the feminine in kabbalistic symbolism. I have concluded on the basis of the very same passages that Tishby mentioned that the role assigned to the woman is secondary and subservient to that of the male. The sacral character of carnal intercourse is to be judged exclusively from the vantage point of the man's obligation to procreate and thereby extend and increase the divine image in the world. It is true that the woman has an important role in human sexuality, but it can hardly be said that she occupies an exalted position. Such a claim simply neglects to take into account the socio-cultural dimension of gender symbolism in the theosophic kabbalistic sources.

[49] The androcentrism is also evident in another motif that recurs in zoharic literature, viz. that by virtue of marriage and sexual intercourse the man cleaves to the Presence and is thus situated between two females (his earthly wife and the divine Presence) in the pattern of the sixth gradation, *Tif'eret*, who is lodged between *Binah* and *Malkhut* (for references see Tishby, 1963, pp. 1357–1358).

image in the world through procreation.[50] This divine image, however, corresponds to the phallus. Simply put, through conjugal intercourse the woman provides the vehicle by which man extends his phallus.[51] The point is made with particular poignancy in the following zoharic passage:

> On account of the holy seal in a person he must augment the image of the supernal King in this world.[52] This secret is that the waters of the river that flows and comes forth never stop. Therefore, the river and source of a person should never stop in this world. The river alludes to the holy covenant sealed in his flesh which is in the pattern of that river, an allusion to the [masculine] *Ṣaddiq* who is joined to [feminine] *Ṣedeq* as one above. Therefore, below a man should unite with his wife in holiness in order to be strengthened through her in this world. Whenever a man is not successful in this world, the Holy One, blessed be He, uproots him and plants him several times as before. [*Zohar* 1:186b]

The end of the passage provides the key to the text as a whole: the purpose of sexual union is to produce offspring, so that the man does not have to endure the punishment of transmigration of the soul.[53] The sexual act reflects the union above

---

[50] See Mopsik, 1989, pp. 48–73.

[51] This is the theosophic implication of the interpretation of "The Lord is great and much acclaimed in the city of our God" (Ps. 48:2) in *Zohar* 3:5a:

> When is the Holy One, blessed be He, called great? When the Community of Israel is found together with Him. . . . It may be inferred that the King without the Matrona is not a King, and He is not great or glorious. Therefore, he who is not found as male and female, all praise is removed from him and he is not in the category of an anthropos.

See also *Zohar* 2:38b: "In the place where male and female are found, there is no praise except for the male."

[52] The kabbalistic view is obviously based on the aggadic notion that the one who does not fulfil the obligation to procreate diminishes the divine image (cf. B. Yevamot 63b; *Genesis Rabbah* 34:14, ed. Theodor & Albeck, p. 326, and other sources discussed there in n. 2).

[53] See *Zohar* 1:187a; Tishby, 1963, p. 1362. For the most part the phenomenon of transmigration of the soul or metempsychosis is treated in zoharic passages as a punishment for the man who dies without having fathered children (see Scholem, 1991, p. 209). Interestingly enough, according to ancient Mandaean lore, reincarnation is similarly viewed as

of the ninth and tenth emanations, *Ṣaddiq* and *Ṣedeq*, the man corresponding to the former and the woman to the latter. The ultimate goal of this union, however, is the extension and augmentation of the divine image in the world through reproduction.[54] As Moses de León plainly states in one of his Hebrew theosophic writings:

> Therefore, he who fears his Creator should take a wife and have children from her, to extend his form so that he can enter the palace. You already know that regarding him who does not have a child in this world, his image is cut off from the image of the All (*temunat ha-kol*)[55] and he does not enter the palace. [*The Book of the Pomegranate: Moses de León's Sefer ha-Rimmon*][56]

From yet another perspective, the kabbalistic understanding of sexual intercourse has to be seen as rooted in a cultural androcentrism: the carnal union of masculine and feminine obliterates the essential femaleness of the female insofar as the feminine left is contained in and transformed by the masculine right or, in terms of another metaphor used in the *Zohar*, the feminine judgement is sweetened by the masculine mercy as a result of sexual copulation (see Liebes, 1993b, p. 187, n. 177). I have already alluded to this facet of the kabbalistic understanding of sexuality, but it is necessary to explore it at this juncture in some more detail. Let us consider the following zoharic text:

> The feminine extends in her side and cleaves to the sides of the male until she is separated from his sides and she comes to join with him face-to-face. When they are joined they

---

punishment for childlessness (see Drower, 1962, p. 41). The similarity between the Mandaean and kabbalistic positions was already noted by Yamauchi (1970, p. 41, n. 193).

[54] With respect to this understanding of sexuality, the kabbalists follow the rabbinic tradition that likewise emphasizes the procreative aspect of sexual intercourse (see n. 46).

[55] This designation of the *Shekhinah* is an abbreviated form of the expression used by Ezra of Gerona, *temunah ha-kolelet kol ha-temunot*, "the image that comprises all the images"; see Tishby, 1963, p. 1375 n. 63; Liebes, 1976, pp. 50–51.

[56] Wolfson, 1988, p. 224 (Hebrew section; all subsequent references to this volume are to this part of the text). See ibid., pp. 241–242, and the passage from Joseph of Hamadan cited in n. 85 below.

> appear as one actual body. From here we learn that a man alone appears as half a body, and he is entirely mercy, and similarly the woman.[57] When they are joined as one, everything appears as one actual body. Thus, when the male joins with the female, everything is one body, and all the worlds are in joy for they are all blessed from the complete body. [*Zohar* 3:296a (*'Idra' Zuṭa'*)]

The relationship of man and woman below reflects that of the male and female aspects of the sefirotic pleroma—respectively, the sixth and tenth emanations. Just as the divine male and female together form one complete body, the male half representing the attribute of mercy and the female half the attribute of judgement, so, too, in the case of human beings. In the continuation of the above passage the zoharic authorship emphatically affirms man's ontic status as comprising male and female; the latter is contained in the former. The ontically inferior and derivative status of the feminine is alluded to in the statement that "the beauty of the woman is entirely from the beauty of the male" (*Zohar* 3:296a [*'Idra' Zuṭa'*]).[58] The overriding theological purpose of sexual intercourse is to ameliorate divine judgement by mercy which translates in gender terms to the masculinization of the feminine. The transformation of the female into male ensuing from sexual copulation is affirmed explicitly in one text, as follows:

> R. Yose said, Thus have I heard from the holy lamp [i.e. R. Simeon bar Yoḥai]: When [the male and female forces] are united to show that the female is contained in him as one entity, the female is called by the name of the male, for then the blessings of the *Matrona* are found and there is no separation in her at all. [*Zohar* 3:31a][59]

---

[57] Although not stated explicitly in the text, it is obvious that just as the male is entirely mercy, the woman is entirely judgement. The union of the two results in the amelioration of the feminine by the masculine.

[58] The subordinate position accorded the woman is also in evidence from *Zohar* 1:49a: "Come and see: when a woman is joined to her husband she is called by the name of her husband, *'ish* and *'ishah*, *ṣaddiq* and *ṣedeq*, he is dust and she is dust, he is *ṣevi* and she is *ṣeviyyah*."

[59] This passage is cited by Scholem (1991, p. 186), but as evidence to support the claim that there are active as well as passive elements in the *Shekhinah*. In my view, Scholem's reading misses the point of this text,

The matter is expressed in another zoharic passage as follows:

> R. Eleazar was standing before R. Simeon, his father. He said to him, It is written, "Enjoy happiness with a woman you love all the fleeting days of life" [Eccl. 9:9]. He said to him, Come and see: "Enjoy happiness with a woman you love", this is a great secret, for a person must comprise life in this place,[60] the one without the other does not go, and a person must contain the attribute of the day in the night and the attribute of the night in the day.[61] This is [the meaning of] "Enjoy happiness with a woman you love." What is the reason? For this is your portion in life, for life does not dwell except upon this. [*Zohar* 3:177b]

Man's task in conjugal union is to combine the masculine and the feminine. Yet, a careful reading of the above passage, and of others wherein the same thematic is addressed, indicates that the issue is the containment of the female in the male. Hence, in the continuation of the passage it is emphasized that the left is contained in the right,[62] so that "everything that a person does should be contained in the right" (*Zohar* 3:178a). The point is reiterated in another passage:

> Come and see: R. Eleazar said, every woman is characterized as judgement until she tastes the taste of mercy, as it has been taught: from the side of the man comes white and from the side of the woman comes red. When the woman tastes some of the white, the white dominates. [*Zohar* 3:259b][63]

---

which is to underscore that the feminine is contained in the male and ontically transformed as a result of the sexual union. Hence, the active elements of the *Shekhinah* are in no way related to femininity but derive, rather, from the masculine. The zoharic claim that the female is called by the name of the male signifies the ontological effacement of the feminine in the moment of coitus. See also *Zohar* 3:183b: "In the place where a male is found even the female entity is called masculine."

[60] Life corresponds to the masculine, or, more specifically, the *semen virile*, and place to the feminine.

[61] On the containment of the attribute of the night in that of the day, see *Zohar* 1:120b; *Book of the Pomegranate*, p. 50.

[62] For discussion of this theme, see reference to my study in n. 15 above.

[63] See parallel in *Zohar Ḥadash* (Margaliot, 1978b), 56c.

It is evident that in this context the image of tasting is a metaphorical expression for sexual intercourse.[64] The union of man and woman results in the transformation of the feminine into the masculine, the overpowering of the redness of judgement by the white of mercy, the containment of the left in the right. The point is made explicitly by Joseph of Hamadan as well:

> The pure and holy overflow and the good oil descends upon the attribute of the *Shekhinah* in the pure and holy chain [*shalshelet ha-qedoshah we-ha-ṭehorah*].[65] Therefore it is

---

[64] The use of eating as a metaphor for sexual intercourse is found already in rabbinic sources; see Boyarin, 1993, pp. 70–75, 116–117, 123. As Boyarin astutely notes, this metaphorical field is determined by the fact that in rabbinic thought the very essence of sexuality is procreation, in an analogous fashion to eating, whose essence is the preservation of the life of the body.

[65] The image of the chain [*shalshelet*] is used by Joseph of Hamadan to refer to the sefirotic pleroma on the whole. On the other hand, this image is used more specifically to refer to the aspect of the divine that corresponds to the phallus, which comprises within itself all the divine potencies. See Meier, 1974, pp. 243–244, where the rite of circumcision is said to symbolize the "chain of the image (*shalshelet ha-demut*) that alludes to the glorious form corresponding to the face below". See ibid., p. 251, where the man who has no children is compared to "one who does not establish the image of the chain" [*demut ha-shalshelet*]; cf. pp. 140, 146, 152, 179, 252, 256, 262, 271; "Joseph of Hamadan's *Sefer Tashak*" (Zwelling, 1975), pp. 62, 72, 80, 81. In the latter instance, the beginning of the "holy and pure chain" of emanation, *Keter*, is described in the obviously phallic image of the "holy spring". It should be noted that on other occasions Hamadan describes *Keter* as the skin that covers the head of the supernal form, an image that calls to mind that of the corona of the penis (cf. ibid., pp. 69, 104). See ibid., p. 126, where the rabbinic custom of covering one's head is connected with the theosophic notion that God's head is covered. Cf. ibid., pp. 235–236, where the covering of the head of the *Matrona*—related to the bent shape of the letter *kaf*—is connected with the proper sexual modesty vis-à-vis the Holy King. The same symbolism is linked to the closed *mem* on p. 252. On Sabbath the *Matrona* embraces the Holy King, and head covering is pushed back so that her face is exposed. In the moment of sexual union the *Matrona* is represented by the final *kaf*, which is a straight and extended line: cf. pp. 237–240. On pp. 297–298, the reason given for the woman's covering her head is to prevent the disclosure of the forces of judgement, which are linked to her hair. In the same context the reason given for a woman's cutting her hair when she is pure is to remove all impurity before she has sexual intercourse with her husband. Cf. ibid.,

written, "We will add wreaths of gold to your spangles of silver" (Song of Songs 1:11), so that the judgement [symbolized by the gold] will be mixed with mercy [the silver], and it is one thing like the flame bound to the coal that is unified in its colours. Everything becomes one. ["Joseph of Hamadan's *Sefer Tashak*", Zwelling, 1975, p. 51][66]

---

pp. 298–299: "Each and every hair from those holy hairs of the Matrona are inscribed with names that are called other gods, and they arouse all kinds of magic and all kinds of sorcery." Cf. ibid., pp. 301:

> The holy hairs of the Matrona are harder than the hairs of the Holy One, blessed be He, because the skull of the Holy One, blessed be He, is completely merciful without any hairs of judgement from various sides; therefore it is soft. The skull of the Matrona has an aspect of judgement from various sides and thus [the hairs of Matrona] are harder and darker than the hairs of the Holy One, blessed be He.

On the other hand, Joseph of Hamadan emphasizes the masculine, and indeed phallic, aspect of hair, which serves as a channel to transmit the flow of divine energy. Cf., ibid., e.g., pp. 298–300:

> Through these holy hairs the holy dew descends from the head of *'Arikh 'Anpin* to the head of the Matrona . . . and she is sweetened. . . . These holy hairs of the Matrona are intertwined with the head of the Holy One, blessed be He. . . . The holy hairs of the Matrona are called the thread of mercy that the Holy One, blessed be He, extends to the righteous.

Needless to say, many more examples from this text and other works of Joseph of Hamadan could be adduced. Liebes (1993b, pp. 124–125) contrasts this aspect of Joseph of Hamadan's writings with the zoharic view that relates the growing of hair to the augmentation of the forces of judgement and impurity. He did not, however, take into account the passages that I mentioned, which are much closer to the negative valorization of hair according to the *Zohar.* On the symbolic implication of the image of enveloping in Joseph of Hamadan, see reference in Wolfson, 1995c , p. 181 n. 353. Finally, mention should be made of the passage in "Joseph of Hamadan's *Sefer Tashak*", Zwelling, 1975, p. 132: "When the seventh millennium comes the holy name will not be seen except for the letter *yod*, and nothing will be seen except for the Supernal Crown that resembles the letter *yod*." It is evident from the context that the *yod* also symbolizes the sign of the covenant. It follows, therefore, that a connection is made between the *yod*, *Keter*, and the corona of the phallus.

[66] Cf. Joseph of Hamadan's description of sexual copulation in Meier, 1974, p. 243: "When a man unites with his wife and he enters the sign of the covenant in the attribute of judgement, the judgement is mixed with mercy (*mit'arev ha-din 'im ha-raḥamim*), and this is the secret of the *'aravot*, and he sweetens the efflux from above and causes the unity of the bridegroom and the bride." On this symbolic connotation of the word *'aravot*, cf. ibid., pp. 133 and 137.

In the final analysis, the affirmation in theosophic kabbalistic sources of sexual mating sanctioned by marriage did not imply metaphysical or social equality between the sexes. The literary evidence proves just the opposite: the positive valorization of human sexuality must be interpreted within a social framework that is thoroughly androcentric.[67] The point is epitomized in the late-thirteenth-century treatise on marital relations, the *'Iggeret ha-Qodesh* ["The Holy Epistle"].[68] According to this text, both man and woman are assigned specific intentions during coitus that help determine the character of the offspring: the task of the man is to be mentally bound to the upper realm so that he can draw down the efflux of divine light onto the *semen virile*, whereas the task of the woman is to synchronize her thoughts with her male partner. Although the language of this text does not explicitly affirm the transformation of the female into a male, it is evident that the role of the woman is to become integrated in the man so that she gains indirect access to the divine realm. While the male directly contemplates the sefirotic entities and is thereby conjoined with them, the female can hope to form a mental image of her male partner and thereby assist in the shaping of the foetus. The intention [*kawwanah*] of the woman is entirely directed towards and subsumed under the male (*Kitve Ramban*, 2, pp. 331–335). To be sure, the man and woman are said to correspond, respectively, to the divine hypostases of *Ḥokhmah*, Wisdom, and *Binah*, Understanding—and the offspring they produce corresponds to *Da'at*, Knowledge, representing the union of the two. This symbolic correspondence, however, does not signify the attribution

---

[67] A similar point is made by Boyarin, 1993, pp. 75–76, with respect to rabbinic Judaism: "The commitment to coupling did not, however, imply any reduction of the radically unequal distribution of power that characterized virtually all of the societies of late antiquity. That inequality not only remained a fact of life for rabbinic Judaism but was confirmed in a whole conceptual apparatus, along with a complex tangle of emblematic stories, articulated in the talmudic literature."

[68] This work has been the object of several scholarly discussions. See Scholem, 1944–45, pp. 179–186, and the additional note of Scholem in *Kiryat Sefer* 22 (1945–46), p. 84; Harris, 1962, pp. 197–220; Cohen, 1976, pp. 7–27; Guberman, 1984, 1, pp. 53–95; Mopsik, 1986. See also discussion of the epistle in Biale, 1992, pp. 102–109.

of an equal social role to the earthly man and woman.[69] On the contrary, primary emphasis is placed on the man whose intentions and thoughts produce and determine the nature of the semen. The goal is for the man to harmonize his intention with that of his wife, so that she produces the seed first and, following the rabbinic dictum (B. Berakhot 60a; Niddah 25b, 28a, 31a.),[70] gives birth to a male (*Kitve Ramban*, p. 336).[71] The logical implication is drawn explicitly by the anonymous author of this kabbalistic work, commenting on the statement in B. Berakhot 20a concerning R. Yohanan's sitting by the bathhouses so that the women exiting from ritual immersion could look upon his face and be blessed with offspring as beautiful as he:

> Thus with the key that we have placed in your hand you can understand the action of that pious one who would sit at the gates of the bathhouses so that the thought [of the women] would cleave to his form, and his form would cleave to the supernal entities. [*Kitve Ramban*, p. 334]

Expressed in slightly different terms, the androcentric perspective is also evident in the following zoharic passage:

> When is a man called one? When there is male and female, and he is sanctified in the supernal holiness and he has the intention to be sanctified. Come and see: when a man is in

[69] See Biale, 1992, p. 107. While Biale duly notes the subordinate role of women in sexual intercourse according to the *'Iggeret ha-Qodesh*, his statement that "[s]ince each partner is connected symbolically with the male and female *sefirot*, the thought or intention of each is equally powerful", needs to be qualified in light of the explicit claims that women are never directly connected to the divine realm. The intention of the woman is vital, but not nearly as powerful as that of the man.

[70] The view of the rabbis reflects the Hippocratic and Galenic (as opposed to the Aristotelian) notion that both parents produce sperm. See Atkinson, 1991, pp. 47–49.

[71] Cf. Judah ben Solomon Campanton, *'Arba'ah Qinyyanim*, Ms. JTSA Mic. 2532, fol. 45a: "This actual matter you find [in the case of] Abraham and Sarah who gave birth in their good thought to Isaac who resembled his father, as it is written, 'Abraham fathered Isaac', the expression 'fathered' (*holid*) has the numerical value of resembled (*domeh*). Thus every man must sanctify himself in the time of intercourse." See ibid., fols. 49a–b.

> the union of male and female, and he intends to be sanctified as is appropriate, then he is complete and he is called one without any blemish. Therefore, a man should gladden his wife at that time, to invite her to be of one will with him. The two of them together should have the same intention for that matter. When the two are found as one, then they are one in soul and body. [*Zohar* 3:81a–b][72]

The intent of the female must be synchronized with that of the male so that the male will be unified and completed by her participation and cooperation in the sexual act. As a result of the sexual union, the woman may be impregnated and hence empowered to procreate. Through the process of reproduction the femaleness of the woman is transformed into a male, since she becomes an active potency that gives birth.[73] The point is underscored in one zoharic passage that describes the *Shekhinah*, on the basis of Eccl. 5:8, as the king who dwells upon a house inhabited by a man who unites with his wife in order to procreate. In her capacity as the active power that gives birth to the souls that are joined to the body produced by the union of a husband and wife, the feminine *Shekhinah* is masculinized (*Zohar* 1:122a).[74] One may assume that this gender transformation also applies to the earthly female when she gives birth.

---

[72] See Tishby, 1963, p. 1360.

[73] My approach is to be contrasted sharply with that of Scholem, who sees the active and passive aspects as related to the feminine nature of the *Shekhinah*, the former consisting of the woman's capacity to give birth (see Scholem, 1991, pp. 165, 174–175). I am suggesting, by contrast, that the gender of femininity is valorized exclusively as passive, and that the more active role associated with the feminine is dependent upon the metamorphosis of the female into a male. See further discussion below on the kabbalistic symbol of the mother. It should be noted, however, that in another passage (p. 183) Scholem takes a position closer to my own when he says that in the *Zohar* there is an attribution of "active and, in Kabbalistic terms, masculine aspects" to the lower *Shekhinah*, previously considered quintessentially feminine. See also p. 186, where Scholem speaks of the "active, masculine aspects" that are applied to the *Shekhinah* alongside the feminine symbols.

[74] The masculine valence of the woman's ability to bear children is underscored in the following passage in Ḥayyim Vital, *'Eṣ Ḥayyim*, 39:7, 72b–c:

> It is known that when *Ze'eir* and *Nuqba'* copulate, he imparts the male waters and she imparts the female waters. It is known what the rabbis,

blessed be their memory, said, "a woman does not make a covenant except with him who makes her into a vessel" [B. Sanhedrin 22b]. The rabbis, blessed be their memory, also said that "a woman does not get pregnant from the first sexual intercourse" [B. Yevamot 34a]. . . . The explanation of these matters is as follows: it is known that *Nuqba'* does not take any light except by means of *Ze'eir 'Anpin*, and it is known that the two crowns are in *Da'at*, and they are called *Ḥesed* and *Gevurah*, and they are the forty-five-letter name and the fifty-two-letter name. Even though *Nuqba'* was [attached] back-to-back with *Ze'eir 'Anpin*, she could not be perfected and become a configuration (*parṣuf*) until she received the crown of strengths, which are the five forces of strength. She does not take the five forces of strength by themselves but only their illumination as they pass through the hinder parts of *Ze'eir 'Anpin*. The five forces of strength descend after the completion of the [forces of] mercy, and they stand in the phallus of *Ze'eir 'Anpin*, and from there they transmit their illumination to *Nuqba'*. These stand in her permanently and they are her life-force, and they are called the soul of *Malkhut*. Since her substance only comes to be from their illumination, she was not fit to give birth, for the female is only fit to give birth when she is complete, and if she is deficient she cannot give birth. All the perfection comes to be only when the five forces of strength, which are the fifty-two-letter name, are in her . . . for this is verily the soul of *Nuqba'*. This is the reason why the woman does not get pregnant from the first sexual intercourse, for the first intercourse turns her into a vessel to receive the drop of semen, and after that vessel receives [the semen] from the first intercourse from that point on she can become pregnant and she receives the drop of semen in other copulations.

According to this passage, the soul of the female, which allows her to give birth, consists of the five forces of judgement that derive from the male and that are implanted in the female in the first act of coitus. That act transforms the female into a vessel, which is endowed with the task of receiving the seminal fluid. One will readily admit that the nature of the female is represented exclusively from the vantage point of the phallus.

To highlight the extent to which the androcentric understanding of parturition informed the kabbalistic mentality, I will briefly analyse some key passages in an important treatise by the seventeenth-century Sabbatian theologian, Abraham Miguel Cardoso, *Derush ha-Shekhinah*. (I am currently preparing a full-length study on the role of the feminine in Cardoso's thought. What is presented here is a preliminary discussion of one aspect that is most relevant to the theme of the masculinization of childbirth.) On the one hand, Cardoso insists that the *Shekhinah* occupies a unique position because she alone is endowed with the capacity to create, and thus she manifests the full intention of the first *sefirah*. On the other hand, Cardoso recognizes that the feminine cannot give birth without the masculine: "Certainly one will comprehend that there is no woman without a man, according to [the verse] 'for from man she was taken' (Gen. 2:23). Then you will discern the secret of divinity (*sod ha-'elohut*)" (Ms.

In support of my last claim, I will cite a passage that conveys the idea that the transformation from femaleness to maleness represents the ideal movement for the earthly woman during intercourse, emulating thereby the progression in the divine realm. The text is an anonymous kabbalistic exposition on the commandment of levirate marriage, *sod ha-yibbum*, whose provenance, I surmise, is thirteenth-century Catalonia:

NYJTSA Mic. 1677, fol. 2a). The secret of divinity, which Cardoso reiterates in many of his compositions, entails the androgynous nature of the Creator, who is distinguished from the hidden First Cause. Part and parcel of the theological secret is the acceptance of the ontically secondary status of the female as that which is taken from the male. Yet, in spite of this recognition, Cardoso attributes supreme value to the female. In fact, so enamoured is Cardoso of the feminine that he even turns the biblical conception of the woman's derivative status into a positive:

> The intent of what we say that Eve was contained in Adam is that she was with him in order to emerge afterward in a complete disclosure. The Holy One, blessed be He, constructed the feminine from the rib [or side] of Adam. She is the last of all created beings and she comprises everything that was in Adam, and in addition she comprises the essential being of Adam for she was not made from the dust [of the earth] as he was but rather from the flesh and bone of Adam. . . . Thus the greatness of Eve over Adam is clarified, she comprises everything that he comprises and in her is the existence of the masculine for she is flesh of his flesh. [Ms. NYJTSA Mic. 1677, fols. 5a–b]

In the final analysis, Cardoso cannot shed the androcentric bias of mediaeval kabbalah. The feminine is extolled as the creative force in the universe, but that power ultimately derives from the masculine.

> Eve was complete and she was called "woman" [*'ishah*] since she was taken from the man [*'ish*], and his being and his power are comprised in her. Therefore she is called *'ishah* for she is ready to give birth. It is appropriate that each and every female is taken from the male . . . for a man imparts to her the spirit, which comprises his essence and his power, by means of the first intercourse, and through that his wife becomes a vessel that is suitable to bear sons and daughters. . . . When the female does not [carnally] know a male it is written in relation to her *na'ar*, but after she has had intercourse she is called *na'arah*, for prior to the intercourse she is like a male who cannot give birth and after the intercourse she becomes a vessel and she is called *na'arah*, the complete female that comprises the power of the male (*neqevah shelemah she-kolelet koaḥ ha-zakhar*). This is clear proof that the female must contain the being [of the male] in order to give birth in his image and in his likeness. . . . The woman comprises the man, "for from man she was

It is written in *Sefer ha-Bahir*[75] that the Holy One, blessed be He, created seven holy forms, and the forms are divided into two hands, two legs, a head and the body. Thus there are six, and these six [are male]. [It is written] "male and female He created them" [Gen. 1:26] . . . the seventh form is the female. Thus the woman completes the seven forms. When the Holy One, blessed be He, created Adam, He combined all seven forms together, and afterward He separated the seventh so that the woman would be the seventh form of the man, and the man is not complete without her, as it is written, "it is not good for man to be alone",[76] and it is written, "they will be as one flesh".[77] . . . Just as Sabbath is rest for the six days so too the woman is rest for the six forms, for without her a man is not stationary, he wanders to and fro. As the rabbis, blessed be their memory, said, "the one who dwells without a wife dwells without goodness".[78] And this is what the rabbis, blessed be their memory, said, "a person is not exempt from [the commandment] to procreate until he has a boy and a girl",[79] so that what is born to him corresponds to the seven forms. This is also what they alluded to by the fact that a man and not a woman is commanded with respect to procreation, for most of the forms and their essence are in the male, and the woman is but the completion. This is [the intent of] what the rabbis, blessed be their memory, said, "a woman who produces seed first gives birth to a male", for the seed of the man, in which there are the six forms, annuls the seed of the woman which has but one form. The male comes by way of the male and the female by the power of the female. [Ms. VBAE 236, fols. 76a–b.][80]

---

taken" (Gen. 2:23), and they are one flesh and one substance. The blemish of one harms the other [Ms. NYJTSA Mic. 1677, fols. 8a–b]

The feminine becomes fully herself only after she has had intercourse with the male and she becomes a vessel to receive the semen. Cardoso falls short of explicitly affirming the gender transformation of the female to the male, but it is quite obvious that he locates the procreative power of the female in the male.

[75] *Sefer ha-Bahir*, § 172.

[76] Gen. 2:19.

[77] Gen. 2:25.

[78] B. Yevamot 62b.

[79] Ibid., 61b.

[80] See also Ms. PBP 2704 (De Rossi 68), fol. 87a.

The feminine potency is here portrayed as the seventh form that completes or perfects the other six. That this completion involves the female being reintegrated into the male is obvious from the examples adduced in the realm of human relationships. The lack of autonomy of the feminine is underscored in the continuation of the text that elaborates on the biblical law that the male child and not the female inherits the property of the father. Most significantly, the woman is depicted as the vehicle that allows the man to produce offspring. While the talmudic opinion that a man fulfils his obligation of procreation by having a child of each sex is theosophically reinterpreted,[81] it is clear from the end of the passage that having male children is privileged, for the female ontically is only the completion of the masculine. Indeed, conjugal intercourse replicates the structure above: the seminal fluid symbolizes the six male forms and the vaginal secretion the seventh female form. Following the rabbinic view, which, in turn, reflects the Hippocratic and Galenic standpoint,[82] conception requires the mixing of two seeds, but the desired situation involves the domination and superiority of the male so that a male child is conceived. By secreting her fluids first, the woman allows the sperm of the man to dominate, and thus the embryo that is conceived is male. Through the production of male progeny, the woman's task to complete the male structure is accomplished.

Masculine transvaluation of motherhood: the phallic womb

By giving birth in general, and to male offspring in particular, the female assumes the role of the engendering male. Although pregnancy and childbirth are generally thought to be the exclusive burden (perhaps even curse) of the woman, following the explicit claim of Gen. 3:16, in kabbalistic literature they are valorized as positive, masculine traits. The biological woman assumes the male gender through these bodily functions. The point is alluded to in the following zoharic text:

[81] Cf. *Zohar* 3:7a, discussed in Tishby, 1963, p. 1361.
[82] See Preus, 1977, pp. 65–85; Boylan, 1984, pp. 83–112.

> R. Yose said: from the time a woman gets pregnant until the day she gives birth there is nothing in her mouth but that her child should be a male. Thus it says, "When a woman brings forth seed and bears a male" (Lev. 12:2). [*Zohar* 3:42b]

The intention of the woman expressed verbally to bear a male child has the effect of masculinizing her so that she produces seed like a man and gives birth to a boy. According to the zoharic exegesis, the bringing forth of the male seed on the part of the woman is accomplished through the orifice of the mouth that corresponds to the procreative organ of the male, a parallelism that is a foundational structure in Jewish esotericism. By uttering her desire to have a boy, the woman takes the place of a male who procreates.

It can be shown from still other zoharic sources that the female who gives birth is depicted as male. In his discussion of the feminine element of divinity in kabbalistic symbolism, Scholem already noted that one must distinguish between two aspects of femininity—corresponding to the upper and lower *Shekhinah*—the active energy and creative power, on the one hand, and the passive receptivity, on the other. The former is associated more specifically with the image of the "upper mother", the third gradation or *Binah*, and the latter with the "lower mother", the tenth gradation or *Malkhut* (Scholem, 1991, pp. 174–175). Scholem comes close to realizing the complex inversion of gender that this symbolism presupposes when he remarks that the "male symbol" of the Creator or Demiurge (applied to *Binah*) "represents that aspect of the feminine that is in principle denied to the lower *Shekhinah*" (ibid., p. 176). Analogously, Scholem remarks that "when the *Shekhinah* functions as a medium for the downward flow of life-giving energies, it is understood in male symbols" (ibid., p. 186). In spite of these momentary insights, however, Scholem's analysis in general (as most other scholars who have written on the subject) suffers from a lack of attentiveness to the dynamic of gender metamorphosis. That is, he too readily describes the symbolic valence of motherhood as a feminine trait, assuming that the biological function reflects the meaning of the theosophic symbol. Thus, when describing the active forces of the *Shekhinah*, Scholem speaks of the "maternal, birth-giving, and creative element that comes about as a result of the very act of receiving". The dual role of giving and receiving is designated by Scholem as the "dialectics of femininity" (ibid., p. 187). In my view, the idea of motherhood in kabbalistic symbolism is decidedly masculine, for the womb that gives birth is valorized as an erectile and elongated phallus.[83] One would do better, therefore, to refer to the creative and maternal element of the female as the transvaluation of the feminine into the masculine.[84]

In light of this gender transformation one can appreciate the active characterization of the divine gradation that corresponds to the upper mother. Indeed, as I have already noted above, in zoharic literature and other texts influenced thereby, *Binah*, the feminine counterpart to the second emanation, *Ḥokhmah*, is called the world-of-the-masculine [*'alma' di-dekhura'*] as opposed to the lower *Shekhinah* which is called the world-of-the-feminine [*'alma' de-nuqba'*], for *Binah* is the womb whence the other emanations that constitute the divine anthropos derive. Many of the images and symbols that are employed in the *Zohar* and related sources to depict the ninth gradation, *Yesod*, which corresponds to the divine phallus, are also used in relation to *Binah*, the gradation that is referred to as the mother or the womb that receives the seed from *Ḥokhmah*, the father. To be sure, the attribute of *Binah* is empowered to give birth by virtue of the semen that she receives from *Ḥokhmah*, but that reception transforms her phallically into a spring that overflows. As Moses de León in one of his writings expresses the matter:

> She is called *Binah* when the concealed Thought emanates, and this is the source of life, for from there is the issue of life, for the secret of the Mother, the supernal well, hidden in her secret and her character, the hidden world, the conceal-

---

[83] On portrayals of the uterus as the penis in Renaissance anatomical material, see evidence adduced by Laqueur, *Making Sex*, pp. 79–98. The kabbalistic transformation of motherhood into a masculine ideal is also predicated on a one-sex model that viewed the female genitals as internal analogues to the male genitals. The womb, therefore, is characterized in terms of a penis-like extension.

[84] On the androgynous character of the archetype of the Great Mother, see Neumann, 1954, p. 46. On the phenomenon of the phallic mother, or the uroboric snake woman that combines begetting and child-bearing, see Neumann, 1963, pp. 13, 170, 308–310.

> ment of His strength. [Scholem, 1976, p. 375; cf. *Zohar* 1:229a; 3:78a]

The archetype of the mother, *Binah*, is here portrayed as simultaneously concealing the masculine strength (i.e. the phallus) and revealing it in the overflow that issues forth from her. The dialectic of hiddenness and disclosure, passive receptivity (symbolized by the image of the well) and active creativity (symbolized by the image of the source of life), characterizes the lower feminine, *Malkhut*, as well, in relation to *Yesod*. To cite again Moses de León, who succinctly conveys the point: "When the holy sign is revealed it overflows and the perfect bride, [of whom it is said] 'the glory of the princess that is inward' (Ps. 45:14), stands in her completeness and illuminates her portion" (*Book of the Pomegranate*, p. 229). The feminine can be productive only to the extent that she receives the overflow from the masculine and is thereby transformed from a passive receptacle to an active agent. The gender metamorphosis is epitomized in the mystical interpretation of Noah's entry into the ark:

> When the Righteous joins the ark then all the beings issue forth to be established and the souls fly out from there. When everything comes forth from the ark . . . by means of the power of the Righteous, there is existence for all the beings that issue forth from the ark by the power of the covenant of the living Righteous. [Ibid., p. 166; cf. *Zohar* 1:59b–60a]

The uterus that contains the fecundating phallus is transformed thereby into an instrument of the male principle.

The phallic nature of *Binah* is underscored in a striking way in the following comment of Isaac of Acre (active in the early part of the fourteenth century) on the passage in *Sefer Yeṣirah* that speaks of the covenant of unity set in the middle of the ten *sefirot* corresponding to the mouth or tongue that is set in the middle of the ten fingers and the penis that is set between the ten toes:

> All the functioning limbs are in pairs except for the mouth and the penis. . . . These two are single to inform you that even though you find opposites in the world you should not say that they could not derive from a simple thing, for you already see that the mouth is one and it comes from

> another, and similarly the penis is an opening to bring forth the semen but it is one. Corresponding to the penis in a man is the *sefirah* called *Yesod* for from there the souls emerge, and *Binah* corresponds to the mouth in a man for from it comes forth the issue of life. The two of them correspond to one another. The two of them are called *Shekhinah*, the upper one *Binah* and the lower one *Malkhut*. *Yesod* and *Malkhut* are bound together, and *Binah* is the tongue . . . *Yesod* is the penis and it is called *qeshet* for it throws with strength and vigor below. . . . He who sins with respect to these two is called one who "alienates his friend", *mafrid 'alluf* [Prov. 16:28] or cuts the shoots, *meqaṣṣeṣ ba-neṭi'ot*,[85] for he separates (*mafrid*) *Yesod* from *Malkhut* or *Binah* who is the "mother of the children" [Ps. 113:9]. *Binah* is called *yod-he'* and *Yesod* is *waw-he'*, and the one who creates a division in *Binah* is called *'eryah*, and the secret is "All bared and ready is your bow", *'eryah te'or qashtekha* [Hab. 3:9], and the one who creates a division in *Yesod* is called *'ervah*.[86] The *sefirah* of *Yesod* binds together the upper *Shekhinah* and the lower one, and similarly the tongue is the bond of love through speech between a man and his wife or between two lovers. Therefore lovers kiss one another through their mouths. [Scholem, 1955–56, p. 386]

The union of the Godhead, represented by the Tetragrammaton, depends upon the binding of *Binah* (signified by the first two letters of the name) and *Yesod* (signified by the last two letters), which correspond, respectively, to the orifice of the mouth above and the penis below. The structural and functional homology between the two is disrupted when they are separated, an act that is compared to the uncovering of the genitals. Moreover, just as *Yesod* is bound to *Binah*, so, too, is it bound to *Shekhinah*, upon which it overflows like the penis that discharges semen. Interestingly enough, however, the heterosexual imagery of the kiss used at the end of the citation depicts symbolically the union of *Binah* and *Malkhut* rather than of

[85] This is the technical expression used in some rabbinic sources to refer to the apostasy of Elisha ben Abuyah. For references and discussion, see Halperin, 1980, pp. 90–91.

[86] Both words, *'eryah* and *'ervah*, have the connotation of nakedness and can refer more specifically to the uncovering of the genitals.

Yesod and *Malkhut*. The bond of love between the upper and lower *Shekhinah* is secured by the tongue of speech that corresponds to the phallic *Yesod*.

In the zoharic corpus, too, the very concept of motherhood is shaped by the parallelism set between the divine grades of *Binah* and *Yesod*. Thus, for instance, another designation of *Binah* in zoharic literature is the "concealed world" (*'alma' de-itkkaseya'*, corresponding to *'olam ha-nistar* in Moses de León's Hebrew writings), a term that relates specifically to the character of *Binah*, the divine mother, as that which encompasses and encloses her offspring.[87] The aspect of concealment, frequently associated with the phallic *Yesod*, is linked to the image of *Binah* as the mother who sits upon her children (see *Zohar* 1:158a). The masculine element is especially highlighted in those contexts where the image of the mother hovering over her children is combined with that of the mother nursing her babes (*Zohar* 2:9a). Breast-feeding, too, is valorized as a phallic activity (the milk obviously taking the place of the semen) insofar as anything that sustains by overflowing is automatically treated as an aspect of the phallus.[88] The point is underscored in one zoharic

[87] See, e.g., *Zohar* 1:219a and *Book of the Pomegranate*, p. 138:

> Behold I will reveal you a true secret. Know that there is no male in Israel who is married that does not stand between two women, one hidden and the other revealed. When a man is married the *Shekhinah* above his head becomes in relation to him a hidden world, and his wife stands next to him in the matter that is revealed. Thus, he stands between two women, one hidden and the other revealed, to be in the pattern that is above.

The biblical model recalled in this context is Jacob, who stands between his two wives, Leah and Rachel, symbolically corresponding to *Binah* and *Malkhut*. See parallel in *Zohar* 1:50a, already noted by Liebes (1993b, pp. 72–73). In line with the gender dynamic operative in this text, the upper female in relation to the male is a concealed world and the lower female is the revealed world. The upper feminine, however, in this posture is valorized as male.

[88] See *Zohar* 1:184a, where the image of nursing from the mother's breast (cf. Song of Songs 8:1) is interpreted as a reference to the unity and love between *Yesod* and *Shekhinah*. In that context, therefore, breast-feeding assumes a sexual connotation. The breasts can also symbolize masculine and feminine potencies; cf. *Zohar* 1:44b and 2:253a (both interpreting Song of Songs 4:5). In the latter instance it is evident, moreover, that the divine name *shaddai*, etymologically connected to

passage that reflects on the word *'eḥad* in *shema' yisra'el yhwh 'elohenu yhwh 'eḥad* [Hear, O Israel, the Lord is our God, the Lord is one] (Deut. 6:4). In line with earlier kabbalistic sources,[89] the zoharic authorship interprets the three letters of this word as a reference to the ten *sefirot*: the *'alef* corresponds to the first *sefirah*, *Keter*, the letter *het* to the eight *sefirot* from *Ḥokhmah* to *Yesod*, and the *dalet* to the *Shekhinah*, who is the impoverished [*dal*] emanation. According to the masoteric orthography, however, this *dalet* is enlarged, and this theosophically signifies that the *Shekhinah* cleaves to the upper gradations. In this state the *Shekhinah* is "augmented and all the world suckles from her, and the breasts 'were like towers, so I became in his eyes as one who finds favor' (Song of Songs 8:10)" (*Zohar* 1:256b). The *Zohar* contrasts the existential situation of the *Shekhinah* in exile and in a state of blessing and augmentation: the first instance is depicted by the verse, "We have a little sister, whose breasts are

---

shadayim, breasts (on the possibility of this philological connection in the biblical text itself, see Biale, 1982, pp. 240–256) signifies the phallic activity of the feminine potency, which supplies sustenance for all things below her in accord with what she receives from the right side of mercy. See also *Zohar* 2:257a, where the celestial palace [*hekhal*] is called *'el shaddai* because it sustains the world like breasts and

> God will fill it and establish it in the future, as it is written, "That you may suck from her breast consolation to the full, that you may draw from her bosom glory to your delight" (Isa. 66:1). The breast of consolation and the splendor of her glory are all in this palace, and at that time it is written, "Who would have said to Abraham that Sarah would suckle children!" (Gen. 21:7), for suckling is dependent upon Abraham.

Hence, it is evident from this passage that the nursing of the breasts is valorized as a male trait, related specifically to the attribute of mercy personified in the figure of Abraham. The masculine valorization of nursing that one finds in kabbalistic literature should be contrasted with the application of the maternal imagery of breast-feeding to Jesus and the prelates that one finds in twelfth-century Cistercian devotional texts; see Bynum, 1982, pp. 110–169. In the case of the Christian authors, there does not seem to be any transvaluation of the feminine into the masculine, but, rather, the appropriation of maternal metaphors—especially breasts and nurturing—to describe aspects of the relationship of Jesus and the prelates to individual souls. In the kabbalistic literature, by contrast, the application of the maternal images to God is predicated on the gender transformation of the concept of motherhood. Images of giving birth and nursing are valenced as specifically phallic activities.

[89] See Idel, 1988b, p. 55.

not yet formed" (Song of Songs 8:8), whereas the latter is conveyed in the aforecited verse, "My breasts are like towers, so I became in his eyes as one who finds favor" (Song of Songs 8:10). The maturation of the *Shekhinah* from a woman without breasts to one with full-grown breasts in effect symbolizes her gender transformation from a female to a male.[90] Thus the breasts are described in the obvious phallic image of a tower whence all beings are sustained.[91] The phallic function of the breasts is also alluded to in the expression, "as one who finds favor"—*ke-moṣ'et*

---

[90] In the continuation of the zoharic text, the growth of the breasts is linked more specifically to the righteous and meritorious activities of Israel. That is, when the Jewish people cleave to the Torah and go in a truthful path, then the *Shekhinah* is fortified like a wall and develops towering breasts. The allegorical depiction of Israel's deeds as the breasts of the *Shekhinah* is also found in *Zohar* 2:80b. See also 1:45a, where the beauty of a woman is tied especially to her breasts.

[91] The phallic signification of the mature breasts is also evident in *Zohar* 3:296a (*'Idra' Zuta'*):

> The beauty of the female is entirely from the beauty of the male. . . . This female [*Shekhinah*] is called the smaller wisdom in relation to the other one, and thus it is written, "We have a little sister, whose breasts are not yet formed" (Song of Songs 8:8), for she tarries in the exile. "We have a little sister", certainly she appears as little, but she is big and great. for she is the completion of what she has received from everyone, as it is written, "I am a wall, my breasts are like towers" (ibid., 10). "My breasts" are filled to nurse all things. "Like towers", these are the great rivers that issue forth from the supernal mother.

The phallic characterization of the breasts is drawn explicitly in Menahem Azariah of Fano, *Yonat 'Elem*, ch. 57, 45a:

> The blessings of the breasts that lactate milk according to the secret of "And the Lord passes," wa-ya'avor YHWH (Exod. 34:6), for these [letters allude to] the 72 [letter name, i.e. 'ayin-bet], the 216 [letters comprised in that name, i.e. reish-yod-waw], and 26 [the numerical value of YHWH]. In this manner [are the letters arranged]: the 72 on the right side of Binah, the 216 on the left side and YHWH in the middle. The numerical value of them all is equivalent to the sum of Shaddai [i.e. 72 + 216 + 26 = 314], which is from the word shadayim. . . . When the Mother nurses Ze'eir and Nuqba' [she] is called El Shaddai on account of the breasts (shadayim) that are in her median line.

The breasts, therefore, are aligned in the phallic position of the middle and it is on account of them that the maternal potency of God assumes the name *El Shaddai*. Compare the explanation of impregnation [*'ibbur*] in the Lurianic text preserved in Ms. NYJTSA Mic. 2155, fol. 69a: "After birth *shalom*—the term *shalom* serving in zoharic literature as in other kabbalistic compositions as one of the designations for the divine phallus.

The motherly quality of brooding over the offspring is also connected with the concept of *Teshuvah* [literally, "return"]—that is, the emanations are in stationary position in relation to their source (*Zohar* 2:85b).[92] This, too, is the theosophic symbolism of Yom Kippur, the Day of Atonement: on that day all things return to their ontic source, to be sustained by the overflowingness of the primal concealment. Thus, on that very day, there is an aspect of disclosure, for the fifty gates of *Binah* open up to every side, but there is also an aspect of concealment, for the Mother remains covered and hidden. The latter motif is connected with the prohibition of uncovering the nakedness of the father and mother (Lev. 18:7), the precise Torah portion that is read in the afternoon service of Yom Kippur (*Zohar* 3:15b).[93] In a profound inversion of symbolism, the concealment of the Mother enables her to sustain her offspring, and in that act of nourishing she is masculinized. Theosophically interpreted, the sin of disclosing the genitals of the mother creates a blemish above that separates the Mother from her children; repentance

---

[*Binah*] nursed him in the secret of the milk until he grew up and was weaned (cf. Gen. 21:8) and this is [the significance of] *'el 'elyon gomel* [the supernal God bestows goodness] from the expression *wa-yigmol sheqedim* [it bore almonds] (Num. 17:23). During the time of the nursing she is called El Shaddai from the expression *shadayim*." Finally, let me note that the symbolic correlation of the penis and the breasts that I have delineated in kabbalistic literature represents the reverse of what one finds in Freudian psychoanalytic theory. That is, according to Freud, the penis becomes heir to the nipple of the mother's breast when sucking comes to an end (see Freud, 1916–17, p. 565). Although Freud evaluates the sexuality of the breast entirely from the vantage point of the penis, he does not, as the kabbalists, interpret the biological functions of the breasts in phallic terms.

[92] Cf. *Book of the Pomegranate*, p. 163. The nexus between the motif of returning and the role of *Binah* as that which overflows in blessings is underscored in the anonymous kabbalistic text, influenced by zoharic traditions and the writings of Moses de León, the *Sefer ha-Ne'elam*, Ms. PBNH. 817, fol. 57a.

[93] On the paradoxical nature of this passage, see the marginal notes in Scholem, 1992, p. 2232.

is, quite literally, causing the Mother to return to her place wherein she continues to assume the masculine role of feeding and sustaining the offspring in a manner that is concealed.[94] When the Mother and children are united, the genitals are covered, and the children nurse from her in a pattern that resembles the primary opening of the womb through the attribute

---

[94] The nexus of Repentance, Yom Kippur, and illicit sexual relations, especially uncovering the genitals of the father and mother, in the zoharic text is also evident in the following comment of Joseph of Hamadan in his commentary on the *sefirot*, Ms. OBL 1628, fol. 67b:

> From there [*Binah*] begins the drawing-forth of the genitals (*yeniqat 'arayot*), and thus on Yom Kippur we read at the time of Minhah [the afternoon service] the matter of illicit sexual relations (*'arayot*), for they draw forth from the attribute of *Binah* which is called *Teshuvah* in every place. On Yom Kippur we stand in the strength of *Teshuvah*, and you find that the beginning of the [section on] illicit sexual relations is 'the nakedness of the father and mother' (Lev. 18:7), which is the attribute of *Binah* on account of the beginning of the secret of illicit sexual relations (*sitre 'arayot*).

For a parallel to this explanation, cf. Joseph of Hamadan's *Sefer Ṭa'ame ha-Miṣwot*, positive commandments (no. 48) in Meier, 1974, p. 196: "We read the section on *'arayot* in the Minhah prayer on Yom Kippur because we comprehend [at that time] the attribute of *Binah*, and from there we begin to draw forth the *'arayot*, the secret of the wife and her husband, the secret of unity." For a slightly different formulation, cf. "Joseph of Hamadan's *Sefer Tashak*", Zwelling, 1975, p. 109, where it is emphasized that from *Binah* is the drawing-forth of the golden bowl [*yeniqat golat ha-zahav*], i.e. the phallus, that overflows to all the attributes. Cf. Joseph of Hamadan's *Sefer Ta'ame ha-Miṣwot*, negative commandments (no. 30), Ms. PBNH 817, fol. 155a, where a connection is made between the custom to read the section on *'arayot* during the afternoon service of Yom Kippur and the tannaitic treatment of illicit sexual relations as an esoteric discipline (according to M. Ḥagigah 2:1). In that context, moreover, Hamadan offers a slightly different nuanced explanation for this commandment:

> Know that the matter of the *'arayot* all relates to the fact that one should not make use of the sceptre of the glorious king, for he who has intercourse with his mother it is as if he actually had intercourse with the *Shekhinah* for she is the mother of all living things. Therefore, it is written [in Lev. 18:7] "your mother" twice, corresponding to the mother above and the mother below. Not for naught did the rabbis, blessed be their memory, say [B. Berakhot 57a], the one who has intercourse with his mother in a dream should anticipate understanding. . . . This is the attribute of *Binah* that is called mother. Therefore, he who has intercourse with his mother makes use of the sceptre of *Binah* who is called

of mercy. By contrast, when the Mother and children are separated, the genitals are uncovered, and the attribute of judgement dominates.[95]

That the divine Mother is described in the same or proximate terms used to describe the phallus indicates that the female who gives birth is valorized as a male, for the act of birthing is treated as a form of expansion or ejaculation that is characteristically

---

> mother, and he who makes use [of the sceptre] of the glorious king is guilty of death. Therefore the Torah says, "Your father's nakedness and the nakedness of your mother, you shall not uncover", corresponding to *Ṣaddiq* and *Malkhut* who are called father and mother, and [the continuation of the verse, "she is your mother—you shall not uncover her nakedness"] corresponds to *Binah*.

According to an alternative symbolic explanation, on Yom Kippur there is a reunion of mother and daughter, i.e. *Binah* and *Malkhut* are conjoined in a union that has no precise analogue in the anthropological sphere. On the contrary, sexual relations between husband and wife are prohibited precisely because in the divine realm this mating occurs. Cf. *Book of the Pomegranate*, pp. 162–163; *Sefer ha-Ne'elam*, Ms. PBNH 817, fol. 57b.

[95] The complex symbolism and dialectic of concealment and disclosure is well captured in the following passage of Isaac Luria copied by Samuel Vital and printed in *Sha'ar Ma'amere Rashbi* (Jerusalem, 1898), 23b:

> Just as *Neṣaḥ*, *Hod*, and *Yesod* of the Mother are clothed in the head of *Ze'eir 'Anpin*, so *Neṣaḥ*, *Hod*, and *Yesod* of *Ze'eir 'Anpin* extend and enter into the point of Zion of the foundation of *Malkhut*, her femaleness [i.e. the uterus; cf. ibid., 28b], and they are joined in the secret of union. . . . Then the womb of the female of *Ze'eir 'Anpin* that is below opens up, but she also is concealed and hidden. It follows that the beginning of that key is united with and is closed in relation to the Mother and its end is closed and united below with the Female. . . . Thus the two genitals, that of the Mother and that of the Daughter, are concealed, and then there are no complete judgements. But when, God forbid, Israel sin they cause the Mother to depart from her children and consequently the Mother removes her *Neṣaḥ*, *Hod*, and *Yesod* from the skull of *Ze'eir 'Anpin*, and thus her foundation was revealed. This causes the *Ze'eir 'Anpin* also to depart above and he is not with his Female. Consequently, the foundation of the Female was also revealed, and this is the matter of the uncovering of the genitals. This causes the judgements of the Mother and Daughter to come forth from there and they extend below. . . . But you should know that when their wombs open up this is the secret of the opening of the womb (*peter reḥem*) at the time of childbirth, and then, by contrast, is the aspect of mercy and not the aspect of judgement. Understand this distinction.

masculine.[96] The act of procreation is decidedly phallic. Hence, the tenth of the emanations, the *Shekhinah*, which is characterized as feminine vis-à-vis the upper emanations, is masculine in relation to what is beneath her, and indeed is referred to frequently as *malkhut* on account of this procreative quality.[97] According to one text in the *Zohar*, interpreting the verse, "Drink water from your cistern, running water from your own well" (Prov. 5:15), when the *Shekhinah* receives the influx from the upper masculine divine potencies, she is transformed from an empty cistern [*bor*] that has nothing of its own into a well [*be'er*] that is full and overflows to every side: the impoverished *dalet* becomes an open *he'* (*Zohar* 1:60a).[98] In the aspect of overflowing, the queen becomes king, and the open womb symbolically assumes the role of a phallus; thus one of the most common and influential symbols of the feminine Presence is King David. The appropriateness of this symbol is not due to a feminization of David, but, rather, to the masculinization of the *Shekhinah*.[99]

---

[96] With respect to this quality of motherhood, there is an obvious discrepancy between the social and religious duty of the woman and the theosophic symbolism. That is, the symbolic valorization of the mother as masculine stands in marked contrast to the exclusive (secondary) social and religious role accorded the woman related to the biological functions of motherhood. This process is to be contrasted sharply with that of Christianity, wherein the construction of spiritual motherhood (related to the ideology of monasticism) replaced biological motherhood as the most efficacious role of women. See Atkinson, 1991, pp. 64–100. The situation of Christianity is also to be distinguished from Judaism insofar as in the case of the former, ideas about the motherhood of God were shaped around texts and rituals connected to the figure of Mary. See Atkinson, 1991; Benko, 1993.

[97] See passages from Joseph of Hamadan cited in n. 94, above.

[98] In other contexts a distinction is made between *be'er* and *be'erah*, the former referring to the *Shekhinah* before she receives water from the masculine attribute of *Ḥesed* and the latter once she has received it; cf. *Zohar* 3:183b. The former expression is used in particular in contexts that describe the relationship of Isaac, who represents the attribute of judgement, and the *Shekhinah*: cf. *Zohar* 1:60b, 135b; 3:103a, 115a, 156b.

[99] See, e.g., *Zohar* 1:60b, 3:84a. The latter context is particularly interesting insofar as the topic of discussion is the gaze of the Holy One upon David: "When the Holy One, blessed be He, wants to have mercy upon the world He looks upon that David, and shines His face upon him, and he illuminates the worlds and has pity on the world. The beauty of this David illuminates all the worlds." It is possible that this passage implies an element of homoeroticism in the divine realm. That is, even

It is in light of this masculine quality, moreover, that the *Shekhinah*, too, is called mother—or, to be more precise, the lower mother in relation to *Binah*, the archetypal image of the great mother. To cite one textual illustration: "From this Female are united all those that are below, they are sustained from her and to her they return, and she is called the mother of them all" (*Zohar* 3:296a [*'Idra' Zuta'*]). The concept of motherhood is predicated on the quality of overflowing and sustaining. In relation to the world, then, the *Shekhinah* assumes male characteristics and is thus depicted as a mother.

> The upper world of the masculine is bound to the lower one, which is the world of the feminine, and the lower is bound to the upper, and the one is like the other. It is said that there are two worlds . . . and even though the two are feminine one is adorned as a male and the other as a female. . . . The one is a mother and the other is a mother. One is called the "mother of the children" (Ps. 113:9) and the other is called the "mother of Solomon" (*Zohar* 1:248b).

In this connection, it is also of interest to note the interpretation of the verse,

> On the third day, Esther put on royal apparel and stood in the inner court of the king's palace, facing the king's palace, while sitting on his royal throne in the throne room facing the entrance of the palace. [Esther 5:1]

in the following zoharic passage:

> "On the third day," when the power of the body was weakened and she existed in spirit without a body, then "Esther put on royal apparel" [*wa-tilbash 'esther malkhut*]. . . . She was adorned in the supernal, holy *Malkhut*, she most certainly was clothed in the Holy Spirit. [*Zohar* 3:183b]

---

though David is a standard symbol for the Presence, usually valorized as female, in this context the issue seems to be the masculine deity gazing upon the aspect that sustains the world. That aspect is the male dimension of the Presence, indeed the corona of the phallus. See *Zohar* 1:168a, where the zoharic authorship reworked the older motif of God gazing upon the icon of Jacob and having pity upon the world. For discussion of this theme see Wolfson, 1995c.

The text goes on to record that Esther was granted to be clothed in the Holy Spirit as a reward for her reticence to disclose information about her upbringing to Ahasuerus (see Esther 2:20). The significant point for this analysis is that Esther takes on, or is united with, the aspect of God referred to as *Malkhut*, the tenth emanation that corresponds to the feminine *Shekhinah*, only when she overcomes her own physical status. To become the divine feminine involves a denial of biological womanhood. The underlying conceptual point here is identical to the issue that I raised before—namely, that the engendering aspect of the *Shekhinah*, designated as *Malkhut*, is related to the masculine potency of God; hence, only when the distinctive bodily characteristics of the woman are subjugated by the spirit that is related to the masculine can she receive the overflow (or the Holy Spirit) from the divine realm. Ironically enough, according to the complex gender system of theosophic kabbalah, conception, pregnancy, birthing, and nursing are all seen as male traits. A perfect homology thus exists between the divine and mundane spheres: just as the divine feminine can assume the qualities of the male, so, too, the earthly biological woman can be gendered as masculine. One may speak, therefore, of a kind of spiritual transvestism that is logically implied by kabbalistic myth: a woman actualizes her fullest potential *qua* human when she is adorned with the qualities of the male, realized principally through conception and procreation. The point is affirmed in the following zoharic text:

> The Mother [*Binah*] lends her garments to the Daughter [*Shekhinah*] and adorns her in her ornamentation. When does she adorn her in her ornamentation as is appropriate? When all the males appear before her, as it is written, "[Three times a year all your males shall appear] before the Sovereign, the Lord", *'el pene ha-'adon yhwh* [Exod. 23:17], and this [the *Shekhinah*] is called Sovereign (*'adon*), as it says, "the Ark of the Covenant of the Sovereign of all the earth", *hinneh 'aron ha-berit 'adon kol ha-'areṣ* [Josh. 3:11]. Then the *he'* goes out and the *yod* enters, and she is adorned in the garments of the male corresponding to all the males in Israel. [*Zohar* 1:2a]

The gender transformation of the feminine *Shekhinah*, the Daughter, into a male is here depicted in terms of the reception of the garments and adornments of *Binah*, the Mother. This process ensues when the Israelite males appear before the *Shekhinah* during the three annual festivals. On those occasions, the *Shekhinah* assumes the role of the Ark of the Covenant, for she is a receptacle that contains the phallus like the ark that contains the tablets of the covenant. In this containment, however, the feminine is masculinized or becomes part of the phallus. This ontic transformation is characterized in terms of letter symbolism as well: the *he'*, symbolic of the feminine, departs, and the *yod*, symbolic of the masculine, enters. The masculine overtakes the feminine, and in the process the feminine is itself transformed. At this point the *Shekhinah* can properly be described as putting on the garments of *Binah*, which are referred to as the garments of the male. The visual participation of the lower males transforms the *Shekhinah* such that she takes the position of *Binah* in relation to the lower realm.

The implications of the zoharic symbolism are succinctly expressed by the sixteenth-century master, Isaac Luria, in the following passage, commenting on the aforecited zoharic text:

> With the arousal of the lower beings and the appearance of all the males of Israel in the Temple,[100] which alludes to her,

---

[100] Cf. Exod. 23:17 (34:23): "Three times a year all your males shall appear before the Sovereign, the Lord" [*shalosh pe'amim ba-shanah yera'eh kol zekhurkha 'el pene 'adon yhwh*]. The meaning of this biblical idiom according to many kabbalists is linked to the phallomorphic gaze that binds God and the male mystic. That is, the divine phallus is the object of vision, and the human phallus is the faculty of vision. See Wolfson, 1994e, pp. 369–370. Cf. Azulai, 1986, § 33, 15b: "This is the secret of the verse, 'all your males shall appear before the Sovereign, the Lord,' for the male should imagine His form and His existence in the *Shekhinah* who is standing there. Even though the comprehension of God is in every place, nevertheless a person should not contemplate in order to engrave His image in the *Shekhinah* as He is seen in the sacred place." Azulai thus limits the imaginative visualization of God to the Temple, the *hagios topos*. From a philosophical perspective God is omnipresent and therefore he can be comprehended everywhere, but from a phenomenological perspective the iconic representation of God's image in the imagination should occur only within the spatial confines of the sacred space. The nature of that vision, moreover, entails contemplation of God's form within the *Shekhinah*. In my opinion, this relates to the fact that the *Shekhinah* is the *'aṭeret berit*, the corona of the phallus. Hence, the divine form can be seen through the *Shekhinah*.

> she turns into a male in actuality, adorned in the garment of a male, to disclose in her the holy covenant (*berit qodesh*, i.e. the phallus) in the image of *Binah*, for even though she is female she ends with the masculine. When she is clothed in the six extremities of the masculine whose end is *Yesod*, then she is called *Binah*, *ben yah*, and she is one with the All. Similarly, in the case of *Malkhut* by means of the arousal of the lower beings . . . she becomes male and is called Lord (*'adon*), and this is [the import of the biblical idiom] the "face of the Lord", *pene 'adon* [Exod. 23:17, 34:23]. She becomes Elohim, "like mother, like daughter" [Ezek. 16:44]. [*Sha'ar Ma'amere Rashbi*, 7b][101]

According to this Lurianic text, the *Shekhinah* is transformed into a male when the Israelite males enter into the Temple, which is one of the symbolic representations of the *Shekhinah*. The males who appear before God in the Temple constitute the phallus that transforms the feminine *Shekhinah* into a male and thus endows her with the titles "Lord" and "Elohim". The phallic transference, moreover, is alluded to in the biblical idiom, to "appear before the Sovereign", which should be rendered quite literally to appear before the face of the Lord—that is, the phallus.[102] Through this gender transformation the *Shekhinah* emulates the attribute of *Binah*, which likewise is characterized as a female that becomes male. In the case of *Binah*, this transformation occurs as a result of the production of the six emanations from *Ḥesed* to *Yesod* that collectively represent the male divine anthropos; hence the name *Binah* is decomposed into the form *ben yah*, for the Mother is named *Binah* on account of the male form that she produces, and in so doing she is herself transmuted into the masculine. More specifically, it is on account of the last of those six emanations, *Yesod*, that *Binah* receives its phallic character. As it is expressed in another Lurianic text:

> Even though the point of the supernal Zion that is within *Binah* is not discernible, there is found in it the concealed potency of femininity and the revealed potency of masculin-

---

[101] See Meroz (1988).

[102] On the essential connection of masculinity and the face, see Vital, *Eṣ Ḥayyim*, 31:5, 34c.

> ity, and through this aspect *Yesod* is called Zion. . . . These two aspects are Joseph and Benjamin, one is the female waters, and this the spring of the well that is never separated from the well, and the other is the male waters in the secret of Joseph the Righteous, one is above and the other below, entering and exiting, entering to bring in the male waters and exiting to bring forth the female waters corresponding to the male waters. [*Sha'ar Ma'amere Rashbi*, 28c]

According to this text, the womb of the divine Mother, referred to by the technical expression, the "point of the supernal Zion",[103] is depicted as a parallel to the phallus below. Even though that aspect of Binah is treated as bi-sexual—that is, it comprises the potencies of masculinity and femininity—it is clearly the latter that assumes the central position insofar as it is the male element that is disclosed. The male element of *Binah* is homologous to the phallic *Yesod*. Indeed, we are to distinguish two aspects of the phallus: the upper one, named Joseph, and the lower one, Benjamin. These two aspects, moreover, correspond respectively to the seminal secretions of the male and female waters, a motif to which I return in the concluding part of this chapter. The important point to note in this context is the gender transformation implied in this text: the uterus of the divine Mother is depicted as the upper aspect of the phallus and is correlated with the male waters, whereas the penis of the divine Son is depicted as the lower aspect of the phallus and is correlated with the female waters.

Homoeroticism as a mystical ideal of transvaluation

One of the obvious implications of my argument that the feminine is to be localized in the phallus is that the female images related to God must be transposed into a masculine key. That is to say, even when a given text overtly refers to God in feminine terms, it is implicitly speaking about the male deity, and most specifically about the corona of the penis.[104] Thus, in kabbalistic texts, especially evident in the zoharic corpus, the peak mystical

---

[103] For some references, see n. 95 above.

[104] See, e.g., *Zohar* 1:38b: "It is written, 'A capable wife is a crown for her husband' (Prov. 12:4). The secret of faith entails that a man cleaves to

experience of seeing the feminine Presence is transmuted into a visualization of the exposed corona.[105] In light of this gender metamorphosis and hermeneutical transformation, one must wonder whether there is not a latent homoeroticism in the kabbalistic sources. What does it mean to say that the phallus is the ultimate object of the kabbalists' contemplative gaze and devotion?

There is no question here regarding the acceptance and ultimate affirmation of heterosexuality as the required sexual mores in Jewish society. Even if there were occasional instances of homosexual relations in kabbalistic circles, it would not challenge in any serious way the repeated emphasis on heterosexuality as the sole appropriate mode of sexual behaviour, inasmuch as human sexuality within any rabbinic framework is for the most part legitimated by procreation. The negative attitudes towards homosexuality notwithstanding, the issue that I am raising involves the symbolic valence accorded homoeroticism in the larger mythic framework of theosophic kabbalah. That is, if the female is ontically part of the male, and, indeed, anatomically part of the penis, attitudes towards the female would be absorbed in a phallocentrism that may theoretically—if not practically—embrace homoeroticism as the proper means to characterize the relationship of the different members of the mystical fraternity as well as the relationship between that fraternity and God.[106] The stated goal of the enlightened kabbalists [*maskilim*] is to join the *Shekhinah*, the feminine Presence. This communion should be viewed as both theurgical and mystical: that is, on the

---

his Master to fear him constantly without deviating to the right or left." The righteous person is portrayed as cleaving to the aspect of God depicted as the crown. It is evident that this refers to the *Shekhinah* (cf. *Zohar* 2:83b, 3:42b, 96b, 72a, 82b, 136b, 178b, 230a), but precisely through this image the femininity of the *Shekhinah* is transposed into masculinity inasmuch as the crown signifies the corona of the penis.

[105] See my study referred to in n. 32 above, and Wolfson, 1994b.

[106] It is extremely difficult to assess whether these homoerotic tendencies were expressed in overt homosexual behaviour. There is hardly any documentation outside the imaginative literature of the mystics to confirm homosexual practices. A similar theoretical question has been raised by various scholars in relation to the explicit homoerotic imagery used by Andalusian Hebrew poets: does this language signify that the poets actually practised homosexuality? For representative treatments, see Schirmann, 1955, p. 57 n. 4; Allony, 1963, pp. 311–321; Roth, 1982, pp.

one hand, it benefits the divine by enhancing the unity of the male and female aspects of the Godhead, and, on the other, it is the basic datum of the religious experience of the individual mystics. *Prima facie*, it would seem that the kabbalists avoid the issue of homosexual union with God by identifying the *Shekhinah*, the feminine potency par excellence, as the object of

---

33–59; Press, 1989, pp. 12–26; Scheindlin, 1986, pp. 82–83, 86–88. On sexual promiscuities and deviances from traditional norms in Jewish communities of Spain during the time of the flourishing of theosophic kabbalah, see Assis, 1988, pp. 25–60. It is in order here to recall the observation of Biale, 1992, p. 89, that the "mystics may have guarded against sexual license in this world by projecting it into a higher realm". Although in that context Biale does not refer to homosexuality amongst the kabbalists, it is instructive to expand his comments in this direction. On the possible intimation of latent homosexuality in the case of Joseph Caro, see Biale, p. 115. See also p. 147, where Biale discusses the homosexual innuendo of an anti-Hasidic author reflecting on the male fellowship of the Hasidic court. It should be noted that in sixteenth-century kabbalistic material, there are explicit penitential instructions for the sin of homosexuality. Cf. Azikri, *Sefer Ḥaredim* (Jerusalem, 1966), p. 200; *Sha'ar ha-Kelalim*, ch. 11, printed in Vital, *'Eṣ Ḥayyim*, p. 18. The work is associated with three of Luria's disciples, Moses Yonah, Moses Najara, and Joseph Arzin. According to Y. Avivi, however, the text was authored by Ḥayyim Vital on the basis of compositions written by the aforementioned kabbalists. See Meroz, 1988, pp. 90–91. What is most striking is the fact that material related to homosexuality is found in esoteric works that were written only for circulation amongst a small elite, as we find in the *Kanfe Yonah* of Moses Yonah. See extended discussion in Ms. JS 993, pp. 208–217. While there is still not enough evidence to document actual homosexuality, the need to incorporate such a lengthy discussion about the theurgical ramification and ultimate rectification of this sin in this work may be revealing. It is also of interest to note the following comment in a collection of Lurianic materials extant in Ms. OBL 1782, fol. 177b: "The remedy (*tiqqun*) for homosexuality was given by the Rabbi, blessed be his memory [i.e. the Ari] to three people but it is not known if that remedy has the same effect for all Jews." This passage clearly indicates that the discussions about homosexuality in the relevant Lurianic texts were not simply theoretical but had practical applications. Still, it must be emphasized that the Lurianic kabbalists, in consonance with earlier sources, uphold heterosexuality as the only legitimate and authorized form of sexual behaviour. All forms of deviant sexuality outside the relationship of husband and wife are considered detrimental inasmuch as such actions create a division above between male and female. It is for that reason that homosexuality, celibacy, and onanism are all demonized in kabbalistic literature (see Liebes, 1993b, pp. 67–74; 1992, pp. 163–164).

their mystical communion. Erotic language could be appropriated to describe that communion inasmuch as God was imaged as female.[107] But if the feminine *Shekhinah* is, in fact, transmuted into the *'aṭeret berit*, the corona of the penis, what does that say about the sexual quality of the cleaving of the mystics to the *Shekhinah*? The phallocentrism of kabbalistic symbolism so overwhelms the perspective on gender that the female is reduced to an aspect of the male. Does not the logic of the mythos imply that the divine phallus is the ultimate object of the kabbalists' visual contemplation and mystical communion? Is there any need for the female as such when the feminine is ontically localized in the male organ?[108]

In a separate study I have argued that, according to the zoharic text, the mystical fellowship represents the constitution of the divine face. The gathering of the comrades and their master is valorized as a sexual union identified as a face-to-face encounter. In this encounter the comrades represent the feminine persona that stands facing the male, the master who embodies the cosmic foundation and divine phallus.[109] Just as I have argued at length above that the sexual union of male and female is, in truth, an ontological reconstitution of the male—that is, a reintegration of the female into the male—so, too, can male-to-male bonding be understood in heterosexual terms. In either case, the issue is the reconfiguration of the male, but in one instance that reconfiguration involves transmuting heterosexual language into homosexual images and in the other homosexual language

---

[107] For such an approach in twelfth-century Cistercian literature, see Bynum, 1982, pp. 161–162.

[108] In this context it is also relevant to note that kabbalistic authors, especially in the *Zohar* and subsequent texts influenced thereby, viewed masturbation and nocturnal emission as cardinal sins, for the male semen is spilled without any female receptacle to hold it. My suggestion that the peak mystical experience of union is in fact a reconstitution of the androgynous phallus should not be seen as suggesting in any way a legitimation of onanism. The imaging of divine sexuality, reflecting the accepted sexual practices below, is based on the union of male and female. The issue is, however, the gender valence accorded the female in light of an androcentric and monistic ontology. What would be considered illicit sexuality in the anthropological sphere is thus transferred as the mythical structure operative in the divine sphere.

[109] See Wolfson, 1994c.

into heterosexual symbols. In the present context I will cite Joseph of Hamadan, who provides an exemplary illustration of the gender transformation to which I have alluded.

According to one passage written by this kabbalist, the righteous (a cipher for the mystics) are said to "cleave to the *Matrona* like a son to his mother", and they are further described as suckling the splendor of the *Matrona* from her breasts ("Joseph of Hamadan's *Sefer Tashak*", Zwelling, 1975, p. 154). In the continuation of this passage, the overtly feminine images of the breasts and the process of lactation are transformed into masculine traits.

> Moreover, that letter *he'* [symbolic of the Matrona] is a half-moon, and it is a half-circle in the manner that the seventy members of the Sanhedrin sat, and the point in the middle is the head of the court (*'av bet din*), and from there judgement issues from the letter *he'*, as it is written, "God stands in the divine assembly [among the divine beings He pronounces judgment]" [Ps. 82:1], and the *Shekhinah* is in the middle. . . . All the souls of the righteous are crowned by the holy letter, as the sages of old said, "This indicates that the Holy One, blessed be He, in the future shall be a crown on the head of all the righteous."[110] The righteous are crowned by this holy letter and they cleave to the splendor of the *Shekhinah*, the holy Matrona. ["Joseph of Hamadan's *Sefer Tashak*", Zwelling, 1975, pp. 154–155][111]

That the feminine Presence to which the mystics cleave is valorized as masculine is signified by the image of the point in the middle of the half-moon or half-circle.[112] In her function as the midpoint that sustains the righteous, the *Shekhinah* is transformed into a male, symbolized by the technical expression of

---

[110] B. Sanhedrin 111b.

[111] The phallic nature of the breasts seems to be implied in "Joseph of Hamadan's *Sefer Tashak*", Zwelling, 1975, p. 280. In that context the letter *ṣaddi*, which symbolizes the attribute of the phallic *Ṣaddiq*, is applied to the "apples of the Matrona", which clearly represent the breasts. See n. 115, below.

[112] Cf. the description of letter *pe* in "Joseph of Hamadan's *Sefer Tashak*", Zwelling, 1975, p. 272:

> The *yod* in the middle alludes to the head of the Holy One, blessed be He, and the circle that surrounds it is the secret of the knot of the phylacteries and the praying shawl (*tallit*) of the Holy One, blessed be

He, above. . . . Moreover, the secret of this letter *pe* [entails] the circle that surrounds the *yod* within it, which is the Supernal Crown (*keter 'elyon*) that emerges from the tip of the *yod* . . . and this is the secret of the membrane that surrounds the holy head.

On the image of *Keter* as the membrane that covers the head, which I assume corresponds to the corona of the penis, see n. 65, above. On the depiction of the feminine as a half-circle, or the letter *kaf*, cf. ibid., pp. 236–237. When the feminine unites with the masculine, the circle becomes full, and the *kaf* is transformed into a *samekh* (cf. ibid., p. 265). The crown is also associated with a circle in the depiction of the letter *qof* in ibid., pp. 282–283. In fact, this letter symbolizes the coronation of the souls of the righteous who are represented by the line that is encircled by the crown. On the image of the *Shekhinah* as the centre-point of the circle whence all things derive their sustenance, see, e.g., *Zohar* 1:229a–b. In that context it seems that the point in the middle of the circle, identified as the holy of holies, *qodesh qedashim*, symbolically corresponds to the clitoris, the erectile organ of the vulva that is homologous to the penis. See, however, *Zohar* 3:296b (*'Idra' Zuta'*) whence it appears that the holy of holies symbolically corresponds to the vagina in which the head of the penis enters, the latter depicted as the High Priest who alone had access to the inner sanctum of the Temple (concerning this passage, see Liebes, 1993b, pp. 63–64). On the phallic description of the *Shekhinah* as the point in the middle of the circle, see especially *Book of the Pomegranate*, p. 333, where Moses de León writes: "The foundation stone whence the world is established stands in the middle. Indeed, the secret of the lower point is in the middle . . . for just as King Solomon, the secret of the median line, stands in the middle between the upper and lower waters, so too the secret of the lower point stands in the middle. When she stands in the middle she ascends in holiness." The image of ascent here signifies the transformation of the female aspect of the *Shekhinah* into the masculine. It is in light of this transformation that the lower point is the foundation stone that sustains all existence. Precisely such a dynamic underlies the following passage in a Lurianic text in Ms. OBL 1741, fol. 128a:

Malkhut is the secret of the point beneath *Yesod* for she was there from the time that the point came forth. When *Malkhut* ascends to receive the light that is in *Yesod* she is the single attribute comprised of ten (*middah 'aḥat kelulah mi-yod*). When she ascends to *Neṣaḥ* and *Hod* she becomes a distinct configuration (*parṣuf 'eḥad*). When she ascends to the chest she receives the aspects of *Keter* and she becomes a complete configuration (*parṣuf shalem*) and she is called 'my sister, my beloved' (Song of Songs 5:2).

The feminine *Malkhut* becomes a complete configuration only when she ascends to the chest of the masculine and receives the aspects of *Keter*, the divine crown. Although it is not stated explicitly, I presume that this signifies the transformation of the feminine point into a crown, and, more specifically, the corona of the male organ. Ironically enough, it is in this posture that the description of the female beloved of Song of Songs is the head of the court, the *'av bet din*—a title that is appropriately applied to *Shekhinah* inasmuch as that gradation is an expression of divine judgement.[113] To be sure, Hamadan elsewhere affirms that both the masculine and feminine personifications of the divine have breasts that are designated euphemistically as the holy apples.[114] Indeed, the breasts of women are said to be larger than those of men because they have the biological function of nursing ("Joseph of Hamadan's *Sefer Tashak*", Zwelling, 1975, p. 123). The point I am making, however, involves the gender signification of this biological fact. When the physiological issue is viewed from the standpoint of gender, it becomes clear that the lactation of the breasts functionally transforms the female into a male, as I have argued above with respect to the *Zohar*. In the moment that the *Shekhinah* feeds others through her breasts, she assumes the role of the phallus that sustains by means of its seminal overflow.[115]

---

applied to *Malkhut*. The phallic character of the symbol of the point for *Shekhinah* is even more emphatically expressed in another work of Moses de León. Cf. Wijnhoven, 1964, p. 110: "The last point is the secret of the holy phallus (*sod berit ha-qodesh*) and she stands amongst her hosts like the secret of the mid-point . . . within the circle." Cf. also passage from Moses de León's commentary on Ezekiel's vision of the chariot, Ms. NYJTSA Mic. 1805, fol. 20b, cited and discussed in Wolfson, 1994f, pp. 199–200 n. 61.

[113] On the image of the *Shekhinah* as the half-moon with a dot in the middle, cf. "Joseph of Hamadan's *Sefer Tashak*", Zwelling, 1975, p. 134. In that context, moreover, the connection is made between that image and the head of the court who sat with seventy members of Sanhedrin. It is evident from that passage as well that the *yod* is the corona of the penis. Cf. ibid., pp. 167–168.

[114] The motif of the holy apples is also employed in zoharic literature to refer to the three central gradations that correspond to the Patriarchs; cf. *Zohar* 2:207b. In the singular the apple can symbolize the sixth gradation, *Tif'eret*, which corresponds to the Holy One, blessed be He, or the divine son; cf. *Zohar* 3:74a, 286b. Mention should also be made of a common designation of the *Shekhinah* in zoharic literature as the orchard of the holy apples; cf. *Zohar* 1:142b, 147b, 224b; 2:12b, 60b, 84b, 88a; 3:84a, 128b, 271a (*Piqqudin*), 292b (*'Idra' Zuta'*). It is possible that in some contexts the image of the apples refers anatomically to the testicles; cf. *Zohar* 2:15b, 141a (*'Idra' Rabba'*).

[115] The gender transformation is implied in "Joseph of Hamadan's *Sefer Tashak*", Zwelling, 1975, p. 323:

> King Solomon, may peace be upon him, said in his wisdom, "I am a wall, my breasts are like towers" (Song of Songs 8:10), this alludes to the

breasts of the Matrona that are like towers, and from these holy apples of the Matrona the righteous in the Garden of Eden and the holy angels are nourished. . . . From these breasts of the Matrona the upper and lower beings are sustained, and the holy ang‹ ‛.› and souls of the righteous draw forth from there honey and milk. Thus it is written, "Honey and milk are under your tongue" (ibid., 4:11).

Consider Hamadan's statement on p. 124: "Those who do not nurse from the breasts of the mother nurse from the breasts of the Holy One, blessed be He. All the prophets and pious ones suck from the holy apples in the world-to-come and they are illuminated by those holy hairs that surround the holy apples." The homoerotic element here is quite evident: the prophets and the pious suck directly from the breasts of the male aspect of the divine. Although in the physical world the breasts of the woman are generally larger than those of a man (see p. 123), in the spiritual realm, designated the "world-to-come", the traditional eschatological term employed by the rabbis, it is a greater level to be nursed by the breasts of the masculine. From the context, moreover, it is clear that this sucking is the physical depiction of the spiritual state of God teaching Torah to the righteous. It is possible that in these examples the "holy apples" of the male potency symbolically represent the testicles, which are the masculine counterpart to the breasts. Precisely such a point is made by Joseph of Hamadan in the text preserved in Ms. JM 134, fol. 124a:

It has been taught: the secret of hidden secrets concerning these holy apples of the body of the holy King, and they are like breasts. Those holy apples of the holy King produce honey, and from the breasts of the Matrona milk is produced, as it is written, "Honey and milk are under your tongue." Whoever studies Torah in this world merits in his portion [in the world-to-come] to suck honey from the breasts of the holy King and milk from the breasts of the Matrona.

That the holy apples of the male refer to the testicles is stated explicitly in another passage from the same composition, fol. 125a:

It has been taught: from that penis hang two apples and hanging on those [apples] are the holy hairs. . . . Therefore, those holy apples, from which are hanging those holy hairs, are like the holy skull (*moḥa' qaddisha'*) that has two membranes, the upper membrane and the lower membrane, for it is the skull for the lower ones, *Neṣaḥ* and *Hod*, for from there *Ze'eir 'Anpin* receives and from there the upper and lower beings are blessed.

The two apples thus symbolize the testicles, which correspond to *Neṣaḥ* and *Hod*, also identified as the "feet of the Holy One, blessed be He". (On fol. 130b, *Neṣaḥ* and *Hod* are identified as the kidneys of the divine anthropos, but on fol. 131a they are again designated the "holy feet of the Holy One, blessed be He".) In an astonishing exegetical turn, Joseph of Hamadan interprets the first letter of Scripture, the enlarged *bet*, as a reference to these two potencies—the source of the dual Torah and the source of this world and of the world-to-come.

It must be concluded, therefore, that the breast that nurses is functionally equivalent to a penis that ejaculates. If that is the case, then the righteous described as suckling from the splendor of the breasts of the *Shekhinah* are, in fact, cleaving to and drawing from the corona of the divine phallus. This is made explicit in a second passage from Hamadan:

> When a person departs from this world to his world, he is detained in the Garden of Eden below until his mate comes, and they ascend to the heavenly academy, and they are crowned round about in the crowns of the Holy One, blessed be He, within the body of the holy king. The Matrona sits in the middle and the righteous and pious ones are all around and they suckle from that point in the middle that is the *Shekhinah*. From that point they receive food, manna from the dew and the efflux of the supernal heaven. . . . They are nourished from the splendor of the Matrona, all of them encircled on the right and the left. Therefore the beginning of the word *tivu* [goodness] is the letter *tet* for from there the upper and lower entities derive benefit and from there everything is blessed and sustained, and everything is joyous when that holy letter that shines in several supernal holy beings in this world and the world-to-come is revealed. ["Joseph of Hamadan's *Sefer Tashak*", Zwelling, 1975, pp. 174–175][116]

The source of sustenance is depicted in this passage as the corona of the penis (symbolized by the letter *tet*) rather than the breasts of the *Shekhinah*. From a phenomenological vantage point the corona of the penis easily interchanges with the breasts inasmuch as the function of the latter transforms the

[116]The homoerotic aspect of the mystics' communion with God is strikingly evident in the following comment of Joseph of Hamadan in Ms. JM 134, fol. 128a: "It is written, 'And the enlightened will shine [like the splendor of the sky]' (Dan. 12:3), because they derive pleasure from the holy body (*gufa' qaddisha'*) of the Holy One, blessed be He, and they are illuminated by Him and cleave to Him, as it is written, 'and to Him shall you cleave', verily to Him, blessed be He, and to His light." I suggest that in this passage, as is the case in other kabbalistic documents (see Liebes, 1976, pp. 170, 178, 258–260), the word "body" signifies the male organ (cf. Ms. JM 134, fol. 129a). It follows, therefore, that according to Joseph of Hamadan's interpretation of the critical verse from Daniel, the mystics in particular take joy in and cleave to the divine phallus.

evidently female part of the anatomy into a male organ. In light of this transformation it again becomes obvious to what extent there may be a homoerotic underpinning to the kabbalistic representation of the *Shekhinah*. Ostensibly, the cleaving to the *Shekhinah* on the part of the mystics is portrayed as a union of masculine and feminine, but it may signify, rather, the joining of the males to the corona of the phallus, that which bears the sign of the holy covenant. The erotic bond with the *Shekhinah*, therefore, marks the reconstitution of the androgynous phallus, a restoration of the female back to its ontological source in the male.

On becoming female

Do we have evidence in kabbalistic literature for movement in the opposite direction—that is, crossing gender boundaries such that the male becomes female? Is it ever appropriate, according to the kabbalists, for the male to divest himself of his maleness and adopt the characteristics associated with femininity in relation to the masculine God? Given the hierarchical nature of the gender attribution in these sources, one would not expect to find such a reciprocal process. Yet, there is precisely a dynamic of this sort that is most fully articulated in the kabbalistic theosophy of Isaac Luria, as transmitted by his various disciples. In the remainder of this study I would like to explore in some detail the theme of the male becoming female in the myth and ritual of Lurianic kabbalah. It is obviously the case that many of the motifs in this corpus are exegetical elaborations of earlier sources, especially zoharic passages. I will only mention briefly some of the background ideas and images from the *Zohar* that are indispensable for a proper appreciation of the later material.

The motif that serves as the basis for my discussion is that of the upper and lower waters, the former depicted as masculine and the latter as feminine. This motif, briefly alluded to above, is expressed already in classical rabbinic sources,[117] perhaps reflecting some form of Gnostic speculation,[118] where the dual

[117] See P. Berakhot 9:3,14a; *Genesis Rabbah* 13:13, p. 122.
[118] See Altmann, 1942, pp. 23–24.

waters have an exclusively cosmological reference. In later kabbalistic literature, especially the *Zohar*, this motif is developed further and assumes a theosophic connotation as well.[119] The obvious gender symbolism associated with these waters, based on the model of orgasmic secretions, is drawn quite boldly in the following zoharic passage:

> The upper water is male and the lower female, and the lower are sustained by the male. The lower waters call out to the upper like a female who opens up for the male, and she spills water corresponding to the male water that produces semen. The female is nourished by the male. [*Zohar* 1:29b]

Perhaps the most interesting development of this motif in zoharic literature involves the idea of the souls of the righteous entering into the *Shekhinah*, wherein they are integrated into the lower female waters, the *mayyin nuqbin*, that arouse the upper male water, *mayyin dukhrin*. To cite one representative text:

> The desire of the female for the male is not realized except when a spirit enters into her and she discharges fluid corresponding to upper masculine waters. So too the Community of Israel [the *Shekhinah*] does not arouse the desire for the Holy One, blessed be He, except by means of the spirit of the righteous who enter into her. Then the fluids flow within her corresponding to the male fluids, and everything becomes one desire, one bundle, one bond. This is the will of everything, and the stroll that the Holy One, blessed be He, takes with the souls of the righteous. [*Zohar* 1:60b]

In an extraordinary reversal of gender symbolism, the penetration of the souls of the righteous into the feminine Presence results in their stimulating and becoming part of the fluids secreted by the female, which, in turn, arouse the seminal fluids of the upper male potency of the divine. The ontic status of the righteous is determined precisely by this role:

---

119 See Scholem, 1991, pp. 187–188; Liebes, 1993b, pp. 53, 185 n. 157. Although Scholem duly noted that the concept of the female waters involved the active force of the feminine, his attempt to distinguish between the zoharic and Lurianic usage of this motif cannot be upheld. The developments that occur in the Lurianic material must be seen as exegetical transformations of the earlier passages occasioned by distinctive psychological orientations.

> Rachel gave birth to two righteous individuals, and this is appropriate for the sabbatical year is always situated in between two righteous individuals, as it is written, 'The righteous [*ṣaddiqim*, i.e. in the plural] shall inherit the land' (Ps. 37:29), the righteous above and the righteous below. The supernal waters flow from the righteous above and from the righteous below the female flows with water in relation to the male in complete desire. [*Zohar* 1:153b]

It is clear from any number of passages that the zoharic authorship sees this task as the purpose of the nocturnal ascent of the righteous:[120]

> When the soul rises it arouses the desire of the female towards the male, and then the fluids flow from below to above, and the pit becomes a well of flowing water . . . for this place is perfected by the soul of the righteous, and the love and desire is aroused above, and it becomes one. [*Zohar* 1:135a]

The entry of the righteous soul into the *Shekhinah* entirely reverses the gender roles normally associated with each of the relevant agents in this drama, for the masculine soul becomes feminine as it is integrated as part of the feminine waters and the feminine aspect of the Godhead becomes masculine insofar as the pit is transformed into a well of flowing waters. The feminization of the righteous accounts as well for the image of God taking a stroll with the souls of the righteous, an act that is a euphemism for sexual intercourse, based ultimately on the phallic understanding of the feet.[121] This image is entirely appropriate because the souls of the righteous are female partners in relation to the masculine deity. Again we must confront the possibility of an implicit homoeroticism that necessitates the feminization of the human male vis-à-vis the divine who is valorized as masculine.[122] If, however, there is a latent homoeroticism

[120] Concerning this theme, see Wolfson, 1993a, pp. 209–235.

[121] See Wolfson, 1992, pp. 143–181; 1995d, pp. 240–241 n. 112.

[122] Cf. *Zohar* 2:127a, where the *Shekhinah* is described as the Garden of Eden that God planted "for the sake of his pleasure and his desire to take delight in it with the souls of the righteous". Cf. *Zohar* 3:79b: "Praiseworthy are the righteous for several supernal secrets are hidden for them in that world, and the Holy One, blessed be He, takes delight in them in

in the zoharic symbolism, it should be noted that it is still expressed within a purely heterosexual context: the male righteous constitute the feminine waters that arouse the overflow of the masculine waters upon the divine feminine. The issue is rendered that much more complex by the fact that, as I have argued, the divine feminine is itself part of the male organ.

The ideas expressed in the zoharic corpus are elaborated in kabbalistic materials that derived from sixteenth-century Safed, especially those composed by members of the circle of Isaac Luria.[123] Most importantly, in the Lurianic literature this motif is applied to specific rituals wherein it is clear that the goal of the male adept is to become female. Thus, for example, in *Sha 'ar ha-Kawwanot* Ḥayyim Vital offers the following explanation for the gesture of shutting the eyes[124] that is required when the *Shema'*, the traditional proclamation of divine unity, is recited:

> Before you say "Hear O Israel [the Lord, our God, the Lord is one]" [Deut. 6:4] you should close your two eyes with your

---

that world." Needless to say, many more examples that depict God's taking delight with the souls of the righteous could have been cited. The significant point for this study is that the righteous are generally described in these contexts as being crowned in the Garden of Eden, a symbolic reference for the *Shekhinah*. I do not think it is incorrect to suggest that the implicit ontic significance of this symbol is that the righteous constitute the crown itself, i.e. the corona of the penis with which God takes delight.

[123] For Luria's own reformulation of the zoharic conception, cf. *Sha'ar Ma'amere Rashbi* 29a and 30c. The mystical transformation of the male worshippers into the female waters through prayer is affirmed by other sixteenth-century Safedian kabbalistis; cf. R. Moses Cordovero, *Tefillah le-Mosheh* (Prezmysl, 1932), 69b and 112b. The transformative quality of the supplication prayer in the thought of Cordovero and Luria has been discussed by Fishbane (1994, pp. 111–115). On the significance of the symbol of the male and female waters in the various stages of the development of Lurianic kabbalah, see Meroz, 1988, pp. 150–151, 167, 220–222, 230, 258–259, 262–263, 282–287. See also Avivi, 1993, pp. 44–45; Jacobson, 1993, p. 255.

[124] A *locus classicus* for the ritual of closing the eyes during prayer in kabbalistic literature is *Zohar* 3:260b, where it is connected specifically with the prohibition of looking at the *Shekhinah*. Regarding this gesture during prayer, see Zimmer, 1989, pp. 92–94. On shutting the eyes as a contemplative technique in kabbalistic sources, see also Idel, 1988c, pp. 134–136. For discussion of some of the relevant sources and the reverberation of this motif in Hasidic texts, see Gries, 1989, pp. 220–222.

right hand and concentrate on what is written in the [zoharic section] *Sabba' de-Mishpatim* [regarding] the beautiful maiden that has no eyes.[125] We have explained in that context that the meaning [of this expression] is Rachel who ascends at this point [of the prayer] in the aspect of female waters in relation to the Father and Mother. [*Sha'ar ha-Kawwanot*, 21c][126]

To appreciate the complex symbolism underlying this comment, it is necessary to bear in mind that, according to the Lurianic interpretation of the liturgical order, the mystical significance of the *Shema'* is "to raise the female waters from the Male and Female to the Father and Mother so that the Father and Mother will be united and the [influx of the] consciousness (*moḥin*) will come down to the Male and Female" (*Sha'ar ha-Kawwanot*, 20c).[127] The worshiper thus joins the feminine hypostasis so that he may rise with her in the aspect of the female waters to facilitate the union of the lower two masculine and feminine configurations [*parṣufim*] in the Godhead, *Ze'eir 'Anpin* and *Nuqba' di-Ze'eir*, which, in turn, stimulate the union of the upper masculine and feminine configurations, the Father [*'Abba'*] and Mother [*'Imma'*].[128] The latter union results in the overflowing of the male waters [*mayyim dukhrin*] from *Ze'eir 'Anpin* to *Nuqba' di-Ze'eir* during the moment of coupling that is consummated during the *'Amidah*, the standing prayer of the Eighteen Benedictions. What is most significant for this discussion is that, according to the Lurianic interpretation, the male adept ritually covers his eyes to transform himself into the divine grade that is symbolized by the zoharic image of a beautiful maiden without eyes—namely, the configuration [*parṣuf*] called *Nuqba' di-Ze'eir* that corresponds to the last of the ten *sefirot*, the *Shekhinah*. One can speak here of a process of

---

125 *Zohar* 2:95a, 98b–99a.

126 Cf. *Peri 'Eṣ Ḥayyim*, p. 168.

127 Cf. *'Eṣ Ḥayyim* 39:7, 72c: "This is the secret of the unity of the reading of the *Shema'* in truth, for it is already known that it is the aspect of the union of the Father and Mother in order to give *Ze'eir* and *Nuqba'* new consciousness (*moḥin ḥadashim*) so that they too will be able to unite to produce other children." Cf. Avivi, 1985, 4: 82–83.

128 Cf. *'Eṣ Ḥayyim*, 29:2, 84a; *Sha'ar Ma'amare Rashbi*, 53a–b; see also *Sha'ar ha-Kelalim*, ch. 1, p. 10.

effeminization of the worshiper—a motif that has not been sufficiently noted in discussions of Lurianic symbolism and ritual. The motif of the males becoming integrated into the female waters is part of this larger phenomenon of gender metamorphosis. To be sure, the union of the righteous souls with the *Shekhinah* is based on the fact that they correspond to the male aspect of the divine, the *membrum virile*. However, once these souls enter into the *Shekhinah*, they become incorporated as part of her and constitute the female waters that further stimulate coitus in the higher grades of the divine realm.[129] Thus, in another context, Luria describes the righteous in the following terms:

> When they sacrifice their lives in sanctification of God through the verse, 'Hear O Israel,' they unite the Bridegroom and the Bride, and this is one sancitification [*qiddush*], for the Bridegroom betroths [*meqaddesh*] the Bride. When he sacrifices himself he is considered as one who has died and through his soul the union of the female waters is accomplished, and the Other Side is pleased with his body and thus does not enter to separate the Bridegroom and the Bride [*Sha'ar Ma'amare Rashbi*, 26b; Meroz, 1988, pp. 258–259]

In accord with the zoharic precedent, Luria understands the liturgical recitation of Deut. 6:4, as well as the supplication prayer discussed below, as an occasion to enact the spiritual death of the worshiper.[130] The erotic nature of that spiritual death is underscored by the fact that the worshiper penetrates the feminine *Shekhinah*, wherein he is integrated as part of the female waters in an effort to assist the unification of the masculine and feminine potencies of the divine.[131]

The assimilation of the male into the female is characterized as the male closing his eyes in emulation of the beautiful maiden without eyes. The ritual gains its mystical valence from

---

[129] Cf. *'Eṣ Ḥayyim* 39:1, 65a; 49:1, 112d; *Qehillat Ya'aqov*, p. 3.

[130] Cf. *Zohar* 3:120b–121a, 195b; see also *Zohar* 2:200b; *Zohar Ḥadash* 42a; *Book of the Pomegranate*, pp. 83–84; Liebes, 1993b, pp. 52–53.

[131] On the death of the righteous providing the female waters that serve as a stimulus for the union above, cf. Ḥayyim Vital, *Sha'ar ha-Gilgulim*, ch. 24, pp. 176–177; see also further references in *Sha'ar ha-Kawwanot*, 46d.

the fact that the eyes function as a symbol for the male sexual organs while still remaining eyes—or, to put the matter somewhat differently, the eyes are the aspect in the head that function like the genitals in the lower region of the body. Hence, the female persona of the divine is depicted as the beautiful maiden without eyes.[132] The male worshiper must partake of the character of the feminine by emasculating himself, a procedure that is ritually fulfilled through the shutting of the eyes. The interpretation that I have offered is confirmed by a second passage in *Sha'ar ha-Kawwanot*, which deals more generally with the closing of the eyes during prayer (*Sha'ar ha-Kawwanot*, 59c). In this text, Vital has imputed new theosophic meaning to a well-established prayer gesture that has as its purpose the augmentation of intention during worship:[133] by closing his eyes the male worshipper becomes the beautiful maiden without eyes. According to this passage, the mystical significance of prayer in general, enacted by means of this gesture, is connected to the fact that the male is assimilated into the female in order to arouse the unity of the masculine and feminine above. The point is well made in the following passage supposedly written by Luria himself:

> The appropriate intention of a person's prayer is above in the supernal depth, in the secret of the point of Zion, and there is the concealment of the supernal holy phallus, whence there extends two kinds of overflow by means of the supernal union. . . . The union is complete when he is in the path that is not known above or below. . . . The matter is that there must be an arousal of the lower entities in the way of the

---

[132] Cf. the marginal note of Jacob Ẓemaḥ in Ḥayyim Vital, *Mavo' She'arim*, 2:2.6, 8c. According to that passage the eyes are said to correspond to the consciousness of Knowledge that is in the head [*moaḥ ha-da'at she-ba-ro'sh*]. Here, too, one sees the specific linkage of the eyes to a masculine potency, albeit displaced from the genital region of the body to the cranium. In that context the zoharic reference to the beautiful maiden without eyes is also mentioned.

[133] In the Lurianic material one can still find evidence for the more standard kabbalistic approach to the closing of the eyes as a technique to enhance mental concentration; see, e.g., *Sha'ar Ruaḥ ha-Qodesh* (Jerusalem, 1874), 42d, 46d; *Sha'ar ha-Kawwanot*, 4a (regarding Luria's own practice of shutting his eyes during the private and public recitation of the Eighteen Benedictions).

> lower union, to elevate the female waters. Therefore, one must direct one's prayers there, and consequently that path will elevate the female waters to the male waters. This path is not known above or below, neither in the secret of the female waters nor in the secret of the male waters. . . . The union is not complete except by means of that path. When there is no arousal below, there is no union by means of that path, for there are no female waters. [*Sha'ar Ma'amere Rashbi* 29a]

The mandate for the male worshiper, therefore, is not simply to act as a stimulus to arouse the secretions of the female, but, rather, to be integrated into them.[134] It is evident, however, that the crossing of gender boundary implied here is not predicated on any ambiguity regarding, or open challenge to, the status accorded the respective genders in kabbalistic thought. On the contrary, the hierarchy of gender roles in classical kabbalah is only reinforced in the Lurianic material. That is, the male's becoming female is necessary so that the female may become male through the activation of the masculine principle of beneficence. Vital expresses this in the context of describing the supplication prayer [*nefillat 'appayim*] that succeeds the *'Amidah* in the traditional morning liturgy on Monday and Thursday:

> Now is the time of the descent of the drop of male waters of grace into the female Rachel. One must first raise the female waters in order to receive afterwards the male waters, according to the secret, "When a woman brings forth seed and

---

[134] The point is underscored with respect to the righteous in the following Lurianic text extant in Ms. OBL 1551, fol. 135b: "The secret of the female waters is the merit of our prayers. . . . And also the souls of the righteous that ascend . . . they arouse these male waters, i.e. the consciousness (*moḥin*) of *Ze'eir* and his *Nuqba'*. After they arouse the male waters of *Ze'eir* they too are called female waters in relation to the *'Abba'* and *'Imma'*, *Yisra'el Sabba'* and *Tevunah*, which are also joined together." The principle is stated by Vital in *'Eṣ Ḥayyim*, 39:1, 66c:

> When *miṣwot* and good deeds are found in Israel, through them *Ze'eir* and *Nuqba'* can unite face-to-face, and by means of them she can raise the female waters towards the male waters in the masculine. But if, God forbid, there is no merit in Israel, there is no power in the *Nuqba' di-Ze'eir 'Anpin* to raise her female waters to her husband, for it is known that the female waters do not rise except by means of the lower souls.

> bears a male" [Lev. 12:2]. And the rabbis, blessed be their memory, said,[135] "a woman who produces seed first gives birth to a male." [*Sha'ar ha-Kawwanot*, 46d]

Without entering further into the complicated symbolism articulated in the continuation of the above passage, related specifically to the descent of the righteous into the realm of the demonic shells to liberate the entrapped sparks,[136] suffice it to say that for Luria the male fulfils an essential religious task by becoming female, by being assimilated into the female waters that rise to stimulate the male waters that in turn inseminate the female so that she gives birth to a male. To translate this web of symbols grammatologically: he becomes she so that she arouses he to turn she into he. This circular process of reconstituted masculinity is referred to in Lurianic kabbalah as the secret of impregnation [*'ibbur*]. To cite one textual witness:

> Just as the souls of the righteous elevate the female waters each night during sleep to *Malkhut*, and she renews them, according to the secret, "They are renewed every morning" (Lam. 3:23), and the explanation of this renewal is that she illuminates them in the aspect of expanded consciousness [*moḥin de-gadlut*] . . . so too when Ze'eir 'Anpin ascends in the secret of the female waters he is renewed by means of the Father and Mother. [*'Eṣ Ḥayyim* 29:3, 21d].[137]

The stimulation of the female waters has the sole purpose of assisting in the rebirth of the male through the masculinized feminine in a state of increased consciousness. In the final

---

[135] See n. 70, above.

[136] In this context, then, the female waters comprise demonic forces, aspects of judgement, that need to be purified. Cf. *Kanfe Yonah*, Ms. JS 993, pp. 23–24, 26–27; *Sha'ar ha-Kelalim*, ch. 1, p. 10; Joseph ibn Tabul, *Kawwanat Beri'at ha-'Olam*, Ms. Columbia x893/M6862, fols. 95b–96a, 114b (concerning this composition, see Meroz, 1988, pp. 81–82); *'Eṣ Ḥayyim* 39:1–2, 65a–68a; *Mavo' She'arim*, 2:3:9, 16d–17d. See Tishby, 1942, pp. 89–90; Meroz, 1988, pp. 262–263, 282–287.

[137] Cf. *Sha'ar Ma'amere Rashbi*, 17d–18a. According to that complex passage, *Ze'eir 'Anpin* constitutes the female waters also identified as the encompassing light [*'or ha-maqif*]. The male is contained in the female in the secret of impregnation [*sod ha-'ibbur*]. This containment signifies the masculinization of the feminine rather than the feminization of the masculine.

analysis, the androcentric and phallocentric orientation adopted by kabbalists is so pervasive that even the positive values normally associated with the feminine are assigned to the male. This is captured in the brief comment of Vital that "there are five aspects of grace (*ḥasadim*) of the Mother and five aspects of grace of the Father, and the aspects of grace of the Mother are the acts of strength of the Father" (*'Eṣ Ḥayyim* 39:11, 76a).[138] As noted above, according to standard kabbalistic symbolism, grace is associated with the masculine and strength with the feminine. It follows, therefore, that the male attributes in the Mother must be transposed into female attributes of the Father.

In conclusion, it can be said that there is a psychodynamic model in the classical texts of theosophic kabbalah of the male becoming female just as there is one of the female becoming male. It is, indeed, appropriate—in fact, mandatory—for the male to divest himself of his maleness and assume the posture of the feminine. For sixteenth-century kabbalists, especially the followers of Lurianic kabbalah, this gender transformation is the essential dynamic enacted in the structure of the liturgy. This movement, however, reifies the standard binary hierarchy of gender symbolism: the male becomes female only in order to add strength to the female to renew herself as male. The female must either be restored to the male or turned into a male by the male becoming female. From the vantage point of kabbalists, this is the secret that establishes the covenant of unity.

The logical implications of this gender symbolism are explicitly drawn in the Lurianic corpus: the ultimate rectification of the break in the Godhead is attained when there is a reconstitution of the female as male—that is, the ultimate purification of the demonic forces involves a restoration of judgmental forces into mercy. As Vital expresses the matter in one context:

> Thus there are two aspects to the female of *Ze'eir 'Anpin*, one when she is contained initially in the male, and the second when she is separated from him, and he gives her the crown of strength. . . . And thus you can understand why the aspect of the female is always judgments for her root is the aspect of the kings that died. They are called kings (*melakhim*) from the word kingship (*malkhut*). When she

[138] See Meroz, 1988, pp. 177–178.

> sep-arates from him and becomes an autonomous aspect, then the two of them are in the secret of a husband and his wife, the male alone and the female alone. [*'Eṣ Ḥayyim* 10:3, 49a–b][139]

At the core of the zoharic myth of the Edomite kings, who symbolize the forces of impurity within the Godhead, is the ontological problem of the feminine. The death of the kings thus represents the purification of the feminine. Again to quote Vital: "These are the kings who ruled in the land of Edom' (Gen. 36:31), for when they emerged the aspect of these kings immediately began to be purified to produce the aspect of the feminine for Him" (*'Eṣ Ḥayyim*, 10:3, 48d). The purpose of the divine catharsis is to purify the feminine aspect of the divine, but the ultimate purification is attained only when the feminine is restored to the male, when the other is obliterated in the identity of sameness. The messianic era is thus described as the final obliteration of the evil force (related exegetically to Isa. 25:8), which entails a restitution of the world to a primeval state of chaos. In that stage the feminine is completely integrated in the masculine, a point represented symbolically by the overcoming of the divine name that numerically equals fifty-two (the force of the feminine operating independently of the male) by the names that equal sixty-three and seventy-two, which correspond to the feminine and the masculine, respectively (*'Eṣ Ḥayyim*, 10:3, 49a–b). The reconstitution of the female as male is also represented by the image of the female being the crown of her husband (*Sha'ar ha-Haqdamot*, 28c) or the eschatological teaching of the rabbis (B. Berakhot 17a) that in the future the righteous sit with their crowns on their heads (*Mavo' She'arim*, 2:3:2, 12a; see Meroz, 1988, pp. 244–245). The eschaton signifies the reintegration of the feminine as part of the masculine, an ontic unity that was rendered asunder in the beginning of creation. The mythical element of the Lurianic cosmogony is predicated on the notion that fission of the Godhead is a cathartic process by means of which the (feminine) "other" is discarded so that it may be purified and ultimately restored to its ontological source in the male androgyne. Both the image of the woman

[139] A parallel to this passage is found in *Mavo' She'arim* 2:3:2, 12c. The latter source is cited by Jacobson, 1993, p. 251.

being the crown of her husband and that of the righteous sitting with their crowns on their heads signifies the ultimate unification that involves the recontextualization of the feminine as part of the phallus, a mystery related by Vital to the eighth of the Edomite kings who survived—namely, Hadar, who corresponds to "*Yesod* that comprises male and female, which is the crown that is in him" (*'Eṣ Ḥayyim*, 10:3, 48d).

The full force of this mythic conception will be appreciated if we bear in mind that in other contexts Vital tries to preserve the relatively autonomous aspect of the feminine by distinguishing between the feminine as the corona of the phallus and the feminine as a separate configuration. Thus, for example, he writes:

> This is [the intent of] what is written, "under His feet there was the likeness of a pavement of sapphire" [Exod. 24:10], for *Yesod*, which is called the pavement of sapphire (*livnat ha-sappir*), is underneath His feet, which are *Neṣaḥ* and *Hod*. . . . *Yesod* is the aspect that is appropriate to hide and to conceal, and on account of His glory, blessed be He, they did not publicize it but only explained its place, which is beneath His feet. *Yesod* itself is comprised of male and female in the secret of the phallus (*yesod*) and the corona (*'aṭarah*) that is in him, as I have already informed you that the corona (*'aṭarah*) is not the secret of *Malkhut* in itself but rather the containment of the masculine in all ten sefirot, and this [*'aṭarah*] is the aspect of *Malkhut* in him [*Yesod*]. But the essential *Malkhut* is Rachel, *Nuqba' di-Ze'eir 'Anpin*, and this is simple for [it is written] "But I would behold God from my flesh" [Job 19:26], the corona (*'aṭarah*) is one matter and the female (*neqevah*) is another independent matter. [*Sha'ar ha-Kawwanot*, 18d][140]

We find a similar approach in the following passage in *'Eṣ Ḥayyim*:

> The aspect of *Malkhut* in each and every configuration (*parṣuf*) of these five configurations is in this manner: *Malkhut* that is in the masculine configuration, such as *'Abba'* and *Ze'eir 'Anpin*, is in the aspect of the corona (*'aṭarah*) that is on the *ṣaddiq* who is called *Yesod*, in the

---

[140] Cf. parallel in *Peri 'Eṣ Ḥayyim*, p. 158.

> secret of "Blessings light upon the head of the righteous", *berakhot le-ro'sh ṣaddiq* [Prov. 10:6]. . . . *Malkhut* in the feminine configuration, such as *'Imma'* and *Nuqba' di-Ze'eir 'Anpin*, is also in the aspect of the corona of the phallus (*aṭeret yesod*) that is in her, for the phallus (*yesod*) in her is the womb and the corona in her is the aspect of the pulp of the apple (*besar ha-tapuaḥ*) that is over her, which is called in the language of the sages, blessed be their memory, *shippule me'ayyim* [the lower part of the abdomen], in matters pertaining to the signs of barren women, as is known.[141] However, the comprehensive *sefirah* of *Malkhut*, the final configuration of the five configurations, which is called *Nuqba' di-Ze'eir 'Anpin*, is a complete configuration like the other configurations. [*Eṣ Ḥayyim* 1:1, 14c]

Here again Vital tries to preserve some ontological autonomy of the feminine. The aspect of *Malkhut* in the male configurations [*'Abba'* and *Ze'eir 'Anpin*] is the corona of the penis, and in the upper female configuration [*'Imma'*] the aspect of *Malkhut* is the part of the womb that corresponds to the phallus. Only in the case of the final configuration [*Nuqba' di-Ze'eir 'Anpin*] can one speak of a fully formed feminine that compliments the male.

These examples, and others that could have been cited, do not challenge my presumption that the female in an originary and ultimate sense is part of the male organ. Indeed, the aforecited passages in which Vital describes the autonomous character of the feminine relate to the ontic situation of *Malkhut* before the final *tiqqun*, a process, as I have argued, that is predicated on the restoration of the female to the male, principally in the image of corona of the phallus. The ontological containment of the female in the male is expressed in another context by Vital in which he relates the four species of plants used on Tabernacles (citron, palm branch, myrtle, and willow) to the letters of the Tetragrammaton:

> *Yod* [alludes to] *Ḥesed*, *Gevurah*, and *Tif'eret*, and they are the three myrtle branches (*hadassim*); *he'* [alludes to] *Neṣaḥ* and *Hod*, and they are the two willows of the brook (*'arve nahal*); *waw* [alludes to] *Yesod*, and this is the palm branch (*lulav*); the final *he'* is the citron (*'etrog*), and this is the

---

[141] Cf. M. Niddah 9:8.

> [aspect of] *Malkhut* that is in him, which is the corona of the phallus (*'aṭarah she-ba-yesod*) called the head of the righteous one (*ro'sh ṣaddiq*), but it does not refer to *Nuqba' di-Ze'eir 'Anpin*, as many have thought. This is a well-known mistake for the *Malkhut* of *Ze'eir 'Anpin* himself, which is united with him, is symbolized by the union of the secret of the final *he'* of the Tetragrammaton. However, the feminine has its own complete name, which is Elohim or Adonai, as is known. Therefore [the citron] is called the "fruit of the tree of splendor", *peri 'eṣ hadar* [Lev. 23:40], that is to say, the fruit of the phallus (*peri shel ha-yesod*), which is called *'eṣ hadar*. The fruit that is in him is the corona (*'aṭarah*). The phallus (*yesod*) is also called *hadar* according to the mystery of "show deference to the elderly", *hadarta pene zaqen* [Lev. 19:32]. . . . [The citron] is the [aspect of] *Malkhut* in the phallus of *Ze'eir 'Anpin*, and this is the reason for the prohibition of separating the citron from the palm branch when it is lifted up. One must unite them together for the palm branch is the phallus and the citron is the corona that is conjoined to it without separation. [*Sha'ar ha-Kawwanot*, 105c]

As an autonomous entity, the feminine has her own name—either Elohim or Adonai—but as part of the male she is the final *he'* of the Tetragrammaton. The independent position attributed to *Malkhut* signifies a subsidiary state that is overcome by the unification of male and female and the consequent restoration of the female to the male. When the feminine is evaluated from the vantage point of the unique divine name, which represents the essential and elemental force of God's being, she is the completion of that name rather than a distinct potency. The Tetragrammaton represents the male androgyne, the perfect male who comprehends within himself both masculine and feminine characteristics. The mythic structure is instantiated by the ritual of lifting up the palm branch in the right hand and the citron in the left. To separate the two is to create a division between the masculine and the feminine. When the two are joined together, the female is reintegrated into the male in the form of the corona of the phallus.

That this was the ontic situation of the *Ein Sof* prior to the process of emanation is stated explicitly by Menaḥem Azariah of Fano:

The head that is no head is in relation to them [the head that is nothing and the head of *'Arikh 'Anpin*] in the secret of Ein-Sof on account of His great concealment. . . . Here He is called in truth the head that does not know and that is not known for He does not know the root of His essence from a higher place just as a man does not know the essence of his soul. He is not known at all to anyone outside Him. . . . He is the world of the masculine, and *Malkhut* is not discernible in Him except in the secret of the crown that is included in *Yesod*. [*Yonat 'Elem*, ch. 29, 24a–b][142]

---

[142] Cf. Moses Yonah, *Kanfe Yonah*, Ms. JS 993, p. 35: "The point of *Malkhut* is now in the place of the head of *'Arikh 'Anpin*, for this place is her root and source. . . . Insofar as her place is in the head of *'Arkih 'Anpin*, we have the power through our good actions and our prayers that we pray with intention to raise *Malkhut* above until the place of the head of *'Arikh 'Anpin* . . . since this was the place where she was in the beginning." The elevation of *Malkhut* to the head of *'Arikh 'Anpin* through pious behaviour is a prolepsis of the final *tiqqun*, which involves the restoration of the feminine to the masculine. The depiction of the *Shekhinah* as the corona of the phallus of *Ein-Sof* is expressed in earlier kabbalistic sources, which no doubt served as the basis for the Lurianic material. Consider, for example, *Tiqqune Zohar* 10, 24b: "When [the *Shekhinah*] ascends to Ein-Sof, she is the *yod* in the head of the *'alef*. Through what does she ascend? Through the middle column, which is a *waw*. [She is] the diadem on his head when she ascends. . . . It is said concerning her, 'a capable wife is a crown for her husband' (Prov. 12:4)." The ascent of the *Shekhinah* to *Ein-Sof* through *Tif'eret* results in her transformation into the *yod* in the head of the *'alef*, which must be understood as the corona of the phallus. On the masculine character of *Keter* and the need to masculinize the feminine or left side, see Nathan of Gaza, "Derush ha-Taninim", in Scholem, 1934, p. 25. On the one hand, Nathan categorically rejects the attribution of the feminine at the highest levels of the divine. Thus he states that there is no aspect of the feminine in *Keter*, and therefore there is no blessing. On the other hand, he affirms precisely such an aspect, but he attempts to transform the gender dialectically from feminine to masculine.

> You already know that the left side that is in *Keter* is the feminine, and the feminine is always forming, and by means of her three drops emerge, and each drop [divides] into three drops so there are the nine channels that are the vessels. . . . The drops come out from the phallus of Understanding (*yesod de-Binah*) from the right side, for since she is the feminine she brings forth from the right side in order to be contained in the secret of the male.

It is of interest to note that in the same work Nathan portrays Shabbatai Sevi as the feet of God (based on Exod. 24:10), which in turn are identified as the "corona of the phallus of the Father" [*'aṭeret yesod*

The Infinite is entirely masculine, for the feminine aspect is located ontically in the corona of the penis. From the vantage point of the kabbalists, history is moving towards a state wherein the feminine will be restored to the masculine so that the androgynous quality of the Godhead will be reconstituted in the manner that it was before the independent force of the feminine was operative in the concatenation of worlds. The ultimate purpose of religious ritual is to serve as a catalyst to transform the feminine into the masculine, but to attain that goal it is necessary for the male to become female. The dialectics of gender transformation are succinctly expressed by Pinehas of Korets:

> The one that bestows is garbed in the garment of the one that receives and by means of this the one that receives becomes equal to the one that bestows. By this means the aspect of *Malkhut*, which is the aspect of the one that receives, becomes equal in her stature to the one that bestows as it was

---

'*abba*']. When this aspect of the divine ascends, it assumes the position of the diadem on the head of the masculine potency [*'aṭeret ba'alah*, according to the locution of Prov. 12:4]. The messianic figure is thus portrayed as the corona of the phallus that rises until it becomes ontically integrated into the highest realms of the Godhead (cf. Nathan of Gaza, "Derush ha-Taninim", Scholem, 1934, p. 16). Alternatively, Nathan relates that revelation of the Messiah represents the restoration of the feminine to the masculine. Cf. ibid., p. 20:

> The root of the King Messiah is in the corona of the phallus of the Father (*'aṭeret yesod 'abba'*) . . . and the Messiah, son of David . . . his place is in *'Atarah*, he is in the corona of the phallus of *Ze'eir* (*aṭeret yesod di-ze'eir*). Therefore it says concerning him, "The crown was taken from the head of their king [and it was placed on David's head]" (2 Sam. 12:30) . . . and it says, "Mordecai left the king's presence in royal robes [of blue and white] with a magnificent crown of gold" (Esther 8:15). "Mordecai left", this is the secret of the phallus of the Father (*yesod 'abba'*) that protrudes. It says a "crown of gold" (*aṭeret zahav*) . . . for when the phallus of the Father goes out he takes the crown of gold . . . and when that phallus projects he contains that crown in him, according to the secret of [the verse] "I have set my bow in the clouds" (Gen. 9:13).

This text affirms the structural dynamic that I discussed in the body of the chapter: the messianic moment is marked not by the sacred union of a man and a woman, but rather by the reintegration of the feminine to the masculine, symbolically portrayed by the corona of the extended phallus. I have elaborated on this theme in a lecture, "The Rite of Sabbatai Sevi's Coronation and Sabbatian Myth" (Wolfson, 1994d).

> prior to the indictment of the moon. This is the aspect of the righteous sitting with their crowns upon their heads. That is, the aspect of *Malkhut* becomes the aspect of the crown . . . surrounding the head, for she ascends to the aspect of the head since the one who bestows receives pleasure from the one that receives. . . . Thus it is written "Mordecai left the king's presence in royal robes" [Esther 8:15], that is, Mordecai is the aspect of the one that bestows who is garbed in the garment of the one who receives, that is, *Malkhut*, which is the aspect of the one who receives. By means of this the two of them are of equal stature, for from the one who receives is made the aspect of the one who bestows and from the *shoshanah*, which is the aspect of the feminine, the aspect of *Malkhut*, is made the aspect of *shushan*, the aspect of the masculine. And this is [the meaning of the continuation of the verse] "And the city of Shushan rang with joyous cries." [*Devarim Nehmadim*, cited in *Imre Pineḥas ha-Shalem*, ed. Y. Frankel (Jerusalem, 1988), p. 41][143]

The secret of redemption consists of the female's becoming the corona of the male organ, but that can be achieved only when the male puts on the garment of the female. Despite the reference in the above passage to the attainment of an equal stature on the part of the male and female, the fact of the matter is that the gender hierarchy is not fully overcome. The female is rendered equal to the male when she rises from the status of the one who receives to the one who bestows—a process that is facilitated by the descent of the one who bestows to the status of the one who receives. In the redemptive moment the female is transformed into an aspect of the male, and the original androgynous state is reconstituted.

---

143 See ibid., pp. 5–6.

Comments

Peter B. Neubauer

ON WOLFSON'S "CROSSING GENDER BOUNDARIES"

The themes of crossing gender boundaries, of rituals, and of myths immediately evoke psychoanalytic interest. The issue of gender reminds us of propositions of the psychoanalytic theory of development. Rituals are shared behaviour contrived to protect continuity; myths are shared pre-conscious and unconscious group fantasies, which encourage group cohesion, and a collective system of cognitively acceptable explanations, whereby they influence ego and superego functions.

The kabbalistic view of gender crossing—or, better, the belief that genders may be joined so that male and female are united—assumes the possibility of the transformation of gender characteristics.

The study of kabbalistic literature has led Wolfson to two propositions: (1) that the female is contained or absorbed in the male force which represents the ideal anthropos; and (2) that the historically later view of Luria assumes that the male is to become female, which then is a larger phenomenon of "gender metamorphosis".

We agree with Wolfson's proposition that sex is biologically determined and that gender expresses environmental influence, which assigns sociocultural roles to male and female. We would add here that individual "psychological" shaping of gender identity interacts with the biological and sociocultural factors.

Wolfson calls attention to the difference between the formulation that the ideal anthropos *comprises* both masculine and feminine traits and the formulation that "depicts woman . . . as secondary and derivative and therefore the female is ontically inferior to the masculine". He opts for the latter. Careful examination of the kabbalistic texts that he quotes seems to suggest both propositions, or favours that of male superiority. As we shall explain, these differences gain importance when viewed in the context of theories of psychoanalytic development and the onto- and epigenetic transformations.

General development theories assume that development proceeds from simple behaviour to more and more differentiated behaviour; from global reaction to more specificity. The infant does not as yet distinguish between external and internal stimuli. In his symbiotic world there is unity between his internal biological imperative and the external source of gratification. Biologically determined sex differences exist from infancy on, and even prenatally; the awareness of gender is a later development. Social and cultural determinants reach the infant and toddler only via the influence of the parents, who, in the first three years of life, are not perceived with gender characteristics.

The basic and primary bonding between the infant and the mother, the caretaker, leads at two months to the social smile and at seven months to the beginning awareness between the known and the strange, the unfamiliar. The next developmental step demands the control of body function, the acceptance of routines, of sleep and feeding schedules and toilet training; and only then do the essential differences emerge.

Both the theory of development and clinical experience therefore guide us to the distinction between the pre-oedipal and phallic–oedipal constellations. When we follow Mahler's work about separation and individuation, we understand it to imply that there is a strong developmental pull towards the establishment of autonomy, towards the consolidation of developmental differentiations which should finally lead to individuation and individuality. Separation, or better, separateness is achieved only in the presence of the mother; she is the guarantor of progressive differentiations.

We can therefore postulate a continuous human conflict between the wish to belong, to be taken care of, to *return* to the original state of *unity*, on the one hand, and the need to achieve a consolidated self and to fulfil the promise of each individual aspiration and achievement on the other. The ideal concept of the self, which often corresponds to the idealized image of the loved person, continuously reinforces the wish to return to the earlier state of comfort; this longing is never fully relinquished. Thus we can understand the interminable search for a world in which the earlier unity is longed for; and symbolism, legends, and the exploration of the transmission of magic power are instruments to achieve it.

There are two ways to achieve freedom from conflictual desires: (1) to progress towards sublimations where higher goals transcend individual needs, or (2) to follow the path of regression in order to return to a state of comforting unity.

Can we find in kabbalistic literature both paths: elevation of the *act* of union to a symbol of the divine; and regression to a non-differentiated union?

It may be helpful to introduce now the notion of *identification* and of *phallic-gender primacy*. We assume that the earliest interaction of the baby with the mother proceeds from imitation of the mother to identification and finally to incorporation. These steps facilitate independence and mitigate the experience of loss of the earlier unity between the infant and the mother. Thus Freud proposes the line of development that leads from the fear of the loss of the mother as the nurturing, need-satisfying object to the fear of the loss of the *love* of the mother, to the fear of castration—that is, the fear of losing the integrity of the emerging gender identity due to the oedipal struggle.

We assume that at the age of about three years the child has achieved individuation not because he or she has separated from the mother, but because he has internalized her, has achieved "object constancy"—a sense of permanence of identity and of relationship.

As I read it, the kabbalistic literature does not reflect these issues directly, although they are implied in many explanations offered. It seems that this is also true of the difference between losing nurturing—the water, the breast—and the fear of losing the love of the nurturing person.

Progressive differentiation continues as the psychic organization proceeds from the phase of object constancy to the evolution of gender identity. We assume that normal development demands the consolidation of identity that gives primacy to the phallic gender role. Previous undifferentiated or mixed male or female characteristics now integrate into a consolidated gender identity. Only when this is achieved can the child enter the *triadic* relationship to his parents, as all three are experienced with their gender characteristics. The male child turns towards the mother and the female child towards the father in their desire to unite now on the basis of *gender differences*, of gender polarity. The unity with the opposite sex may mitigate the fear of castration by the father or the fear of penis envy, and thereby secure gender integrity. I will not elaborate here on the implications of Freud's formulation of castration fear of the boy and penis envy of the girl, a formulation that appears to emphasize the centrality of the phallus for both sexes. While this is operative in the phallic phase of development, the oedipal constellation and conflict resolution proceed beyond this constellation; for during the oedipal stage, the boy needs to identify with the father—receive his love—and the girl needs to identify with the mother—needs her love—in order to consolidate their gender. The fear of retaliation is therefore avoided. The girl can turn to the male because she is like the mother, and the boy can turn to the female because he has identified with the father. Thus, *this taking in of the same sex is a step in the strengthening of the gender identity*, which then leads to a secure turning to the opposite sex. On this level of development the internalization of the same gender allows for a unity with the opposite sex without losing gender identity, without the danger of sex "transformation". On this developmental level the female confirms the maleness as the male confirms the femaleness of the partner.

In *Group Psychology and the Analysis of the Ego*, Freud (1921c, p. 105) proposes that the boy

> . . . then exhibits, therefore, two psychologically distinct ties: a straightforward sexual object cathexis towards his mother and an identification with his father which takes him as a

> model. The two subsist side by side for a time without any mutual influence or interference. In consequence of an irresistible advance towards a unification of mental life, they come together at last; and the normal Oedipus complex originates from their confluence.

A psychoanalytic study has arrived at the surprising conclusion that circumcision, the removal of the foreskin, is perceived by some men as the removal of femininity, as if the foreskin were a female appendage like the labia (see Nunberg, 1949). Similarly, clitoridectomy removes a phallic element from the female genitalia. It is as though in both cases a mixture of gender elements is not tolerated. Even if these procedures are interpreted as religious sacrifice, they act so as to purify the individual from cross-gender contamination.

In *Group Psychology*, chapter 7, Freud (1921c) speaks about the two confluent identifications. One is the pre-oedipal identification, the primary identification, when the father represents what the boy wishes to be or wishes to become. A similar identification occurs for the girl and her wish of "what one would like to be", taking her mother as a model. There is furthermore the discrepancy between the finding of the object and the reaction to the loss of the object. In the *New Introductory Lectures*, Freud (1933a, p. 63) states: "If one has lost an object or has been obliged to give it up, one often compensates by identifying oneself with it and by setting it up once more in one's ego, so that here object-choice regresses, as it were, to identification." We have here the notion of a regressive identification. The finding of the object on a mature level of gender definition counteracts or leads away from the regressive identification, which is the response to the loss of an object or the forward pull towards the abandonment of the object. The forward pull will reach a condition of sublimation, a reaching beyond sexuality, a desexualization. In *The Ego and the Id*, Freud writes that this desexualization is

> a kind of sublimation, therefore. Indeed the question arises and deserves careful consideration; whether this is not the universal road to sublimation, whether all sublimation does not take place through the mediation of the ego, which begins by changing sexual object-libido into narcissistic libido and then, perhaps goes on to give it another aim. [1923b, p. 30]

The change of the aim implies the giving up of sexual pleasure in order to find a sublimated state.

As we refer here to the progressive function of sublimation, I would like to return to the regressive pull towards the formation of a unit based on de-differentiation, de-identification, and the pre-gender condition. The ego is not active, and the qualities of the id prevail. Freud (1933a, p. 74) characterizes these in this way:

> There is nothing in the id that corresponds to the idea of time; there is no recognition of the passage of time, and a thing that is most remarkable and awaits consideration in philosophical thought, no alteration in its mental processes is produced by the passage of time. Wishful impulses which have never passed beyond the id, but impressions, too, which have been sunk into the id by repression, are virtually immortal.

We can now attempt to apply these psychoanalytic assumptions to the propositions of various authors about the theosophic Kabbalah:

1. When one translates the principle of multiple determinants to the developmental point of view, one can state that any discussion of gender must take into account the multiple levels of gender formation, or that what may be a reasonable deduction on one epigenetic level may be inappropriate for the preceding or successive one. Gender formation and transformation are part of a continuous process.
2. We have noted the developmental conflict between the desire to unite and the developmental progression towards individuation and therefore of the shaping of gender identity.
3. In order to defend against the loss of the object, there is the regressive pull to the earliest non-differentiated unity and the forward pull towards a sublimated transcendence of the gender difference and the sexual aim. Thus it is required to assess kabbalistic intent as to the position it takes regarding these divergent tendencies.
4. If one argues that on a theosophic level of discourse or abstraction these developmental considerations are not relevant, then one has to examine the kabbalistic text more

> carefully, because we find here a mixture of more abstract formulations and then again reference to poetic symbolism, which demands the assignment of multiple meanings to it. It is this complexity that makes the finding of and the placement of meaning of the human condition and, specifically, of the role of mysticism so challenging and fascinating.

An example often referred to may illuminate these principles. Wolfson, in note 91, quotes *Zohar* 3:296a:

> "We have a little sister" [Song of Songs (8:8)]. . . . Certainly she appears as little, but she is big and great, for she is the completion of what she has received from everyone, as it is written, "I am a wall, my breasts are like towers" (ibid. 10). My breasts are filled to nurse all things. "Like towers" these are the great rivers that issue forth from the supernal mother.

What did the author of this comment have in mind? Did he leave open the multiple meanings of these images, or has he selected one that dominates this construction? Without knowing his intentions, we are invited to suggest multiple meanings. Has sister become big and great from all she has received because she has been nurtured by all (female and male) and therefore she can become the nurturer for all? Or is she big because of her fullness in pregnancy and womanhood? Are the breasts like towers, a fort that needs protection, a sign of power of the giving mother? Or is it justified to understand the tower to be a symbolic expression of male power of the phallus within the female, a "completion" by the incorporation of male attributes? From the verse, "I am a wall, my breasts are like towers", may we infer that this alludes to the breasts of the *Matrona* that are like towers? Basic elements of human function are translated into preferred *higher* levels of meaning. Thus the use of eating as a metaphor for sexual intercourse eliminates the meaning of eating for self-preservation and equates it with sexuality as procreation and therefore as preservation of life. But procreation and eating equated in this way lose their specificity, the difference between self- and other-orientedness. When, in clinical terms, eating becomes a substitute for sexuality (in the sense of gender, not libido) then there is a regression to earlier pregender gratification. Since a significant factor of development rests on the recognition of the forces that demand differentiation, such equations appear one-sided.

The examination of the text alone does not permit a choice with a sufficient degree of certainty. One can argue that the kabbalistic reading of it reveals a preference, but even here the opinions are divided.

Such explanations may elicit the accusation that I offer an interpretation of the original text instead of examining the interpretations that the kabbalistic text offers, such as the statement that "the dual sexuality of the divinity is the very foundation of all the doctrine of the Kabbalah" (Liebes, 1993b, p. 106). This formulation, too, leaves open the question whether this duality refers to a composite of the sexes or whether one gender asserts dominance over the other. Unable to achieve a scholarly reading of the kabbalistic texts, I have to be content to refer to the various readings of it by competent interpreters and show which of them conforms to developmental principles. Therefore, we cannot determine the correctness of one explanation over another, but, rather, define the position of each that leads to a preferred reading of the text of the Kabbalah.

E. R. Wolfson's (1994f) proposition describes the Infinite [*En Sof*] as seen by Kabbalists as a transcendence of gender. It is not clear whether such assumptions rest on a transcendence of gender by sublimation or whether it is an expression of a regression to an undifferentiated, pre-gender state of unity with the timelessness of id characteristics. To be sure, cultural and political factors polarize the character of gender as outlined by C. Walker Bynum (1986, p. 257): "A male and female were contrasted and asymmetrically valued as intellect/body, active/passive, rational/irrational, reason/emotion, self-control/lust. . . ." Surely cultural, economic, and political factors account more for such assignments of values linked to gender than careful observation. These assumptions are not based on theosophic abstractions and must therefore be judged on other levels of relevance. This does not imply that gender difference in personality formation and behaviour do not exist, but that the distribution of power of aggression and libido, of the influence of female and male primary persons in the child's life, does not justify such differences. Thus the reason for such polarization must stem from other sources.

If one assumes that a gender composite occurs on a phallic level, then one has to decide whether the thrust of the literature of the Kabbalah intends a transformation of the gender—that is, an absorption of the female into the male by simultaneously modifying the maleness. The other choice is that it establishes phallic dominance, that the female is absorbed under the centrality of phallic power. Such a position does not represent a composite or transformation of gender difference—it does not transcend gender, but increases the significant characteristics of the phallus, thus establishing male gender superiority. At different periods of kabbalistic history, different models may have been considered, unless there are inherent contradictions between the proposal of a transcendental unity side by side with the glorification of a phallic presentation of the divine so that women are never directly connected with the divine realm.

The composite approach may apply to the position of Gershom Scholem (1991, p. 174–175) when he avoids the polarization of the gender characteristics by ascribing active aspects to the female for her ability to give birth and he also refers to the masculine aspects of the lower *Shekhinah*—that is, to the feminine. This suggests an interchange between male and female images, as we found during the pre-gender phase of development. It is not quite understandable, when we apply developmental sequences, that the maternal image of "God" is predicated on the gender transformation of the concept of motherhood, that images of giving birth and nursing are valenced as specific phallic activities (ibid., p. 93). Scholem proposes that female waters represent the active of the feminine, and therefore he must separate the images proposed by the zoharic usage from that posited by Isaac Luria.

Luria's view that the male enters the feminine Presence, with the resulting interaction between the male and the female, comes closer to the psychoanalytic assumption of early development. The return to unity with the first primary object, the mother, symbolizes the longing for a non-differentiation, a pre-gender state. But this formulation may not correspond to the Lurianic assumption of the male penetration of the female—that is, the maintenance of gender power—when the masculine soul becomes feminine. This suggests a role reversal or transsexuality, and thus Wolfson speaks about the effeminization of the worshipper. What is not clear is the proposal that thereby "the motif of the male's becoming integrated into the female waters is part of this larger phenomenon of gender metamorphosis", for Luria assumes the dominance of the female gender. At the same time, Luria speaks of a path to the union, which is not known above or below, neither in the secret of the female waters nor in the search of the male waters, implying an elevation beyond gender definitions. Thus, more than an integration, here we can apply the term "metamorphosis". There are therefore different messages: those that refer to unification, those that relate to transsexuality, and then the metamorphosis to new levels of unity.

In the main part of his chapter, Wolfson has documented that in texts of the theosophic Kabbalah there is the theme of the centrality of the male, phallic power. In his summary statement he states that there is a model that the male becomes female, *just as* there is one of the female becoming male. Moreover, the male becoming female intends to renew himself as a male. Thus there is not a covenant of unity, but a transformation of the female.

We have also developmental considerations to show the link between evolving humanness and mysticism. The earliest desires, wishes, and conflicts demand fulfilment on various levels of psychic differentiation. The striving for unity in mysticism has its origin in the developmental strivings towards unity by regression and by an attempt to transcend differentiation and individuation to attain a transcendent unification.

Comments on Idel and Wolfson

Mortimer Ostow

The psychoanalyst is always pleased to discover, in texts that he comes upon for the first time, symbolic equivalences that coincide with the insights that derive from the clinical practice of psychoanalysis. In Wolfson's chapter we encounter the observation that sacral space usually connotes the "female axis of divinity"—or, generally in our practice, the mother or a female surrogate for her. Wolfson also explains a comment of the *Zohar* that God strolls with the souls of the righteous as a euphemism for sexual intercourse, based upon the symbolic equivalence of the feet with the genital. Note that the word *coitus* is derived from the Latin *co-ire*, to go together.

As I observed above, we read in a number of different places that "everything is one", that entities combine to form integrated unities. Union and integration is the essence of mysticism. The tendency to regress to the presumed infantile experience of being one with the mother results in the striving to unite with a current representation of the earliest mother image. Sexual union recreates both the emotional and the physical experience of union. But the Kabbalah goes one step further. It posits a supernal sexual union that parallels, influences, and resonates with human conjugal unions. It shows the individual adept that his conjugal union can obtain not only his own access to the world of the *Sefirot*, but actually reinforces the vigour of the Divine (or infradivine, depending upon our definition).

But what are we to do with the strange gender transformations to which Wolfson calls our attention? As psychoanalysts we know that we each possess attitudes and complexes of both sexes—that we are each, in a psychological sense, bisexual. The phallic woman is a well-known archetype of a hostile, unloving, unreceptive, punitive, unwilling, and unappetizing sexual partner. And the castrated male is the converse archetype, of the passive, fearful, unaffectionate, and ineffectual sexual partner, an unmasculine man. But the Kabbalah gives us multiple and frequently changing gender identities. Moreover, it is striking to read that unmodified femininity tends towards stern judgement, whereas unmodified masculinity tends towards compassion: an idea contrary to common belief and incompatible with the derivation of the Hebrew word *rahamim*, compassion, from the word *rehem*, womb. And what could be the consequence of the *Shekhinah*'s intruding into our bedroom and bed? For those of us who are not comfortable with the prospect of orgy or even exhibitionism, the idea can have a chilling rather than an aphrodisiac effect.

At first sight, the explicit sexuality of the Kabbalah seems to be an instance of liberalism in orthodox religious practice, consistent with the Jewish tendency to place a positive religious value on marital sexual activity. However, what is described in the material that Idel and Wolfson place before us is a strange and unappetizing variant of what modern Western culture considers satisfying sexual behaviour. In the first place, the male is encouraged to focus on divine influences rather than his own and his partner's pleasure. In fact the idea of sexual pleasure appears only once in the many quotations that are cited—that is, in Idel's report of Abulafia's comment. Second, mentally, the female partner is expected to attempt to unify her thoughts with those of her male partner, in the hope of engendering male progeny. Of course, she has to hope that that's what he is thinking about.

Wolfson presents more than adequate documentation of his thesis to the effect that the female is valorized as the male—

specifically, that she is conceptually associated with the *corona*[1] of the penis; and that the male, when he enters the female, becomes feminized; and that the pregnant, the parturient, and the lactating woman are all valorized as masculine. Why the kabbalists should wish to have it so is not self-evident.

I suspect that the answer can be found in Wolfson's repeated observation that the Kabbalah is so andro– and phallocentric that even the positive values normally associated with the feminine are assigned to the male.

Why is the female partner valorized as male, and folded into the corona of the penis? Because, at the height of intercourse, the male is concerned only with the pleasurable sensations emanating from the head of his penis and with the concurrent divine experience, so that he becomes almost unaware of his female partner. Psychologically, she disappears into his penis.

Why is the pregnant, parturient, or lactating female valorized as male? Nothing is accomplished simply by translating active to masculine and passive to feminine. I suspect that the true answer is that anything that the woman does that has positive value for the man is considered a masculine activity. A feminine woman cannot do anything of value; any valued activity must be ascribed to a male agent.

Why is the male entering the female valorized as female? Because at the inception of intercourse, at the point of intromission, the male derives pleasure from the contact with the lubricating vagina (the "lower waters"); it seems to act upon his

---

[1] There is a problem with the word "*corona*". It is used in English translations of Kabbalah, the Hebrew–English Soncino Talmud (Yevamoth 55b), and all translations of the Mishnah that I have consulted (Shabbat 19:6), as the equivalent of the Hebrew *atarah*. Since the Hebrew *atarah* and the Latin *corona* both mean crown, that translation seems appropriate. But is it? The Ben Yehudah dictionary and Rashi to Yevamoth 55b define *atarah* as the *head* of the penis, referring apparently to the *glans*. Alcalay gives "glans" as the English translation of *atarah*. The problem arises from the fact that the term *corona*, in the anatomy of the penis, does not refer to the entire glans but only to the proximal circumferential ridge of the glans to which the foreskin of the penis is attached. It is visible on the uncircumcised penis only when the foreskin is retracted or when the penis is erect. It is always visible on the circumcised penis. Did the kabbalists and the rabbis of the Talmud make this distinction? For them, does *atarah* refer only to the *corona* and not to the whole glans?

penis—it is active, and the penis, at the moment of penetration is acted upon, is stimulated. Paradoxically, from the point of view of sensation, the penetrating penis is acted upon by the receptive and lubricating vagina. What the lubricating vagina does is valued, and so it must be masculine; the penis that is acted upon, then, must be feminine. But shortly the "lower" or female "waters" arouses the "upper" or male "waters", the pleasure becomes localized in the head of the penis and the female and her vagina disappear from psychological view.

It is not that the kabbalist has contempt for women—merely a lack of interest. Wolfson notes that phallocentricity was characteristic of the culture in which Kabbalah appeared: "Gender imagery in the kabbalistic sources reflects the binary ideology of the general mediaeval culture, as well as the specific rabbinic society, which reinforced the division of the sexes along hierarchical lines, delegating to the female a subservient role. The male is valorized as the active, dominant, primary sex, and the female as the passive, dominated, and secondary one" (pp. 279–280). We read nothing in this material about female sexual anatomy (although Wolfson reports [note 8] that at some point Joseph of Hamadan does discuss it explicitly). There are no labia, no vulva, no vestibule, no clitoris, only an opening called Zion. And Zion is applied ambiguously to the opening both of the vagina and of the womb. Seminal potential is attributed to female lubrication, and therefore the latter is taken seriously.

If my guess is correct, what Kabbalah does is to preempt the act of sexual intercourse and deprive it of its bonding function between male and female partners, and of sexual pleasure, converting it into an act of religious ritual, significant for the male who hopes to bond with the divine and who hopes to engender a male child. One is reminded of the way *Midrash Rabba* violates the plain meaning of the Song of Songs, deconstructs its text, and converts it to a religious discussion of God's beneficences to Israel. In return for giving up sexual pleasure, both his own and his partner's, the kabbalist is rewarded by the sense of brief contact, or even unification, with an aspect of the infradivine, the *Sefirot*.

EPILOGUE

CHAPTER NINE

Concluding comments: union and reunion

From the point of view of the individual, the mystical enterprise performs a useful defensive function. It can be construed as a method of reducing the pain of confrontation with an unkind reality or with unhappiness arising internally. The individual, whether by trance automatism or by deliberate concentration, displaces his interest from current reality or current affective state to an imagined return to a gratifying infantile experience or fantasy. This return usually includes a feeling of union with one or both parents, or a close visualization, or the experience of being lifted in parental arms, being fed, being rescued, or even the experience of engaging in some sexual, genital contact.

The transition from normal contact with ordinary reality is effected for the mystic by means of the apocalyptic mechanism—a device that defeats a negative affect by replacing it with a positive one, despair with hope. The mechanism usually involves some kind of revelation, a new view of the universe or oneself—a hallucination, doctrine, or belief. It operates automatically and unconsciously, without conscious intent and even without conscious understanding of what is happening. The apocalyptic mechanism also prevails in other phenomena, such as classical apocalypse, messianism, utopianism, fundamentalism, and millenarianism, so that they and mysticism often appear together.

Classical prophecy, too, may overlap with the other members of the apocalyptic complex. Its message resembles that of classical apocalypse in that both foretell the future, and the communication of the message to the prophet is frequently described as a mystical type of experience. What we learned in Halperin's essay (chapter three) is that we can detect by a psychoanalytic type of analysis the prophet's personal agenda behind his public prophecy. To the extent that it coincides with the agenda of the community, he can entrain community participation; to the extent that it is discordant with the community agenda, its appeal may be limited or restricted. Ezekiel's explicit sexuality presumably both attracted and repelled. (B.T.) Hagigah (13a) records a controversy among the rabbis about whether the book should be withdrawn from circulation.

In Ezekiel's mystical trances, he elaborated an image of God that had two interesting properties. First, God's sexuality is fairly clear to anyone who looks beyond the exoteric message. Second, God is visualized travelling in a chariot, which is carried by four chimerical creatures. Vehicular travel through the heavens is characteristic of classical apocalypse. Moreover, the details of the creatures leads one, by the application of exegetical technique, far into prior biblical accounts and into subsequent elaborations in Talmudic and Midrashic legends and parables. Accordingly, Ezekiel's throne–chariot vision became the symbol for mystical speculation (see Halperin, 1988a).

Using Ezekiel's description of the chariot, the *merkavah* and *hekhalot* mystics of the late pre-Christian and early Christian centuries chose to cultivate the illusion of the possibility of visualizing God in the context of what we understand as early childhood fantasies, in which the child looks upward to the parent, usually the father, or into a claustrum, which represents the mother's body. Just as children are sexually curious but understand sexuality only approximately, so this mystical system only suggests but does not deal explicitly with sexual function.

The kabbalistic system, which began to develop towards the end of the first millennium, responded to the impatience of the Jews with the delay of their salvation and to the remoteness of God with respect to their concerns. They postulated a God who was not only remote but absolutely unknowable—in fact, inconceivable. However, he radiated hypostases that paralleled human feelings and attitudes—almost intentions. The parallel divine and human structures resonated with each other and thus created the possibility of a theurgic function: by behaving in a prescribed way, the Jew could induce similar attitudes and behaviour in the Divine Sefirot. In this way, order and even predictability were either restored or introduced into the conception of the universe, and responsibility for salvation now came under the control of the individual Jew.

As God began to resemble humans, at least in his hypostases, the mystical theology began to resemble what might be considered a divine sociology and psychology. Whereas the *merkavah* and *hekhalot* mystics exploited only the parent–child attachment, the kabbalists exploited also the attraction between the sexes. The human quest for mystical experience with God rode upon these two basic instinctual drives.

How are the mystical systems used? What influence do they have on the lives of the mystics, on their daily conduct and frame of mind? Autobiography and even biography are extremely limited in Jewish materials, and so we have much less information here than about what Jews thought and wrote about.

In the Midrashic studies of the *merkavah* and *hekhalot* mystics, we read how one might prepare for or induce an illusion or trance. But we do not know how many people did engage in such activities, and how often. And if they did, how were the other aspects of their lives affected?

How was the theosophic kabbalah used? What proportion of time was devoted to such studies? Did immersion in these studies influence daily practical life? Did the study of the Sefirot affect practical conduct? When the Kabbalist studied the explicitly sexual materials, was he aroused? Did these speculations affect his sex life?

Since we read only of male Kabbalists—the study of the Holy Books in Judaism was almost exclusively a male preoccupation—how did the mystical enterprise affect women? What did they know about it, and how were they expected to respond to it?

Kabbalism was often associated with the attribution of a special redemptive function to the performance of the ordinary *mitzvot*, to each of which the Kabbalists attributed specific reasons [*ta'amei hamitzvot*]. The performance was no longer a matter of satisfying halakhic requirements; it was an act of mystical communication with God. This communication was promoted by achieving a high level of mental concentration, facilitated by the recitation of a formula of intention. (The cultivation of intention was encouraged in rabbinic times, but the kabbalistic intention [*kavvanah*] was intended to raise the performance of the *mitzvah* to a mystical act.)

The idea that human behaviour influenced the behaviour and attitudes of the Divine made it possible for the individual to imagine controlling his own destiny, to encourage God's mercy to prevail over His stern judgement. It was one step from this idea to ideas of magic—that is, changing things in the real world by invoking God's power. Various techniques were employed, imagining combinations and recombinations of the letters of the Hebrew alphabet and obligating God to intervene by addressing Him by His secret names.

We should note the fact that mysticism was often practised in mystical communities. The subjective experience of union with, or attachment to God, the ecstatic experience, was necessarily an individual matter. But interest in these matters and activity with respect to them could—and probably was—encouraged within mystical communities. It is likely that the elaboration of mystical philosophies was the work of groups, more or less tightly organized. The word *cabal* in English is used to signify a conspiratorial organization. For those who resort to mysticism out of frustration and disappointment, group membership itself provides gratifying relief. One is not alone in an unfriendly universe. The group constitutes a friendly universe and creates the impression that the remote cosmos, too, is hospitable. The group then complements the reparative function of the mystical enterprise.

For the reader who is new to mysticism, we must emphasize how broad the subject is, even when we limit our interest to

Judaism. Within the brief compass of this book, it has not been possible to cover or allude to even a reasonably representative fraction of the history of mysticism and its many varieties. For more adequate information, the reader is again referred to the major references listed in the first chapter.

We have tried to formulate a psychological interpretation of the major mystical matters and themes. As psychiatrists we wonder whether the pursuit of mysticism is a useful or a wholesome exercise. Specifically, what are its virtues, and what are its dangers?

However, we must acknowledge that we have no absolute criteria. It is extremely difficult, if not impossible, to establish criteria of normality for group activities. Those individuals who have indulged in mystical activities, in their own times and their own circumstances, were persuaded that these activities were appropriate and laudable. While we are doubtless better informed than they, how can we be sure that future generations, even better informed than we, may not be able to achieve a more sophisticated and valid appraisal? Does spirituality offer an additional dimension to the flat-world of the purely reasoned life, or does it compromise the truly scientific *Weltanschauung* to which Freud aspired?

The elevated or occasionally ecstatic experience of the individual mystic is almost always perceived as gratifying, though sometimes frightening, even terrifying, as well. The apocalyptic type of mood change offers welcome relief from the discomfort of daily life and replaces it with the pleasure of the feeling of rebirth. On the one hand, the shift may replace discouragement and demoralization with new hope and renewed effort to overcome adversity. On the other hand, two of the three individuals whose spirituality I recorded at the beginning of this book were always looking for extra-rational sources of information and inappropriate sources of encouragement: astrology, fortune-telling media, pseudo-remedies, and pseudo-scientific theories. While the desired spiritual experience did not itself lead them into self-defeating error, the frame of mind that encouraged the spiritual quest also encouraged the openness to superstition and magic. They were looking to unreal or non-rational influences for salvation.

Group mysticism is a different matter. Unfortunately, we know little about the history of mystical groups in Judaism. As we observed above, membership in a group provides the comfort of group support and of dissolving one's uncomfortable solitariness into group identity. But groups are as susceptible to the promise of illusion as are individuals. We do know a little of Jewish messianic movements. The ill-fated Bar Kokhba revolt against Rome, as we saw previously, was nourished by the messianic fervour of Akiba. The Sabbatian adventure was plainly encouraged by the perversion of kabbalistic, specifically Lurianic, mysticism of Sabbatai Sevi himself and of his mentor and agent, Nathan of Gaza. (Wolfson, in a recent lecture [1994d], discussed in great detail the kabbalistic theories regarding Sevi.) Messianic fervour in Israel today is feeding militaristic and perhaps self-defeating adventurism.

Modern Hasidim constitutes one mystical group that is quite visible to us. Since we have not considered Hasidism in his book, it would be inappropriate to offer a critique to assess its virtues and faults.

The mystics and mysticism were usually stringently discouraged by the leadership of the normative Jewish community. (The conference on mystical leadership arranged by Idel and Ostow called attention to a few individuals who both led the normative community and also engaged in kabbalistic study and practice. The same paradox existed in rabbinic times as well.) The reason is that although most mystics took great pains to remain within the law, to avoid antinomian postures, nevertheless their preoccupations have tended to lead them away from normative practice. At times they became a law unto themselves and occasionally seemed to be gradually undermining nomian doctrine and practice. Sabbatai Sevi was an extreme case in point. The individual mystic considers his own mystical experience more valid than normative doctrine when they conflict, and may introduce anomian if not antinomian practice.

Psychiatric and especially psychoanalytic interest in mysticism is aroused by the opportunity to understand and to explain irrational thinking, to determine its origins and its purpose. We started with hypotheses that the characteristic mystical experience could be interpreted as a regression to the child's earliest months when he was uncertain whether or not he was a separate individual or a part of his mother or caretaker. We have not encountered any material that could throw direct light on that proposition, but it seems intuitively attractive, and, as we have not found anything that would contradict it either, it remains an appealing explanation. We also proposed that the several mystical images and fantasies and illusions that appear in the mystical materials that evolved in Jewish history can be understood as projections of almost universal unconscious individual fantasies, most, if not all, based in turn upon childhood experience, real or fantasy. I believe that we have been able to demonstrate that that proposition is indeed consistent with the facts in all of the several materials that we have examined.

The scholar of mysticism would also like to understand the psychological basis for the many unrealistic illusions and fantasies that he reads about, above and beyond the realistic circumstances, the time, the environment, and the people that form the background of the mystical productions. I believe that we have offered some useful hypotheses.

Very few of us can enjoy life in a cosmos that is experienced as indifferent. The indifference of the cosmos becomes especially sharp when we have lost individuals whom we love, when the community is demoralized, when we are confronted with frustration and disappointment without any promise for alleviation. Under such circumstances one may be offered—by the group or by a leader, or from within oneself—any of the variants of the apocalyptic complex, apocalyptic violence, messianism, fundamentalist group formation, political revolution or mystical adventure, individual or group. Of these perhaps quietistic mysticism is the least dangerous and certainly no more irrational than the others. How individuals or groups select among these possibilities is far from clear.

We speak of spirituality short of mysticism when we attempt to enrich our lives in a similar way but not necessarily with the scaffold of a fixed myth and the support by encouragement or compulsion of a congenial group. Neubauer suggests that not every aspiration for union and reunion need be considered a regression to infantile modalities of physical attachment to or incorporation within the mother. A certain spiritualization of daily experience, and especially of creative experiences, might result from sublimation of archaic tendencies and might be considered a progressive step.

There is a story, perhaps apocryphal, that Professor Saul Lieberman, a most distinguished scholar and professor of Talmud at the Jewish Theological Seminary of America, a confirmed *mitnaged*, who is reported to have had only contempt for Kabbalah, was called upon at a formal meeting to introduce Professor Gershom Scholem. The audience waited with some anxiety to hear how this confrontation would work out. Lieberman, with his usual charm and wit, began as follows: "Ladies and Gentlemen. We all know that nonsense is nonsense, but the history of nonsense is scholarship." The unconscious has the power to invade, to instinctualize, to supersede rational thought. Many of us who cannot accept the non-rational assumptions necessary to embrace mysticism might nevertheless find a certain degree of comforting spiritual experience in studying what it is, what it does, how it has influenced the lives of millions of people of every religion over the centuries, and where it might take us in the future.

GLOSSARY

Aggadah or *Haggadah* (from the word *higgid*, "to tell", therefore a narrative): The non-halakhic material of the Talmud, incorporating homilies, legends, history, and discussion. (The word "*Haggadah*" is also used for the text of the Passover Seder service, which consists essentially of the narration of the Passover story and elaboration thereof.)

Cherub (plural *Cherubim*): A winged celestial creature referred to at different points in the Bible. Images of cherubim appeared above the ark in both the desert tabernacle and in Solomon's Temple.

En Sof (also transliterated *Ein Sof* and *Eyn Sof*): literally, "There is no end". The Kabbalistic term for the divine entity, unknown, limitless, and indescribable.

Erez Yisrael: The land of Israel.

D'vekuth: Literally, "clinging". In Jewish mystical literature, it signifies the mystic's aspiration to cling or adhere to God.

Gemara: A collection of rabbinic debates of the second to sixth century C.E. that elaborate and codify the cultic and civil regulations of the Mishnah. It also contains edifying legends. In fact, there are two Talmuds, one developed in Palestine and the other in Babylonia. In many ways they resemble each other and overlap; in other ways they differ.

Gematria: The Hebrew alphabet is used not only to form words, but also as a set of number symbols. Therefore each word has a numerical value, i.e. the sum of the numbers signified by its letters. By magical thought, two or more words having the same numerical value can be declared equivalent to each other, and the equivalence can serve as proof of this or that thesis. This system is called *gematria*, a word probably based upon the Greek antecedent of *geometry*.

Halakhah (from the word *halokh*, "to go", therefore literally "procedure"): Religious law primarily derived from the Mishnaic code and Talmudic debate, elaborated and detailed in various codes incumbent upon observant Jews today.

Hasidic Zaddik or *Hasidic Rebbe* (plural *Rebbeim*): The religious leader of a Hasidic community.

Midrash: Rabbinic homiletic writings that were not included in the Mishnah or Gemara, mostly produced at various points in the Jewish world during the first millennium and a half of the Common Era.

Mishnah: A concise code of cultic and civil law, accumulated during the last two centuries before and the first two centuries after the Common Era. It forms the basis of rabbinic Judaism, which is the Judaism currently practised.

Mitzvah (plural *Mitzvot*): Jewish religious obligations.

Nadav and *Avihu:* The two eldest of Aaron's four sons. Verse 3:4 of Numbers tells us that they died because they introduced alien fire into the cultic service, and it adds that they had no children.

Ophan (plural *Ophannim*): Literally, "wheel". In this context it refers to a category of angels. The term is used to refer to the wheels of Ezekiel's chariot as described in chapter 1 of Ezekiel. Since the wheels in the description have eyes, one may infer that they are animate and therefore perhaps infradivine creatures.

Sefirot (also *Sephirot*): Hypostases expressing aspects of the *En Sof* that are recognizable by humans. They are usually imagined as though they are arranged in the shape of a two-dimensional divine anthropos. That is, they are placed in three vertical columns, four in the centre column and three in each of the side columns. In the centre column, the highest Sefirah, representing the head, is called *keter* or "crown". Under that is *tif'eret* or "beauty". Beneath that the next in line is *yesod* or "foundation", representing the phallus. The lowest Sefirah in the centre column is called *malkhut*, "kingdom" or "kingship". The uppermost Sefirah of the right column, that is, the left of the divine anthropos, is called *binah*, "understanding". Under that is *gevurah*, "strength". The lowest of the three is *hod* or "glory". The column on the right side of the divine anthropos, (the left on the diagram) is arranged from above down as follows: *hokhmah* or "wisdom"; *hesed*, "loving kindness"; *netzah*, "victory" or "eternity".

Sitrah ahrah: Literally, "the other side", referring to the other side of the divine universe—that is, the source of evil, the demonic.

Talmud: This term is often used to refer to the combination of Mishnah and Gemara, especially as these are arranged together in the classic text of the Talmud. The term may also refer to the Gemara alone.

Tanakh: The Jewish biblical scriptures. The word is an acronym for ***T**orah*, ***N**eviim* [Prophets], ***K**etuvim* [Writings].

Tohu vavohu: The mythical primordial chaos of the second verse of Genesis.

Torah: Literally the Pentateuch but, by extension, any or all of Jewish scriptures, whether the Pentateuch alone, or the entire Tanakh, or that as well as the Talmud and other authoritative religious works.

REFERENCES

Manuscript collections

Ms. BPNH: Ms. Paris, Bibliothèque Nationale hébraïque.
Ms. JM: Ms. Jerusalem, Mussajoff.
Ms. JS: Ms. Jerusalem, Sassoon.
Ms. MBS: Ms. Munich Bayerische Staatsbibliothek.
Ms. NYJTSA: Ms. New York, Jewish Theological Seminary of America.
Ms. OBL: Ms. Oxford Bodleian Library.
Ms. PBP: Ms. Parma, Biblioteca Palatina
Ms. VBAE: Ms. Vatican, Biblioteca Apostolica ebraica.

Primary sources

Abraham Azulai, *Hesed le-'Avraham.* Bene-Beraq: p.n.k.,[1] 1986.
Abraham Miguel Cardoso, *Derush ha-Shekhinah.* P.n.k.
Alphabet of R. Akiba. In: S. A. Wertheimer (Ed.), *Bate Midrashot.* Jerusalem: Ktav va-Sefer, 1955.

[1]p.n.k. = publisher not known.

Apocalypse of Adam (tr. G. Macrae). In: J. H. Charlesworth (Ed.), *The Old Testament Pseudepigrapha.* Garden City, NY: Doubleday, 1983.

Apocalypse of Zephania (tr. O. Wintermute). Garden City, NY: Doubleday, 1983.

Avot de-Rabbi Natan, version B (ed. S. Schechter). Vienna: p.n.k., 1887.

Book of Mirrors. Sefer Mar'ot ha-Zove'ot by R. David ben Yehudah he-Hasid (ed. D. C. Matt). Chico, CA: Scholars Press, 1982.

Cordovero, Rabbi Moses, *Tefillah le-Mosheh* (ed. Prezmysl). P.n.k., 1932.

Devarim Nehmadim. In: *Imre Pinehas ha-Shalem* (ed. Y. Frankel). Jerusalem: p.n.k., 1988.

Genesis Rabbah (ed. J. Theodor & C. Albeck). Jerusalem: Wahrman, 1965.

Genesis Rabbah. In: *Midrash Rabbah, Vol. I* (tr. H. Freedman & M. Simon). London: Soncino, 1977.

Hagigah. *Babylonian Talmud* [Heb.–Eng. edition] (tr. I. Abraham; ed. I. Epstein). London: Soncino, 1984.

Hayyim Vital, *'Es Hayyim.* Jerusalem: p.n.k., 1910.

Hayyim Vital, *Mavo' She'arim.* Jerusalem: p.n.k., 1904.

Hayyim Vital, *Peri 'Es Hayyim.* Jerusalem: p.n.k., 1980.

Hayyim Vital, *Sefer Ta'ame ha-Miswot.* Jerusalem: p.n.k., 1963.

Hayyim Vital, *Sha'ar ha-Gilgulim.* Jerusalem: p.n.k., 1981.

Hayyim Vital, *Sha'ar ha-Haqdamot.* Jerusalem: p.n.k., 1909.

Hayyim Vital, *Sha'ar ha-Kawwanot.* Jerusalem: p.n.k., 1902.

Hayyim Vital, *Sha'ar ha-Kelalim.* In: Hayyim Vital, *'Es Hayyim.*

Hayyim Vital, *Sha'ar Ma'amere Rashbi.* Jerusalem: p.n.k., 1898.

Hayyim Vital, *Sha'ar Ruah ha-Qodesh.* Jerusalem: 1879. Reprinted Jerusalem: p.n.k., 1976.

Hekhaloth Rabbati. In: *Bet ha-Midrasch, Vol. 1*, Part 3 (coll. & ed. A. Jellinek). Jerusalem: Wahrman, 1967.

Iggeret ha-Kodesh, The Holy Letter (ed. & tr. S. J. Cohen). New York, KTAV, 1976. In: H. Chavel (Ed.), *Kitve Ramban.* Jerusalem: Mosad ha-Rav Kook, 1967.

Imre Pinehas ha-Shalem (ed. Y. Frankel). Jerusalem: p.n.k., 1988.

Isaac of Acre, *Sefer Me'irat 'Einayim* (ed. A. Goldreich). Jerusalem: Akademon, 1981.

Jacob ben Sheshet, *Sefer Meshiv Devarim Nekhohim* (ed. G. Vajda).

Jerusalem: Israel Academy of Sciences and Humanities, 1968.

Joseph Gikatilla, *Sha'are 'Orah* (ed. J. Ben-Shlomo). Jerusalem: Bralik Institute, 1981.

Joseph Gikatilla, *Sod Yod-Gimmel Middot ha-Nove'ot min ha-Keter 'Elyon. Kitve Yad ba-Qabbalah.* Jerusalem: Scholem, 1930.

Joseph ibn Tabul's Sermons on the *Kawwanot* (ed. Y. R. Avivi). In: *Studies in Memory of the Rishon le-Zion R. Yitzhak Nissim* [Heb.] (ed. M. Benayahu). Jerusalem: p.n.k., 1985.

Joseph of Hamadan's *Sefer Tashak.* Critical Text Edition with Introduction (ed. J. Zwelling). Ph.D. dissertation, Brandeis University, 1975.

Kabbalah of the Gra, The [Heb.] (ed. Y. R. Avivi). Jerusalem: p.n.k., 1993.

Kethuboth. *Babylonian Talmud* [Heb.–Eng. edition] (tr. S. Daiches & I. W. Slotki; ed. I. Epstein). London: Soncino, 1971.

Kitve ha-Ramban (ed. C. D. Chavel). Jerusalem: Mosad ha-Rav Kook, 1967.

Lamentations Rabbah. In: *Midrash Rabbah, Vol. IV* (tr. & ed. H. Freedman & M. Simon). London: Soncino, 1977.

Ma'arekhet ha-'Elohut. Mantua: p.n.k., 1558. [Reprinted Jerusalem: Maqor, 1963.]

Maimonides, *Guide of the Perplexed* (tr. S. Pines). Chicago & London: University of Chicago Press, 1963.

Maimonides, *Mishnah Torah. The Book of Judges* (Shofetim). Issued by Jerusalem: Mosad ha-Rav Kook, 1987.

Menahem Azariah of Fano, *Yonat 'Elem.* Amsterdam: p.n.k., 1948.

Midrash Rabbah (tr. & ed. H. Freedman & M. Simon). London: Soncino, 1977.

Midrash Tadshe. In Epstein (Ed.), *Beitrage zur Jüdischen Alterthumskunde.* Vienna: p.n.k., 1887.

Miqra'ot Gedolot. [Contains the text of the Hebrew Bible, with Targums and a selection of the major medieval commentaries (e.g. Rashi, Kimhi, Ibn Ezra). Reprinted Jerusalem: Etz Hayyim, 1974.]

Moses de León, *Sefer ha-Rimmon, The Book of the Pomegranate* (ed. E. R. Wolfson). Atlanta, GA: Scholars Press, 1988.

Moses de León, *Sheqel ha-Qodesh* (ed. W. A. Greenup). London: p.n.k., 1911.

Nachmanides (Moses ben Nahman), *Commentary on Exodus* (tr. C. B. Chavel). New York: Shilo, 1973.

Natan ḥa-Azati, *Treatise on the Menorah*. In: G. Scholem, *Be-Iqvot Mashiah*. Jerusalem: p.n.k., 1944

Nathan of Gaza, *Derush ha-Taninim*. In: *Be-'Iqvot Mashiah* (ed. G. Scholem). Jerusalem: p.n.k., 1944.

Pesiqta' Rabbati (ed. M. Friedmann). Vienna: Kaiser, 1880. [Reprinted Tel Aviv: p.n.k., 1963.]

Pirke Avoth. In: *The Living Talmud, the Wisdom of the Fathers, and Its Classical Commentaries* (tr. & ed. J. Goldin). New York: Heritage, 1955.

Qehillat Ya'aqov. Jerusalem: p.n.k., 1992.

Sanhedrin. *Babylonian Talmud* [Heb.–Eng. edition] (tr. J. Shachter & H. Freedman; ed. I. Epstein). London: Soncino, 1969.

Sefer ha-Bahir. (ed. R. Margaliot). Jerusalem: Mosad Ha-Rav Kook, 1978.

Sefer ha-Mishkal: Text and Study (ed. J. Wijnhoven). Ph.D. dissertation, Brandeis University, 1964.

Sefer ha-Peli'ah. Korets: p.n.k., 1784.

Sefer ha-Zohar (Zohar) (ed. R. Margaliot). Jerusalem: Mosad Ha-Rav Kook (3rd edition, 1960; 6th edition [3 vols.], 1984).

Sefer Haredim (ed. E. Azikri). Jerusalem: p.n.k., 1966.

Sefer Hit'abekut (ed. J. Emden). Lvov: p.n.k., 1877.

Sefer Yesirah (ed. I. Gruenwald). *Israel Oriental Studies 1* (1971): 132–177.

Shir ha-Shirim Rabbah III (ed. S. Dunski). Jerusalem & Tel Aviv: p.n.k., 1980. [Song of Songs Rabbah. In: *Midrash Rabbah, Vol. IV* (tr. H. Freedman & M. Simon). London: Soncino, 1977.]

Shiur Komah. Jerusalem: p.n.k., 1966. [Tr. M. S. Cohen, *The "Si'ur Qomah": The Critical Edition of the Text with Introduction, Translation and Commentary*. Ann Arbor, MI: Universal Microfilms International, 1982.]

Tuviah ben Eliezer, *Lekah Tov on Genesis* (ed. S. Buber). Lemberg: p.n.k., 1888.

Zohar Hadash (ed. R. Margaliot). Jerusalem: Mosad ha-Rav Kook. 1978.

MODERN SOURCES

[Recent publications of primary sources have been included here, listed by editor, as well as under the Primary Sources section.]

Aaron, D. (forthcoming). Imagery of the Divine and the Human: On the Mythology of Genesis Rabba 8 § 1. *Journal of Jewish Thought and Philosophy*.

Agus, A. (1980). Some Early Rabbinic Thinking on Gnosticism. *Jewish Quarterly Review, 71*: 18–30.

Albright, W. (1942). *Archaeology and the Religion of Israel: The Ayer Lectures of the Colgate-Rochester Divinity School, 1941*. Baltimore, MD: Johns Hopkins University Press.

Allony, N. (1963). The Zevi in the Hebrew Poetry of Spain [Heb.]. *Sefarad*, 23.

Altmann, A. (1942). Gnostic Themes in Rabbinic Cosmology. In: I. Epstein, E. Levine, & C. Roth (Eds.), *Essays in Honour of the Very Rev. Dr. J. H. Hertz, Chief Rabbi . . . on the Occasion of His Seventieth Birthday*. London: Edward Goldston.

Anderson, G. (1989). Celibacy or Consummation in the Garden? Reflections on Early Jewish and Christian Interpretations of the Garden of Eden. *Harvard Theological Review, 82*: 121–148.

Angus, S. (1975). *The Mystery Religions. A Study of the Religious Background of Early Christianity*. New York: Dover. [Original, London: Murray, 1929.]

Arlow, J. A. (1951). The Consecration of the Prophet. *Psychoanalytic Quarterly, 20*: 374–397. [Reprinted in: M. Ostow, *Judaism in Psychoanalysis*. New York: KTAV, 1982.]

Arlow, J. A. (1960). Fantasy Systems in Twins. *Psychoanalytic Quarterly, 29*: 175–199.

Arlow, J. A. (1972). The Only Child. *Psychoanalytic Quarterly, 41* (4): 507–536.

Arlow, J. A. (1987). Guilt. In: *Contemporary Jewish Religious Thought* (ed. A. A. Cohen & P. Mendes-Flohr). New York: Scribner's.

Assis, Y. T. (1988). Sexual Behaviour in Mediaeval Hispano-Jewish Society. In: A. Rapoport-Albert & S. J. Zipperstein (Eds.), *Jewish History: Essays in Honour of Chimen Abramsky* (pp. 25–59). London: Peter Halban.

Atkinson, C. W. (1991). *The Oldest Vocation: Christian Motherhood in the Middle Ages*. Ithaca, NY & London: Cornell University Press.

Augustine: The Confessions of St. Augustine (tr. E. B. Pusey). London & Toronto: Dent: New York: Dutton, 1907.

Avivi, Y. R. (1985). Joseph ibn Tabul's Sermons on the *Kawwanot*. In: *Studies in Memory of the Rishon le-Zion R. Yitzhak Nissim* [Heb.] (ed. M. Benayahu). Jerusalem: p.n.k.

Avivi, Y. R. (1993). *The Kabbalah of the Gra* [Heb.]. Jerusalem: p.n.k.

Azikri, E. (1966). *Sefer Haredim*. Jerusalem: p.n.k.

Azulai, A. (1986). *Hesed le-'Avraham*. Bene-Beraq: p.n.k.

Badè, W. (1933). The Seal of Jaazaniah. *Zeitschrift fuer die alttestamentliche Wissenschaft, 51*: 150–156.

Baer, I. (1975). The Service of Sacrifice in Second Temple Times [Heb.]. *Zion, 40*.

Baer, R. A. (1970). *Philo's Use of Categories Male and Female*. Leiden: E.J. Brill.

Ben Sheshet, J. (1968). *Meshiv Devarim Nekhohim* (ed. Georges Vajda). Jerusalem: Israel Academy of Sciences and Humanities.

Ben-Shlomo, J. (Ed.) (1981). Joseph Gikatilla, *Sha'are 'Orah*. Jerusalem: Bialik Institute.

Benayahu, M. (Ed.) (1985). *Studies in Memory of the Rishon le-Zion R. Yitzhak Nissim* [Heb.]. Jerusalem: p.n.k.

Benko, S. (1993). *The Virgin Goddess: Studies in the Pagan and Christian Roots of Mariology*. Leiden: E. J. Brill.

Bergmann, M. S. (1992). *In the Shadow of Moloch: The Sacrifice of Children and Its Impact on Western Religions*. New York: Columbia University Press.

Biale, D. (1982). The God with Breasts: El Shaddai in the Bible. *History of Religions, 20*: 240–256.

Biale, D. (1992). *Eros and the Jews: From Biblical Israel to Contemporary America*. New York: Basic Books.

Bird, P. A. (1991). Sexual Differentiation and Divine Image in the Genesis Creation Texts. In: K. E. Børresen (Ed.), *Image of God and Gender Models in Judaeo–Christian Tradition*. Oslo: p.n.k.

Bloch, R. H. (1991). *Medieval Misogyny and the Invention of Western Romantic Love*. Chicago & London: University of Chicago Press.

Bodenheimer, F. (1962). Fauna. In: *The Interpreter's Dictionary of the Bible: An Illustrated Encyclopedia, Vol. 2*. New York: Abingdon Press.

Bogoras, W. (1965). Shamanistic Performance in the Inner Room. In: W. Lessa & E. Vogt (Eds.), *Reader in Comparative Religion: An*

Anthropological Approach (2nd edition). New York, Evanston, IL, & London: Harper & Row.

Boman, T. (1960). *Hebrew Thought Compared with the Greek* (tr. J. L. Moreau). Philadelphia, PA: Westminster Press.

Boyarin, D. (1993). *Carnal Israel: Reading Sex in Talmudic Literature.* Los Angeles, CA, & Berkeley, CA: University of Californa Press.

Boylan, M. (1984). The Galenic and Hippocratic Challenge to Aristotle's Conception Theory. *Journal of the History of Biology, 17*: 83–112.

Branneman, W. L. Jr., Yarian, S.O., & Olson, A.M. (1982). *The Seeing Eye.* University Park, PA: Pennsylvania State University Press.

Brisson, L. (1986). Neutrum utrumque: La bisexualité dans l'antiquité gréco-romaine. In: *L'Androgyne dans la littérature (Cahiers de l'hermétisme).* Paris: A. Michel.

Broome, E. (1946). Ezekiel's Abnormal Personality. *Journal of Biblical Literature, 65,* 277–292.

Brown, P. (1988). *The Body and Society: Men, Women, and Sexual Renunciation in Early Christianity.* New York: Columbia University Press.

Brownlee, W. (1986). *Ezekiel 1–19 (Word Biblical Commentary, Vol. 28).* Waco, TX: Word Books.

Buber, M. (1947/1975). *Tales of the Hasidim. Vol. 1, The Early Masters; Vol. 2, The Late Masters* (ed. L. I. Newman). New York: Schocken.

Buber, S. (Ed.) (1888). Tuviah ben Eliezer, *Lekah Tov on Genesis.* Lemberg: p.n.k.

Bynum, C. W. (1982). *Jesus as Mother: Studies in the Spirituality of the High Middle Ages.* Berkeley, CA: University of California Press.

Bynum, C. W. (1986a). ". . . And Woman His Humanity": Female Imagery in the Religious Writing of the Later Middle Ages. In: C. W. Bynum, S. Harrell, & P. Richman (Eds.), *Gender and Religion: On the Complexity of Symbols.* Boston: Beacon Press.

Bynum, C. W. (1986b). Introduction: The Complexity of Symbols. In: C. W. Bynum, S. Harrell, & P. Richman (Eds.), *Gender and Religion: On the Complexity of Symbols.* Boston: Beacon Press.

Cadden, J. (1993). *Meaning of Sex Difference in the Middle Ages: Medicine, Science, and Culture.* Cambridge History of Medicine Series. Cambridge & New York: Cambridge University Press.

Carley, K. (1975). *Ezekiel among the Prophets*. Naperville, IL: Alec R. Allenson.

Cassem, N. (1973). Ezekiel's Psychotic Personality: Reservations on the Use of the Couch for Biblical Personalities. In: R. Clifford & G. MacRae (Eds.), *The Word in the World: Essays in Honor of Frederick J. Moriarty, S.J.* Cambridge, MA: Weston College Press.

Charlesworth, J. H. (Ed.) (1983). *The Old Testament Pseudepigrapha. Vol. 1: Apocalyptic Literature and Testaments*. Garden City, NY: Doubleday.

Chasseguet-Smirgel, J. (1985). *The Ego Ideal* (tr. P. Barrows). London: Free Association Books.

Chasseguet-Smirgel, J. (1986). The Archaic Matrix of the Oedipus Complex. In: *Sexuality and Mind*. London: Karnac Books.

Chavel, C. D. (Ed.) (1967). *Kitve ha-Ramban*. Jerusalem: Mosad ha-Rav Kook.

Chavel, H. (Ed.), *Kitve Ramban*. Jerusalem: Mosad ha-Rav Kook.

Chomsky, W. (1933). *David Kimhi's Hebrew Grammar (Mikhlol): Systematically Presented and Critically Annotated. Part One*. Philadelphia, PA: Dropsie College Press.

Chomsky, W. (1952). *David Kimhi's Hebrew Grammar (Mikhlol): Systematically Presented and Critically Annotated. Part Two*. New York: Bloch.

Cline Horowitz, M. (1979). The Image of God in Man—Is Woman Included. *Harvard Theological Review, 72*: 190–204.

Cohen, G. D. (1991). *Studies in the Variety of Rabbinic Cultures*. Philadelphia, PA: Jewish Publication Society.

Cohen, M. S. (Tr.) (1982). *The "Si'ur Qomah": The Critical Edition of the Text with Introduction, Translation and Commentary*. Ann Arbor, MI: Universal Microfilms International.

Cohen, S. J. (Ed. & Tr.) (1976). *Iggeret ha-Kodesh, The Holy Letter: A Study on Medieval Jewish Sexual Morality*. New York, KTAV, 1976. [In: H. Chavel (Ed.), *Kitve Ramban*. Jerusalem: Mosad ha-Rav Kook, 1967.]

Cohn, N. (1970). *The Pursuit of the Millennium*. New York: Oxford University Press.

Cooke, G. (1936). *A Critical and Exegetical Commentary on the Book of Ezekiel* (*International Critical Commentary, Vol. 21*). [Reprinted Edinburgh: T. &. T. Clark, 1951.]

Cordovero, Rabbi Moses (1932). *Tefillah le-Mosheh*. Prezmysl: p.n.k.

Dan, J. (1980). Sammael, Lilith, and the Concept of Evil in Early Kabbalah. *Association for Jewish Studies Review, 5*: 17–25.

Dan, J., & Milch, R. J. (1983). *The Teachings of Hasidism.* New York: Behrman House.

Davis, E. (1989). *Swallowing the Scroll: Textuality and the Dynamics of Discourse in Ezekiel's Prophecy.* Sheffield, UK: Almond Press.

Delcourt, M. (1958) *Hermaphrodite: mythes et rites de la bisexualité dans l'antiquité classique.* Paris: Presses Universitaires de France.

Dement, W., & Wolpert, E. (1958). Relationships in the Manifest Content of Dreams Occurring on the Same Night. *Journal of Nervous and Mental Disease, 126*: 568–578.

De Silva, R., & Lown, B. (1978). Ventricular Premature Beats, Stress, and Sudden Death. *Psychosomatics, 19* (11): 649–661.

Dodds, E. R. (1951). *The Greeks and the Irrational.* Berkeley, CA: University of California Press.

Dresner, S. H. (1960). *The Zaddik, The Doctrine of the Zaddik According to the Writings of Rabbi Yaakov Yosef of Polnoy.* London, New York, & Toronto: Abelard–Schuman.

Dresner, S. H. (1986). *The World of a Hasidic Master, Levi Yitzhak of Berditchev.* New York: Shapolski.

Drower, E. S. (1962). *The Mandaeans of Iraq and Iran.* Leiden: p.n.k.

Dunski, S. (Ed.) (1980). *Shir ha-Shirim Rabbah* III. Jerusalem & Tel Aviv: p.n.k. [Song of Songs Rabbah. In: *Midrash Rabbah, Vol. IV* (tr. H. Freedman & M. Simon). London: Soncino, 1977.]

Eilberg-Schwartz, H. (1994). *God's Phallus and Other Problems for Men and Monotheism.* Boston: Beacon Press.

Eliade, M. (1963). *Patterns in Comparative Religion.* New York: World Publishing.

Eliade, M. (1969). *The Two and the One.* Chicago, IL: University of Chicago Press.

Eliade, M. (1971). *Yoga, Immortality and Freedom.* Princeton, NJ: Princeton University Press.

Elior, R. (1993). *The Paradoxical Ascent to God: The Kabbalistic Theosophy of Habad Hasidism* (tr. J. M. Green). Albany, NY: State University of New York Press.

Emden, J. (1877). *Sefer hit'abekut.* Lvov: p.n.k.

Encyclopedia Judaica (1972) (ed. C. Roth & G. Wigoder). Jerusalem: Keter.

Engel, G. (1971). Sudden and Rapid Death during Psychological Stress: Folklore or Folk Wisdom? *Annals of Internal Medicine, 74*: 771–782.

Epstein (Ed.) (1887). *Midrash Tadshe. Beitrage zur Jüdischen Alterthumskunde*. Vienna: p.n.k.

Epstein, I. (Ed.) (1969). Sanhedrin. *Babylonian Talmud* [Heb.–Eng. edition] (tr. J. Shachter & H. Freedman). London: Soncino.

Epstein, I. (Ed.) (1971). Kethuboth. *Babylonian Talmud* [Heb.–Eng. edition] (tr. S. Daiches & I. W. Slotki). London: Soncino.

Epstein, I. (Ed.) (1984). Hagigah. *Babylonian Talmud* [Heb.–Eng. edition] (tr. I. Abraham). London: Soncino.

Epstein, J., & Straub, K. (1991). Introduction: The Guarded Body. In: *Body Guards: The Cultural Politics of Gender Ambiguity*. New York & London: Routledge.

Farber, L. & Fisher, C. (1943). An Experimental Approach to Dream Psychology through the Use of Hypnosis. *Psychoanalytic Quarterly, 2*: 202–216.

Feldman, S. (1949). Fear of Mice. *Psychoanalytic Quarterly, 18*, 227–230.

Fenton, P. (1989). Abraham Maimonides (1186–1237), Founding a Mystical Dynasty. In: M. Idel & M. Ostow, *Leaders and Leadership in the Jewish Mystical Movements of the 13th Century*. Conference at the Jewish Theological Seminary, unpublished.

Fine, L. (Ed. & Tr.) (1984). *Safed Spirituality: Rules of Mystical Piety, the Beginning of Wisdom.* New York & Ramsey, Toronto: Paulist Press.

Finkelstein, L. (1940). *The Pharisees: The Sociological Background of Their Faith.* Philadelphia, PA: Jewish Publication Society.

Fischel, H. A. (1973). *Rabbinic Literature and Greco-Roman Philosophy.* Leiden: E. J. Brill.

Fishbane, M. (1994). *The Kiss of God: Spiritual and Mystical Death in Judaism.* Seattle, WA, & London: University of Washington Press.

Fisher, C. (1965). Psychoanalytic Implications of Recent Research on Sleep and Dreaming. Part I: Empirical Findings. *Journal of the American Psychoanalytic Association 13*, 197–270.

Fowler, J. (1988). Theophoric Personal Names in Hebrew: A Comparative Study. *Journal for the Study of the Old Testament* (Supplement Series), *49*. Sheffield, UK: JSOT Press.

Frankel, Y. (Ed.) (1988). *Imre Pinehas ha-Shalem.* Jerusalem: p.n.k.

Freedman, H., & Simon, M. (Trs.) (1977a). *Genesis Rabbah.* In: *Midrash Rabbah, Vol. I.* London: Soncino.

Freedman, H., & Simon, M. (Trs. & Eds.) (1977b). *Lamentations Rabbah.* In: *Midrash Rabbah, Vol. IV.* London: Soncino.

Freedman, H., & Simon, M. (Trs.) (1977c). *Midrash Rabbah, Vol. IV.* London: Soncino.

Freud, S. (1900a). *The Interpretation of Dreams.* In: *The Standard Edition of the Complete Psychological Works of Sigmund Freud, Vols. 4–5.* London: Hogarth Press.

Freud, S. (1911c). Psycho-Analytic Notes on an Autobiographical Account of a Case of Paranoia (Dementia Paranoides). In: *S.E., Vol. 12.*

Freud, S. (1912). *Totem and Taboo.* In: *S.E., Vol. 13.*

Freud, S. (1916–17). *Introductory Lectures on Psychoanalysis.* In: *S.E., Vols. 15 & 16.*

Freud, S. (1921c). *Group Psychology and the Analysis of the Ego.* In: *S.E., Vol. 18.*

Freud, S. (1924c). The Economic Problem of Masochism. In: *S.E., Vol. 19.*

Freud, S. (1930a). *Civilization and Its Discontents.* In: *S.E., Vol. 21.*

Freud, S. (1933a). *New Introductory Lectures on Psychoanalysis.* In: *S.E., Vol. 22.*

Freud, S. (1939a). *Moses and Monotheism: Three Essays* In: *S.E., Vol. 23.*

Freud, S. (1941c). A Premonitory Dream Fulfilled. In: *S.E., Vol. 5.*

Friedlaender, S., Holton, G., Marks, L., & Skolnikoff, E. (Eds.) (1985). *Visions of Apocalypse: End or Rebirth?* New York & London: Holmes & Meier.

Friedmann, M. (Ed.) (1880). *Pesiqta' Rabbati.* Vienna: Kaiser, 1880. [Reprinted Tel Aviv: p.n.k., 1963.]

Fromm, E. (1951). *The Forgotten Language.* New York: Rinehart.

Galenson, E., & Roiphe, H. (1971). The Impact of Early Sexual Discovery on Mood, Defensive Organization, and Symbolization. *Psychoanalytic Study of the Child, 26*: 195–216.

Galenson, E., & Roiphe, H. (1974). The Emergence of Genital Awareness during the Second Year of Life. In: R. C. Friedman, R. M. Richart, & R. L. Van de Weiele (Eds.), *Sex Differences in Behavior.* New York: John Wiley.

Galenson, E., & Roiphe, H. (1976). Some Suggested Revisions Concerning Early Female Development. *Journal of the American Psychoanalytic Association, 24* (Suppl.): 29–57.

Galenson, E., & Roiphe, H. (1980). The Preoedipal Development of the Boy. *Journal of the American Psychoanalytic Association, 28*: 805–827.

Garfinkel, S. (1987). Of Thistles and Thorns: A New Approach to Ezekiel II 6. *Vetus Testamentum, 4*: 421–437.

Garfinkel, S. (1989). Another Model for Ezekiel's Abnormalities. *Journal of the Near Eastern Society, 19*: 39–50.

Gårtner, B. (1961). *The Theology of the Gospel According to Thomas.* New York: p.n.k.

Gaster, T. (1941). Ezekiel and the Mysteries. *Journal of Biblical Literature, 60,* 289–310.

Gershenzon-Eliezer Slomovic, R. (1985). A Second Century Jewish–Gnostic Debate: Rabbi Jose ben Halafta and the Matrona. *Journal for the Study of Judaism, 16*: 20–22.

Ginzberg, L. (1970). *On Jewish Law and Lore.* Philadelphia, PA: Jewish Publication Society.

Goldberg, A. M. (1969). *Untersuchungen uber die Vorstellung von der Schekhinah.* Berlin: de Gruyter.

Goldin, J. (1955). *The Fathers According to Rabbi Nathan* (*Yale Judaica Series, Vol. 10*). New Haven, CT: Yale University Press.

Goldin, J. (Tr. & Ed.) (1955). *The Living Talmud, the Wisdom of the Fathers, and Its Classical Commentaries.* New York: Heritage.

Goldreich, A. (Ed.) (1981). Isaac of Acre, *Sefer Me'irat 'Einayim.* Jerusalem: Akademon.

Goodenough, E. (1935). *By Light, Light: The Mystic Gospel of Hellenistic Judaism.* Amsterdam: Philo Press, 1969.

Goodenough, E. (1954). *Jewish Symbols in Greco-Roman Period* (3 vols.). Princeton, NJ: Princeton University Press.

Gospel of Philip (tr. W. W. Isenberg) (1984). In: *The Nag Hammadi Library* (ed. J. M. Robinson). New York: Harper & Row.

Gospel of Thomas (tr. H. Koester & T. O. Lambdin) (1984). In: *The Nag Hammadi Library* (ed. J. M. Robinson). New York: Harper & Row, 1984.

Grant, R. M. (1961). The Mystery of Marriage in the Gospel of Philip. *Vigiliae Christianae, 15*: 129–140.

Greenacre, P. (1956). Experiences of Awe in Childhood. *Psychoanalytic Study of the Child, 11*: 9.

Greenberg, M. (1983). *Ezekiel 1–20: A New Translation with Introduction and Commentary (Anchor Bible, Vol. 22)*. Garden City, NY: Doubleday.

Greenup, W. A. (Ed.) (1911). Moses de León, *Sheqel ha-Qodesh*. London: p.n.k.

Gries, Z. (1989). *Conduct Literature (Regimen Vitae): Its History and Place in the Life of Beshtian Hasidism* [Heb.]. Jerusalem: p.n.k.

Gruenwald, I. (1980). *Apocalyptic and Merkavah Mysticism*. Leiden: Brill.

Gruenwald, I. (Ed.) (1971). *Sefer Yesirah. Israel Oriental Studies, 1*: 132–177.

Guberman, K. (1984). The Language of Love in Spanish Kabbalah: An Examination of the *'Iggeret ha-Kodesh*. In: D. R. Blumenthal (Ed.), *Approaches to Judaism in Medieval Times*. Chico, CA: Scholars Press.

Ha-Azati, N. (1944). *Treatise on the Menorah*. In: G. Scholem, *Be-Iqvot Mashiah*. Jerusalem: p.n.k.

Halkin, A. S. (1950). Ibn Aknin's Commentary on the Song of Songs. *Alexander Marx Jubilee Volume* [Eng. Section] (pp. 389–424). New York: Jewish Theological Seminary.

Halperin, D. J. (1980). *The Merkabah in Rabbinic Literature (American Oriental Series, Vol. 62)*. New Haven, CT: American Oriental Society.

Halperin, D. J. (1984). A New Edition of the Hekhalot Literature. *Journal of the American Oriental Society, 104*: 543–552.

Halperin, D. J. (1987). A Sexual Image in Hekhalot Rabbati and Its Implications. *Proceedings of the First International Conference on the History of Jewish Mysticism. Early Jewish Mysticism. Jerusalem Studies in Jewish Thought, Vol. VI.*

Halperin, D. J. (1988a). *The Faces of the Chariot: Early Jewish Responses to Ezekiel's Vision* (Texte und Studien zum Antiken Judentum, no. 16). Tuebingen: J. C. B. Mohr (Paul Siebeck).

Halperin, D. J. (1988b). Ascension or Invasion: Implications of the Heavenly Journey in Ancient Judaism. *Religion, 18*: 47–67.

Halperin, D. J. (1993). *Seeking Ezekiel: Text and Psychology*. University Park, PA: Pennsylvania State University Press.

Halperin, D. J. (forthcoming). The Hidden Made Manifest: Muslim Traditions and the "Latent Content" of Biblical and Rabbinic Stories. In: D. Wright, D. Freedman, & A. Hurvitz (Eds.), *Pomegranates and Golden Bells: Studies in Biblical, Jewish, and Near*

Eastern Ritual, Law, and Literature in Honor of Jacob Milgrom. Winona Lake, IN: Eisenbrauns.

Hanson, P. D. (1979). *The Doom of Apocalyptic: The Historical and Sociological Roots of Jewish Apocalyptic Eschatology.* Philadelphia, PA: Fortress Press.

Harris, M. (1959). The Concept of Love in Sefer Hassidim. *Jewish Quarterly Review, 50*: 13–44.

Harris, M. (1962). Marriage as Metaphysics: A Study of the *'Iggeret ha-Kodesh. Hebrew Union College Annual, 33*: 197–220.

Hayim Vital. *Peri 'Es Hayyim.* Jerusalem: p.n.k., 1980.

Heider, G. (1985). The Cult of Molek: A Reassessment. *Journal for the Study of the Old Testament, Supplement Series, No. 43.* Sheffield, UK: JSOT Press.

Heschel, A. J. (1985). *The Circle of the Baal Shem Tov, Studies in Hasidism* (ed. S. H. Dresner). Chicago, IL, & London: University of Chicago Press.

Himmelfarb, M. (1993). *Ascent to Heaven in Jewish and Christian Apocalypses.* New York & Oxford: Oxford University Press.

Howie, C. (1950). The Date and Composition of Ezekiel. *Journal of Biblical Literature Monograph Series, No. 4.* Philadelphia, PA: Society of Biblical Literature.

Hundert, G. D. (1991) *Essential Papers on Hasidism: Origins to Present.* New York & London: New York University Press.

Idel, M. (1979). The Commentary on the Ten *Sefirot* and Fragments from the Writings of R. Joseph of Hamadan [Heb.]. *Alei Sefer, 6–7*: 74–84.

Idel, M. (1982). The Magical and Theurgic Interpretation of Music in Jewish Sources from the Renaissance to Hasidism [Heb.] *Yuval, 4.*

Idel, M. (1985a). Hitbodedut qua Concentration in Ecstatic Kabbalah [Heb.]. *Da'at, 14*: 35–82.

Idel, M. (1985b). Kabbalah and Ancient Philosophy in R. Isaac and Jehudah Abrabanel. In: M. Durman & Z. Levy (Eds.), *The Philosophy of Leone Ebreo* [Heb.]. Tel Aviv: ha-kibuts ha-me'u.had veha.Katedrah le-moreshet he-hagut ha-Yehudit be-Universitat Haifa.

Idel, M. (1988a). Additional Fragments from the Writings of Joseph of Hamadan [Heb.]. *Da'at, 21*: 47–55.

Idel, M. (1988b). *Kabbalah: New Perspectives.* New Haven, CT, & London: Yale University Press.

Idel, M. (1988c). *Studies in Ecstatic Kabbalah*. Albany, NY: State University of New York Press.
Idel, M. (1988d). *The Mystical Experience in Abraham Abulafia* (tr. Jonathan Chipman). Albany, NY: State University of New York Press.
Idel, M. (1989a). Kabbalah, Halakhah and Spiritual Leadership. In: M. Idel & M. Ostow (Eds.), *Leaders and Leadership in the Jewish Mystical Movements of the 13th Century*. Conference at the Jewish Theological Seminary, unpublished.
Idel, M. (1989b). Sexual Metaphors and Praxis in the Kabbalah. In: D. Kraemer (Ed.), *The Jewish Family: Metaphor and Memory*. New York & Oxford: Oxford University Press.
Idel, M. (1994). *Hasidism: Between Ecstasy and Magic*. Albany, NY: State University of New York Press.
Idel, M. (forthcoming). Jerusalem in Medieval Jewish Thought [Heb].
Idel, M., & Ostow, M. (Eds.) (1989). *Leaders and Leadership in the Jewish Mystical Movements of the 13th Century*. Conference at the Jewish Theological Seminary, unpublished.
Jacobson, Y. (1993). The Aspect of the Feminine in the Lurianic Kabbalah. In: *Gershom Scholem's Major Trends in Jewish Mysticism 50 Years After* (ed. J. Dan & P. Schäfer). Tübingen: J. C. B. Mohr (Paul Siebeck).
James, W. (1902). *The Varieties of Religious Experience*. New York: Modern Library–Random House.
Janowitz, N. (1989). *The Poetics of Ascent, Theories of Language in a Rabbinic Ascent Text*, Albany. NY: State University of New York.
Jaspers, K. (1947). Der Prophet Ezechiel: Eine pathographische Studie. [Reprinted in: *Aneignung und Polemik: Gesammelte Reden und Aufsaetze zur Geschichte der Philosophie* (pp. 13–21). Munich: Piper, 1968.]
Jastrow, M. (1950). *A Dictionary of the Targumim, the Talmud Babli and Yerushalmi, and the Midrashic Literature*. New York: Pardes.
Jellinek, A. (Ed.) (1967). *Hekhaloth Rabbati*. In: *Bet ha-Midrasch, Vol. 1* (Part 3). Jerusalem: Wahrman.
Jerushalmi, S. (1979). *Commentary of Prayer*. Jerusalem: p.n.k.
Jewish Encyclopedia, The (1906) (ed. I. Singer). New York: Funk & Wagnalls.
Joel, M. (1880). *Blicke in die Religionsgeschichte, I.* Breslau: p.n.k.
Jung, C. G. (1958). Psychology and Religion. In: *The Basic Writings of C. G. Jung* (ed. W. S. de Laszlo). New York: Modern Library.

Jung, C. G. (1959). *The Archetypes and the Collective Unconscious.* Princeton, NJ: Princeton University Press, 1980.

Jung, C. G. (1977). *Mysterium Coniuctionis.* Princeton, NJ: Princeton University Press.

Kahler, E. (1960). The Nature of the Symbol. In: R. May (Ed.), *Symbolism in Religion and Literature.* New York: Braziller.

Kaufmann, Y. (1960). *The Religion of Israel: From Its Beginnings to the Babylonian Exile* (tr. & abr. M. Greenberg). Chicago, IL: University of Chicago Press.

Kautzsch, E. (1910). *Gesenius' Hebrew Grammar* (2nd Eng. edition; tr. A. E. Cowley from 28th German edition, 1909). Oxford: Clarendon Press.

Kellenbach, K. von (1990). *Anti-Judaism in Christian-Rooted Feminist Writings: An Analysis of Major U.S. American and West German Feminist Theologians.* Ph.D. diss., Temple University.

Kerenyi, C. (1955). The Mysteries of the Kabeiroi. In: J. Campbell (Ed.), *The Mysteries, Papers from the Eranos Yearbook. Bollingen Series 30.* Princeton, NJ: Princeton University Press.

Kimhi, D. (1847). *Sefer ha-Shorashim* [*The Book of Roots*]. Berlin: p.n.k. [Reprinted New York: p.n.k., 1948.]

Klijn, A. J. (1962). The "Single One" in the Gospel of Thomas. *Journal of Biblical Literature, 81*: 271–278.

Klostermann, A. (1877). Ezechiel: Ein Beitrag zu besserer Wuerdigung seiner Person und Schrift. *Theologische Studien und Kritiken, 50*, 391–439.

Lachower, F., & Tishby, I. (1989). *The Wisdom of the Zohar: An Anthology of Texts in 3 Volumes* (Eng. tr. D. Goldstein). The Littman Library. Oxford: Oxford University Press.

Lang, B. (1981). *Ezechiel: Der Prophet und das Buch* (*Ertraege der Forschung, Vol. 153*). Darmstadt: Wissenschaftliche Buchgesellschaft.

Langer, M. D. G. (1923). *Die Erotik der Kabbala.* Prague: p.n.k. [Reprinted Munich: p.n.k., 1989.]

Laqueur, T. (1990). *Making Sex: Body and Gender from the Greeks to Freud.* Cambridge, MA, & London: Harvard University Press.

Leuba, J. H. (1925). *The Psychology of Religious Mysticism.* London & Boston, MA: Routledge & Kegan Paul, 1972.

Lewin, B. D. (1973). The Body as Phallus. *The Psychoanalytic Quarterly, 2*: 24–47.

Liebes, J. (1982). The Messiah of the Zohar. In: *The Messianic Idea in Jewish Thought* [Heb]. Jerusalem: p.n.k.

Liebes, Y. (1976). *Sections of the Zohar Lexicon* [Heb.] Jerusalem: p.n.k.

Liebes, Y. (1990). *Het'o shel Elisha': Arba'ah she-Nikhnesu le-Fardes ve-Tiv'ah shel ha-Mistiqah ha-Talmudit* (2nd edition). Jerusalem: Academon.

Liebes, Y. (1992). "Two Young Roes of a Doe": The Secret Sermon of Isaac Luria before His Death [Heb.]. *Jerusalem Studies in Jewish Thought, 10*: 163–164.

Liebes, Y. (1993a). *Studies in Jewish Myth and Jewish Messianism* (tr. B. Stein). Albany, NY: State University of New York Press.

Liebes, Y. (1993b). *Studies in the Zohar* (tr. A. Schwartz, S. Nakache, & P. Peli). Albany, NY: State University of New York Press.

Loraux, N. (1992). What Is a Goddess? In: P. Schmitt Pantel (Ed.), *A History of Women in the West: I. From Ancient Goddesses to Christian Saints* (tr. A. Goldhammer). Cambridge, MA, & London: Harvard University Press.

Lothane, Z. (1992). *In Defense of Schreber: Soul Murder and Psychiatry*. Hillsdale, NJ, & London: Analytic Press.

Lown, B. (1982). Mental Stress, Arrhythmias and Sudden Death. *American Journal of Medicine, 72*: 177–180.

Lown, B. (1987). Sudden Cardiac Death: Biobehavioral Perspective. *Circulation, 76* (Suppl. I): 186–196.

Lown, B. (1988). Reflections on Sudden Cardiac Death: Brain and Heart. *Transactions & Studies of the College of Physicians of Philadelphia, 10*, 63–80.

Lown, B., Temte, J., Reich, P., Gaughan, C., Regestein, Q., & Hai, H. (1976). Basis for Recurring Ventricular Fibrillation in the Absence of Coronary Heart Disease and Its Management. *New England Journal of Medicine, 294* (12): 623–629.

Mahler, M. S. (1967). On Human Symbiosis and the Vicissitudes of Individuation. *Journal of the American Psychoanalytic Association, 15*: 740–763.

Mahler, M. S., Pine, T., & Bergman, A. (1975). *The Psychological Birth of the Human Infant: Symbiosis & Individuation.* New York: Basic Books. [Reprinted London: Karnac Books, 1985.]

Maimon, I. L. (1958). *"Zohar" (Sinai-Jubilee Volume)* [Heb.]. Jerusalem: p.n.k.

Marcus, I. (1981). *Piety in Society, The Jewish Pietists of Medieval Germany*. Leiden: E. J. Brill.

Marcus, I. (1989). Judah the Pietist and Eleazar of Worms: From Charismatic to Conventional Leadership. In: M. Idel & M. Ostow (Eds.), *Leaders and Leadership in the Jewish Mystical Movements of the 13th Century*. Conference at the Jewish Theological Seminary, unpublished.

Margaliot, R. (Ed.) (1978a). *Sefer ha-Bahir*. Jerusalem: Mosad ha-Rav Kook.

Margaliot, R. (Ed.) (1978b). *Zohar Hadash*. Jerusalem: Mosad ha-Rav Kook.

Margaliot, R. (Ed.) (1984). *Sefer ha-Zohar (Zohar)* (6th edition; 3 vols). Jerusalem: Mosad ha-Rav Kook.

Matt, D. C. (Ed.) (1982). *Book of Mirrors*. Sefer Mar'ot ha-Zove'ot by R. David ben Yehudah he-Hasid. Chico, CA: Scholars Press.

May, R. (Ed.) (1960). *Symbolism in Religion and Literature*. New York: Braziller.

McCullough, W. (1962). Rock Badger. In: *The Interpreter's Dictionary of the Bible: An Illustrated Encyclopedia, Vol. 4*. New York: Abingdon Press.

Meeks, W. A. (1974). The Image of the Androgyne: Some Uses of a Symbol in Earliest Christianity. *History of Religions, 13*: 165–208.

Meier, M. A. (1974). *Critical Edition of the "Sefer Ta'amey ha-Mizwoth" ("Book of Reasons of the Commandments"). Attributed to Isaac Ibn Farhi/Section I—Positive Commandments*. Ph.D. diss., Brandeis University.

Merkur, D. (1985). *Becoming Half Hidden: Shamanism and Initiation Among the Inuit*. Stockholm: Almqvist & Wiksell.

Merkur, D. (1988). Prophetic Initiation in Israel and Judah. *The Psychoanalytic Study of Society, 12*, 37–67.

Merkur, D. (1989). The Visionary Practices of Jewish Apocalyptists. *Psychoanalytic Study of Society, 14*: 119–148.

Meroz, R. (1988). *Redemption in the Lurianic Kabbalah* [Heb.]. Ph.D. diss., Hebrew University.

Meyer, M. W. (1985). Making Mary Male: The Categories "Male" and "Female" in the Gospel of Thomas. *New Testament Studies, 31*: 554–570.

Mopsik, Ch. (1986). *Lettre sur la sainteté: Le secret de la relation entre l'homme et la femme dans la cabale*. Paris: Vedier.

Mopsik, Ch. (1989). The Body of Engenderment in the Hebrew Bible, the Rabbinic Tradition and the Kabbalah. In: M. Feher, R. Naddaff, & N. Tazi (Eds.), *Fragments for a History of the Human Body*. New York: Zone.

Mopsik, Ch. (1992). *Les Grands textes de la Cabale: les rites qui font dieu.* Paris: Vedier.

Mopsik, Ch. (1994). *Le Secret du marriage de David et Bethsabée.* Paris: Vedier.

Nachmanides (Moses ben Nahman), *Commentary on Exodus* (tr. C. B. Chavel). New York: Shilo, 1973.

Neumann, E. (1954). *The Origins and History of Consiousness* (fwd. C. G. Jung; tr. R. F. C. Hull). Princeton, NJ: Princeton University Press. [Reprinted London: Karnac Books, 1989.]

Neumann, E. (1963). *The Great Mother: An Analysis of an Archetype* (2nd edition) (tr. R. Manheim). Princeton, NJ: Princeton University Press.

Newman, L. I. (1934/1963). *The Hasidic Anthology, Tales and Teachings of the Hasidim.* New York: Schocken.

Newman, R., Katz, J., & Rubinstein, R. (1960). The Experimental Situation as a Determinant of Hypnotic Dreams: A Contribution to the Experimental Use of Hypnosis. *Psychiatry, 23*: 63–73.

Nunberg, H. (1949). *Problems of Bisexuality as Reflected in Circumcision.* London: Imago Publishing.

Nunberg, H. (1955). *Principles of Psychoanalysis. Their Application to the Neuroses.* New York: International Universities Press.

Nunberg, H. (1961). *Curiosity.* New York: International Universities Press.

Offenkrantz, W., & Rechtschaffen, A. (1963). Clinical Studies of Sequential Dreams. I. A Patient in Psychotherapy. *Archives of General Psychiatry, 8*: 497–508.

Ostow, M. (1955). A Psychoanalytic Contribution to the Study of Brain Function. II The Temporal Lobes. *Psychoanalytic Quarterly, 24* (3).

Ostow, M. (1962). *Drugs in Psychoanalysis and Psychotherapy.* New York: Basic Books.

Ostow, M. (1969). Antinomianism, Mysticism and Psychosis. In: R. E. Hicks & P. J. Fink (Eds.), *Psychedelic Drugs.* New York: Grune & Stratton.

Ostow, M. (1980). The Hypomanic Personality. In: R. H. Belmaker & H. M. van Praag (Eds.), *Mania: An Evolving Concept.* New York:

Spectrum Publications. [Reprinted in: M. Ostow, *Judaism in Psychoanalysis*. New York: KTAV, 1982.]

Ostow, M. (1986). Archetypes of Apocalypse in Dreams and Fantasies and in Religious Scripture. *Israel Journal of Psychiatry & Related Disciplines, 23*: 107–122.

Ostow, M. (1988). Four Entered the Garden: Normative Religion versus Illusion. In: H. P. Blum, Y. Kramer, Arlene Richards, & Arnold Richards (Eds.), *Fantasy, Myth, and Reality: Essays in Honor of Jacob A. Arlow* (pp. 287–301). New York: International Universities Press.

Ostow, M. (1992). The Interpretation of Apocalyptic Dreams. (Read before the American Psychoanalytic Association, May 1989.) *Journal of the Association for the Study of Dreams, 2* (1): 1–14.

Patai, R. (1947). *Man and Temple*. London: Thomas Nelson.

Patai, R. (1978). *The Hebrew Goddess*. Detroit: Wayne State University Press, 1990.

Perry, T. A. (1980). *Erotic Spirituality: The Integrative Tradition from Leone Ebreo to John Donne*. Tuscaloosa: University of Alabama Press.

Pines, S. (Tr.) (1963). Maimonides. *Guide of the Perplexed*. Chicago, IL, & London: University of Chicago Press.

Press, J. (1989). What in the World Is the Sin If I Thrill to Your Beauty? The Homosexual Love Poems of the Medieval Rabbis. *Mosaic*: 12–26.

Preus, A. (1977). Galen's Criticism of Aristotle's Conception Theory. *Journal of the History of Biology, 10*: 65–85.

Reich, P., De Silva, R., Lown, B., & Murawsky, B. (1981). Acute Psychological Disturbances Preceding Life-Threatening Ventricular Arrhythmias. *Journal of the American Medical Association, 246* (3): 233–235.

Robinson, W. C. Jr. (1970). The Exegesis of the Soul. *Novum Testamentum, 12*: 111–117.

Roiphe, H., & Galenson, E. (1981). *Infantile Origins of Sexual Identity*. New York: International Universities Press.

Roth, C., & Wigoder, G. (Eds.) (1972). *Encyclopedia Judaica*. Jerusalem: Keter.

Roth, N. (1982). "Deal Gently with the Young Man": Love of Boys in Medieval Hebrew Poetry of Spain. *Speculum, 57*: 33–59.

Rowland, C. (1982). *The Open Heaven: A Study of Apocalyptic in Judaism and Early Christianity*. New York: Crossroads.

Rowley, H. (1953–54). The Book of Ezekiel in Modern Study. *Bulletin of the John Rowlands Library, 36*: 169–210. [Reprinted in: *Men of God*. London: Nelson, 1963.]

Rubinstein, R., Katz, J., & Newman, R. (1957). On the Sources and Determinants of Hypnotic Dreams. *Canadian Psychiatric Association Journal, 2*: 154–161.

Saperstein, M. (1980). *Decoding the Rabbis*. Cambridge, MA: Harvard University Press.

Schäfer, P. (1992). *The Hidden and Manifest God*. Albany, NY: State University of New York.

Schechter, S. (Ed.) (1887). *Avot de-Rabbi Natan* (version B). Vienna: p.n.k.

Scheidlinger, S. (1964). Identification, the Sense of Belonging and of Identity in Small Groups. *International Journal of Group Psychotherapy, 4*: 291–306.

Scheidlinger, S. (1974). On the Concept of the Mother Group. *International Journal of Group Psychotherapy, 24* (4): 417–428.

Scheindlin, R. P. (1986). *Wine, Women, and Death: Medieval Hebrew Poems of the Good Life*. Philadelphia, PA: Jewish Publication Society.

Schilder, P. (1942). *Mind: Perception and Thought in Their Constructive Aspects*. New York: Columbia University Press.

Schirmann, J. (1955). The Ephebe in Medieval Hebrew Poetry [Heb.]. *Sefarad, 15*:

Scholem, G. (1925–1926). Abraham ben Eliezer ha-Levi's *Masoret ha-Hokhmah* [Heb]. *Kiriat Sefer, 2*: 129–130.

Scholem, G. (1930). *Kitve Yad ba-Qabbalah*, Jerusalem: p.n.k.

Scholem, G. (1931). On the Development of the Concept of Worlds in the Early Kabbalah [Heb.]. *Tarbiz, 3*: 39–41.

Scholem, G. (1934). *Be-'Iqvot Mashiah*. Jerusalem: p.n.k.

Scholem, G. (1941). *Major Trends in Jewish Mysticism*. Jerusalem: Schocken [first paperback Schocken edition 1961; revised edition New York: Schocken Press, 1954].

Scholem, G. (1944–45). Did the Ramban Write the *'Iggeret ha-Qodesh*? [Heb.]. *Kiryat Sefer, 21*: 179–186.

Scholem, G. (1955–56). The Commentary of R. Isaac of Acre on the First Chapter of Sefer Yesirah [Heb.]. *Kiryat Sefer, 31*: 386.

Scholem, G. (1960). *Jewish Gnosticism, Merkabah Mysticism and Talmudic Tradition*. New York: Jewish Theological Seminary of America.

Scholem, G. (1962). *Origins of the Kabbalah* (ed. R. J. Zwi Werblowsky; tr. A. Arkush). Princeton, NJ: Jewish Publication Society, Princeton University Press. [Eng. tr. copyright 1987.]

Scholem, G. (1965). *On the Kaballah and Its Symbolism.* New York: Schocken Books.

Scholem, G. (1972). *The Messianic Idea in Judaism.* New York: Schocken.

Scholem, G. (1973). *Sabbatai Sevi—The Mystical Messiah. 1626–1676.* Princeton, NJ: Princeton University Press.

Scholem, G. (1974). *Kabbalah.* New York & Scarborough, Ontario: Meridian Books, New American Library.

Scholem, G. (1976). Two Treatises of R. Moses de León [Heb.]. *Qoves 'al yad, 8*: 375.

Scholem, G. (1991). *On the Mystical Shape of the Godhead* (tr. J. Neugroschel; ed. & rev. J. Chipman). New York: Schocken.

Scholem, G. (1992). *Annotated Zohar.* Jerusalem: p.n.k.

Schwartz, H., & Bregman, M. (1995). *The Four Who Entered Paradise—A Novella by Howard Schwartz with an Introduction and Commentary by Marc Bregman.* Northvale, NJ: Jason Aronson.

Sevrin, J.-M. (1974). Les Noces spirituelles dans l'Evangile selon Philippe. *Le Museon, 87*: 143–193.

Sevrin, J.-M. (1982). Les rites et la Gnose. In: J. Ries (Ed.), *Gnosticisme et Monde Hellenistique.* Louvain-La-Neuve: p.n.k.

Shinan, A. (1983). The Sins of Nadav and Avihu in the Aggadah of the Sages. In: A. Shinan (Ed.), *The Aggadic Literature—A Reader* [Heb]. Jerusalem: p.n.k.

Soleh, A. (1981). Mivneh ha-Hazon be-Yehezqel 8–11. In: B. Z. Luria (Ed.), *Sefer Doctor Baruch ben Yehudah: Mehqarim be-Miqra ube-Mahshevet Yisrael.* Tel Aviv: The Society for Bible Study in Israel.

Spector, S. A. (1984). *Jewish Mysticism.* New York & London: Garland Publishing Company.

Stroumsa, G. (1981). Le Couple de l'ange et de l'esprit: traditions juives et chretiennes. *Revue biblique, 88*: 46–47.

Suter, D. (1979). Fallen Angel, Fallen Priest: The Problem of Family Purity in I Enoch 6–16. *Hebrew Union College Annual, 50*: 115–136.

Talmage, F. (1975). *David Kimhi: The Man and the Commentaries* (Harvard Judaic Monographs, No. 1). Cambridge, MA: Harvard University Press.

Theodor, J., & Albeck, C. (Eds.) (1965). *Genesis Rabbah.* Jerusalem: Wahrman.

Tinbergen, N. (1951). *The Study of Instinct.* London: Oxford University Press.

Tishby, I. (1942). *The Doctrine of Evil and the "Kelippah" in Lurianic Kabbalah* [Heb.]. Jerusalem: p.n.k.

Tishby, I. (1945). R. Azriel's *Commentary on the Talmudic Aggadot.* Jerusalem: p.n.k.

Tishby, I. (1982). *Studies in Kabbalah and Its Branches* [Heb.]. Jerusalem: p.n.k.

Trosman, H., Rechtschaffen, A., Offenkrantz, W., & Wolpert, E. (1960). Studies in Psychophysiology of Dreams. IV. Relations among Dreams in Sequence. *Archives of General Psychiatry, 3*: 602–607.

Underhill, E. (1961). *Mysticism.* New York: Dutton.

Underhill, E. (1964). *The Mystics of the Church.* New York: Schocken.

Vajda, G. (1957). *L'Amour de Dieu dans la theologie juive du Moyen Age.* Paris: Librairie Philosophique, J. Vrin.

Vajda, G. (Ed.) (1968). Jacob ben Sheshet. *Sefer Meshiv Devarim Nekhohim.* Jerusalem: Israel Academy of Sciences and Humanities.

Vajda, G. (1975). Or Ha-Shekhina. *Révue des Études juives, 134*: 133–135.

Verrier, R., Hagestad, E., & Lown, B. (1987). Delayed Myocardial Ischemia Induced by Anger. *Circulation, 75* (1): 249–254.

Vital, S. (1898). *Sha'ar Ma'amere Rashbi.* Jerusalem: p.n.k.

Vogt, E. (1981). *Untersuchungen zum Buch Ezechiel.* Rome: Pontifical Biblical Institute Press.

Vogt, K. (1991). "Becoming Male": A Gnostic and Early Christian Metaphor. In: K. E. Børresen (Ed.), *Image of God and Gender Models in Judaeo-Christian Tradition.* Oslo: p.n.k.

Von Uexkull, J. (1921). *Umwelt und Innenwelt der Tiere.* Berlin: p.n.k.

Waite, A. E. (1915). *The Way of Divine Union.* London: p.n.k.

Waite, A. E. (1990). *The Holy Kabbalah.* Secaucus, NJ: Carol.

Walsh, R. (1993). Phenomenological Mapping and Comparisons of Shamanic, Buddhist, Yogic, and Schizophrenic Experiences. *Journal of the American Academy of Religion, 61*, 739–769.

Ward, J. (1962). Jaazaniah. In: *The Interpreter's Dictionary of the*

Bible: An Illustrated Encyclopedia, Vol. 2. New York: Abingdon Press.

Wertheimer, S. A. (Ed.) (1955). *Bate Midrashot*. Jerusalem: Ktav va-Sefer.

Wiesel, E. (1978). *Four Hasidic Masters and Their Struggle Against Melancholy*. Notre Dame, IN, & London: University of Notre Dame Press.

Wijnhoven, J. (1964). *Sefer ha-Mishkal: Text and Study*. Ph.D. diss., Brandeis University.

Wind, E. (1967). *Pagan Mysteries in the Renaissance*. New Haven, CT: Yale University Press, 1958.

Wintermute, O. (Tr.) (1983). *Apocalypse of Zephania*. Garden City, NY: Doubleday.

Wirszubski, C. (1975). *Three Studies in Christian Kabbala* [Heb.]. Jerusalem: p.n.k.

Wolfson, E. R. (1986). Left Contained in the Right: A Study in Zoharic Hermeneutics. *Academy of Jewish Studies Review, 11*: 27–52.

Wolfson, E. R. (1987a). Circumcision and the Divine Name: A Study in the Transmission of Esoteric Doctrine. *Jewish Quarterly Review, 78*: 77–112.

Wolfson, E. R. (1987b). Circumcision, Vision of God, and Textual Interpretation: From Midrashic Trope to Mystical Symbol. *History of Religions 27*: 189–215.

Wolfson, E. R. (Ed.) (1988). Moses de León. *Sefer ha-Rimmon, The Book of the Pomegranate*. Atlanta, GA: Scholars Press.

Wolfson, E. R. (1992). Images of God's Feet: Some Observations on the Divine Body in Judaism. In: H. Eilberg-Schwartz (Ed.), *People of the Body: Jewish and Judaism from an Embodied Perspective*. Albany, NY: State University of New York Press.

Wolfson, E. R. (1993a). Forms of Visionary Ascent as Ecstatic Experience in the Zoharic Literature. In: J. Dan & P. Schäfer (Eds.), *Gershom Scholem's Major Trends in Jewish Mysticism: 50 Years After*. Tübingen: J. C. B. Mohr (Paul Siebeck).

Wolfson, E. R. (1993b). The Tree That Is All: Jewish–Christian Roots of a Kabbalistic Symbol in *Sefer ha-Bahir*. *Journal of Jewish Thought and Philosophy, 3*: 31–76.

Wolfson, E. R. (1994a). *The Rite of Sabbatai Sevi's Coronation and Sabbatian Myth*. Read at the Skirball Conference on Myth and Ritual.

Wolfson, E. R. (1994b). Crowning and Visionary Union with the Phallus. In: *Through a Speculum That Shines: Vision and Imagination in Medieval Jewish Mysticism.* Princeton, NJ: Princeton University Press.

Wolfson, E. R. (1994c). Mystical Fellowship as Constitution of the Divine Face. In: *Through a Speculum That Shines: Vision and Imagination in Medieval Jewish Mysticism.* Princeton, NJ: Princeton University Press.

Wolfson, E. R. (1994d). *The Rite of Sabbatai Sevi's Coronation and Sabbatian Myth.* Delivered at a conference on Myth and Ritual in Judaism, sponsored by the Skirball Department of Hebrew and Judaic Studies, New York University, October 23–24.

Wolfson, E. R. (1994e). *Through a Speculum That Shines: Vision and Imagination in Medieval Jewish Mysticism.* Princeton, NJ: Princeton University Press.

Wolfson, E. R. (1994f). Woman—The Feminine as Other: Some Philosophical Reflections on the Divine Androgyne in Theosophic Kabbalah. In: L. Silberstein & R. Cohn (Eds.), *The Other in Jewish Thought and History: Constructions of Jewish Culture and Identity.* New York: New York University Press.

Wolfson, E. R. (1995a). Erasing the Erasure. Gender and the Writing of God's Body in Kabbalistic Symbolism. In: *Circle in the Square: Studies in the Use of Gender in Kabbalistic Symbolism.* Albany, NY: State University of New York Press.

Wolfson, E. R. (1995b). From Sealed Book to Open Text: Time, Memory, and Narrativity in Kabbalistic Hermeneutics. In: S. Kepnes (Ed.), *Critical Jewish Hermeneutics.* New York (in press).

Wolfson, E. R. (1995c). The Image of Jacob Engraved Upon the Throne: Further Speculation on the Esoteric Doctrine of the German Pietists. In: *Along the Path: Studies in Kabbalistic Myth, Symbolism, and Hermeneutics.* Albany, NY: State University of New York Press.

Wolfson, E. R. (1995d). Walking as a Sacred Duty: Theological Transformation of Social Reality in Early Hasidism. In: *Along the Path: Studies in Kabbalistic Myth, Symbolism, and Hermeneutics.* Albany, NY: State University of New York Press.

Yamauchi, E. M. (1970). *Gnostic Ethics and Mandaean Origins* (Harvard Theological Studies, XXIV). Cambridge, MA: Harvard University Press.

Zimmer, E. (1989). Poses and Postures during Prayer [Heb.]. *Sidra, 5*: 92–94.

Zimmerli, W. (1969). *Ezekiel: A Commentary on the Book of the Prophet Ezekiel* [tr. R E. Clements (Vol. 1); tr. J. D. Martin (Vol. 2)]: Philadelphia: Fortress Press, 1979–83.

Zolla, E. (1981). *The Androgyne Reconciliation of Male and Female.* New York: Crossroad.

Zwelling, J. (1975). Joseph of Hamadan's *Sefer Tashak*: Critical Text Edition with Introduction. Ph.D. dissertation, Brandeis University.

Zwi Werblowsky, R. J. (1972). Ape and Essence. In: *Ex Orbe Religionum.* Leiden: E. J. Brill.

Zwi Werblowsky, R. J. (1977). *Joseph Karo, Lawyer and Mystic.* Philadelphia, PA: Jewish Publication Society.

INDEX